CULTURES OF CONTAGION

CULTURES OF CONTAGION

EDITED BY BÉATRICE DELAURENTI AND
THOMAS LE ROUX

The MIT Press
Cambridge, Massachusetts
London, England

This book was set in Adobe Garamond Pro by New Best-set Typesetters Ltd. Printed and bound in the United States of America.

Library of Congress Cataloging-in-Publication Data

Names: Delaurenti, Béatrice, 1972– author. | Le Roux, Thomas, author.
Title: Cultures of contagion / edited by Béatrice Delaurenti, Thomas Le Roux ; afterword by Thomas Piketty.
Description: Cambridge, Massachusetts : The MIT Press, 2021. | Includes bibliographical references.
Identifiers: LCCN 2020040796 | ISBN 9780262045919 (hardcover)
Subjects: LCSH: Communicable diseases.
Classification: LCC RA643 .D44 2021 | DDC 616.9—dc23
LC record available at https://lccn.loc.gov/2020040796

10   9   8   7   6   5   4   3   2   1

Contents

INTRODUCTION

Contagion: Its History and Some Historiographical Examples from Antiquity to Today

Béatrice Delaurenti and Thomas Le Roux

Contagion is in the news. This introduction was being written in March and April 2020, a time when France, following China, along with France's neighbors in Italy, Spain, Great Britain, Germany, with the United States, and almost half the human race, was living through a period of population lockdown, the aim being to fight the advance of COVID-19, the disease caused by SARS-CoV-2. The outbreak and rapid propagation of the epidemic has been a shock, having repercussions for the health, society, politics, economics, environment, intellectual life, and culture of every country as well as for the everyday lives of all. Historians have long understood that epidemics played a significant role in history and viruses have been important agents in human evolution, not least as circulation and exchange increased.[1] This book, already in preparation more than a year ago, nears its publication amid worldwide contagion and general lockdown. For us, to write this introduction at such a time has been a singular experience, which has led us to nuance our perspectives on the subject and its importance.

Now more than ever, contagion has revealed itself to be a powerful interpretative model that is capable of illuminating not only the medical characteristics of a disease's propagation but also a very large number of social aspects and therefore the history of society. The social sciences appear to have established that periods of epidemic have generally been accompanied by a variety of social phenomena, behaviors, and reactions, including changes in theories and ideas.[2] The present-day world's interest in contagion cannot therefore be put down simply to today's glaring headlines.

While the term is now applied most commonly to transmissible diseases, it has also been used to describe situations that go well beyond medicine and entail social relationships at all levels relating to both individual and collective experiences. From the inescapable return of head lice to the scalps of schoolchildren to the generalized pollution of natural environments, from fashionable movements to the conspiracy theories that propagate like spores on social media, from the hacker attacks to the fraudulent use of influence, from the messages that accumulate around places of terrorist attacks to the MeToo movement, contagion is a multifaceted process that runs across all social fields.

Going beyond the immediate environment at the time of writing, the present collection aims to adduce a historical perspective to the notion of contagion. It is not a new field, as it has stimulated research in the human sciences for some decades. In 2011, a special issue of the periodical *Tracés* advocated, with respect to contagion, its "detachment from nature, through historical analysis and working across disciplines, of what stands out as a key to understanding numerous present-day phenomena."[3] Within that perspective, the current volume offers a wide purview of social, cultural, political, and anthropological situations where the concept of contagion has relevance. It points to a number of markers in the history of contagion that reveal the diversity and historicity of the phenomena connoted by the word "contagion" and demonstrates the multiplicity of uses to which it can be put.

A POLYSEMIC NOTION

According to the *American Heritage Dictionary of the English Language*, the primary received sense of the term "contagion" is literal and belongs to medicine. It connotes a "disease transmission by direct or indirect contact" and is complemented by a secondary sense pertaining to the psychological sciences: "the spread of a behavior pattern, attitude, or emotion from person to person or group to group through conscious or unconscious imitation." Two additional meaning are figurative or analogical, "a harmful, corrupting influence" and "the tendency to spread, as of a doctrine, influence, or emotional state."[4] The idea of transmission is common to all of the situations envisaged here, be they in a literal sense or used metaphorically to describe a process amenable to social scientific analysis.

Given the porosity of these definitions, there is a temptation—as has often been the case—to apply the modern medical description to other areas. However, such procedures raise methodological or analytical difficulties. While the medical use of the term prevails today and contagion is often described according to models referencing biology, mathematics, or statistics, this division is not obvious from a historical point of view. That it should appear natural is more apparent than real. The word has enjoyed a great variety of uses over the long term, with an infinity of nuances and an ever-changing balance between medical and other connotations.

In its current medical sense, contagion refers to the transmission from one infected to a noninfected person of a pathogen that attacks the physical organism. The transmission may be direct where there is *contact* between two subjects or indirect where there is an intermediate animal or object that acts as a vector of "contagion." Etymologically, the fundamental idea relates to the phenomenon of "touching" (from Latin, *tangere*), which suggests a necessary proximity. The medical understanding of the term "contagion," however, did not become truly dominant until the end of the nineteenth century, following the discoveries of Pasteur and Koch, which enabled laboratory analysis to reveal the agents of contamination, "bacteria" or "microbes." These had previously been referred to as "corpuscules" or "agents," terms that were used without any medical demonstration of the paths of transmission having yet been provided.[5] The discovery of microbial contamination fundamentally changed conceptions of disease and contagion.

Viewed over the long term, the medical use of the word "contagion" has undergone important changes, depending on learned, cultural, or religious traditions as much as on particular contexts. From antiquity, physicians thought about how diseases were transmitted, even if there was no Greek word to correspond to the notion. In the conceptions of Hippocrates (around 460 to 377 BCE) and Galen (around 129 to 201 CE), which continued to dominate thinking over a long period, disease transmission was not interpreted as a transfer of pathogenic germs but instead was understood principally as the result of the corruption of the air, the one factor common to all individuals affected by contagious illness. The miasmal air was reckoned to be an exhalation from the Earth or from rotting corpses; it was thought to find its way into the body through respiration and then corrupt it. The disease itself was not regarded as an invasive entity but as a disequilibrium of the body and its humors.

In the Latin language, the words *contagio* and *contagium* are attested from the second-century BCE and incorporate the notions of touch and person-to-person transmission; the concept was closely allied to that of pollution, which indicated soiling, but the sense was closer to that of the profanation of a sacred place.[6] Medieval Latin and Arabian physicians were indebted to the Galenic and Hippocratic medical tradition and, along with it, its vocabulary.[7] Thus for some centuries, the notion of contagion had a very wide field of reference; it included any sort of affect transmitted from person to person and placed special emphasis on the influence of the air and more generally the environment.[8] That a particular disease was contagious was not an exclusive diagnosis but was among the elements a physician would identify. Where leprosy was concerned, for example, physicians were prudently reticent about which interpretation to decide on, human transmission or infection coming from the environment.[9]

In the early modern period, medicine continued to envisage the notion of contagion within a Hippocratic and Galenic framework. This was true even of the rare physicians who considered that the plague was borne by corporeal agents, *seminaria* ("seeds"), capable of causing a new infection analogous to a previous one, as is demonstrated by the figure of Girolamo Francastoro in the sixteenth century. While his notion has long been reckoned the precursor of the microbial conception of contagion, he nonetheless professed both "aerism," that is, "miasma," and contagionism. His definition of contagion was not incompatible with the theory of contamination of the air and was not perceived by his contemporaries as a break with tradition.[10] The idea of corrupt air remained a common explanation for plague and even cholera until the end of the eighteenth century, even though it was sufficiently ambiguous to embrace contradictory theories and to not exclude a partial role for direct contagion attributable to circumstances. Medical disagreements at the time were as much politically as scientifically inspired.[11] The word "contagion," in its current medical sense, is thus a *faux ami* for historians. Its present-day connotation has displaced a spectrum of wider meanings and detracts from the religious and moral sense that long dominated the word's use.

Historically, contagion has not been a uniquely medical concept. Far from it. The word's range of meanings in the Middle Ages and early modern period was very extensive, and the word was applied to various phenomena. Speech, for example, was sometimes presented as a form of contagious transmission. In the thirteenth century, the Franciscan Roger Bacon looked into the power wielded by words in politics, in magic, or in any other situation. He offered an explanation based on the multiplication of *species*: the speaker emitted *species*, forms or impressions configured by his body and soul that transmitted a consequent modification through the ambient air to reach, by successive replications, the hearer's body and soul.[12] This could be compared to love sickness, the evil eye, or sexual desire, which were envisaged and explained in the Middle Ages according to a model derived from ophthalmics, as physical affects transmitted by looking: they were the result of contagion through contact with corrupt air, air infected by various emanations.[13] Therefore at the heart of the matter of contagion lie much wider questions of natural philosophy relating to action at distance and the phenomena associated with it.[14]

In the sixteenth century, the sense of the word was just as extensive. The principles of sympathy and antipathy constituted the conceptual framework of medical debate on the plague's contagiousness, particularly in Fracastoro's work.[15] To a twenty-first-century reader, such a construction of contagion might look as if it " hovers between magic and metaphor."[16] But it actually did nothing of the kind. To speak of contagion in connection with love or the evil eye was no metaphor for learned people of the medieval and early modern periods. For them, these were *literally* cases of poisoning with tangible physical effects.

No less literal was the way in which the notion of contagion was used to describe the transmission of sins, and thus that of evil or soiling, even before it was used in a medical sense. This connotation was current from antiquity. In the Middle Ages, thinking about the moral contagiousness of certain behaviors developed independently of that of disease transmission in spite of their continuing to be linked. Medical theorizing about contagion grew out of elements elaborated by medieval theologians' thinking on the propagation of sins.[17] When the long view is taken, the notion is seen to lie at the crossroads of medical, religious, and moral meanings. It assembled an extensive range of manifestations centering on the idea of the transmission of an evil that provoked the corruption of the soul or the body of another.

Today, the word "contagion" is often used metaphorically, to describe a wide range of phenomena entailing imitation, transmission, or suggestion, from the exercise of power to interpersonal exchange, and from social groups to intersubjectivity.[18] The variety of such uses bears witness to the term's "generic plasticity."[19] The word is applicable to science and technology— the way that innovations spread or the proliferation of wavelengths, for instance. Or to economics—the domino effects seen in financial crises, for example. Or to politics, as in areas of influence, manipulation, and rumor. It is similarly applicable to the study of social phenomena, such as crowd behavior, social media, violence, and criminality, as also to religious expressions like mystical ecstasy, heretical movements, demon possession, and trance. In the realm of psychology, we can point to emotional contagion, as in the classic topos of fits of giggling. In the sphere of literary and artistic creation, it is possible to see contagious elements at work in the reception of a motif and changes made to it over time.

In these different areas, it is hard to draw a strict line between the word's literal and metaphorical uses. Contagion blurs the frontiers, not just between the literal and the metaphorical but also between body and soul; between the physical and the spiritual, between explanations that may be natural, demoniac, or divine; or between the transmission of a disease and that of a condition favoring its development. To understand the notion in its diverse uses, which extend well beyond the current sense of microbial contamination, we need to "reimagine" it.[20]

HISTORICAL VARIATIONS AROUND CONTAGION

All of the considerations just outlined, bearing on the term's polysemic character and its malleability as a concept in the humanities and social sciences, point to the usefulness of historians' pooling their approaches to contagion.[21] This is all the more so since the notion is not simply applicable to a variety of situations, but all of them relate to the passage of time and past events. The process of contagion lies somewhere between a creative activity *ex nihilo* and a movement that repeats itself identically. It is the special relationship of contagion to time that provides the present publication with its common thread. A wide variety of social, political, religious, intellectual, and cultural movements are addressed here, all of which can be interpreted through the prism of contagion.

This prism can accommodate many different meanings and uses of the word, be they literal or metaphorical. By "contagion," we mean a process characterized by turns as unremitting, unstable, or unforeseeable and consisting of the transmission of an element or quality, or in the propagation of a phenomenon. The process is one that links a contaminating agent, whose intervention may be spontaneous or deliberate, to a recipient that participates to a greater or lesser extent in the interaction. The contagion may be active or passive, physical or nonphysical, individual or collective. It may be unbridled or, on the contrary, may be the object of efforts to encourage its spread or to control it. It is a notion that encourages shifts and movements toward consequential associations that enrich its polysemy, such as influence, contamination, propagation, or indeed imitation.

The present volume's fifty contributions all describe processes of contagion, exemplifying two distinct approaches. The first examines how the notion of contagion—idea and/or lexis—is employed in the sources and what it signified to contemporaries. This approach helps us to see and understand historic meanings of the term, and accepts them as they present themselves, without preconceptions. Consequently, as Conrad and Wujastyk understand matters, "ideas of contagion emerged from a complex social and cultural matrix of related ideas" differing according to period, place, and context.[22] Some of the contributions therefore offer an investigation of past uses of contagion; they focus on local studies, are anchored in a particular period, and rely on specific knowledge of the sources and the issues that relate to this or that area. They throw light on different facets of the notion.

The second approach corresponds to a different perspective: it considers the notion of contagion as a tool of analysis. This perspective is proper to the task of the historian, providing a model for reading past reality that can sharpen reflection and enrich the gaze. The notion has long been considered a relevant tool for the social and historical sciences, inasmuch as it enables the modeling of certain categories of relationship at different scales; it suggests ways of assembling and interpreting historical data to provide clarity and fresh ideas, stimulate research, and reveal what may previously have gone undetected.[23] The prism of contagion can be revealing, enabling hitherto unnoticed configurations, interactions, and chain reactions to show up that would have otherwise remained invisible. In such instances, it is not the sense that people at the time placed on the word "contagion" that counts so much as the actual process indicated by the word. For example, in some contributions, the notion of contagion avoids too linear a reading of the relationships between art works. In others, it is a crucible that, in articulating the diverse characteristics of a particular society's vision of the world, permits them to be linked together. Yet other contributions distinguish a number of contagious phenomena that were embedded in one another.

The joining of these two approaches means that contagion is examined from both the point of view of individuals in history and that of today's historian. Most often the term is understood negatively. Some of the contributions here particularly emphasize the harm caused by contagion (Cartography, Epidemic, Literature, Microbes, Pollution, Solitude). In other cases, however, it has a positive connotation (Consumption, Manuscripts, Theater). Going beyond this binarity, the conceptual prism of contagion sheds light on a variety of movements, changes, and dynamics in the sources. As will be seen, a number of different lines of inquiry run through the book.

Contagion, as a process, raises the question of the role of the originator or that of the agent responsible for its propagation. This is an especially live question when the notion is applied to artistic and intellectual creation or to technological innovation. Iconography, for example, can be assessed otherwise than as the individual or personal production of a sculptor, painter, or illuminator: artistic creation is then perceived to have a collective dimension revealed by the reappropriation of a procedure or theme. Similarly, the practices of writing bring together copying, reusing, and commentary as just so many forms of intellectual creation. These aspects are especially noticeable in the Middle Ages insofar as the system of copying manuscripts caused texts to shift and fluctuate in a manner very unlike printed texts, which must bow to the "yoke of textual fixity," as Bernard Cerquiglini describes it.[24] In this particular context, but also in other periods, the notion of contagion is relevant to grasping the spread of ideas, arguments and forms of discourse, artistic or literary themes, and techniques.

The contagion model enables scholars to free themselves from hierarchical or genealogical conceptions of works and to adopt a more nuanced, network-oriented view of their links and circulation. It makes it possible to track successive changes and the rise of what might look to have been errors but actually belonged to the freedom of each scribe and each reader. The contributions under Calendar, Iconography, Innovation, Manuscripts, Ritual, and Writing bring these dimensions into the open. A related question is that of deliberation's role in the process: to what extent is the contagion the product of intention? Is the contagious spread a passive affair, a form of active self-affirmation, or is it a mixed process, sometimes active, sometimes passive, of imitation of another? Such matters are discussed in the contributions in Clothing, Crowd, Languages, Luxury, Naming, and Spirituality.

While it is useful to think of contagion as "giving distinct, objectifiable, and detailed life to what is barely visible,"[25] a further difficulty lies in identifying the nature of what is transmitted in the process. What is the entity entailed in contagion? In the modern microbial sense, it comprises infectious germs that pass from one person to another. The history of this interpretation is central to the contributions entitled Cartography, Epidemic, Microbes, and Smallpox. Even so, the question looks different when a wider definition is adopted. What is transmitted may then be a model or a method of doing things (Consumption, Innovation, Solitude, Swamps, Solitude). Sometimes analysis creates a division between what can and cannot be transmitted. In the artistic circles of the Italian Renaissance, for example, it was common to borrow someone's name, without this practice being qualified as a form of contagion; the shift from one kinship model to another, on the other hand, took a form that assimilates it to a contagious phenomenon (Naming).

This question raises another concerning the individual or collective character of contagion. The phenomenon oscillates between these two poles. Sometimes it is the reality of an anonymous crowd made up of people indifferent to one another but manifesting a "collective desire" (Ex-voto and also Crowd, Transnationalism). At other times, it relates to isolated individuals who are nonetheless receptive to the world (Luxury, Spirituality, Yawning). The notion of contagion also helps to describe the shaping of a memory process (Prophylaxis) or the power of religious myth over a long—sometimes very long—period (Myth). In such cases the process under consideration is relevant to a large community and perhaps to a high proportion of the human population.

Modes of spread also raise crucial questions. Is physical contact essential, as the word's etymology suggests? Not always, certainly. In some cases, an object supports the contagion and prolongs the contact, either because it has symbolic value or because it is a repository of transcendence (Ex-voto, Relics). But in many instances, there is no established contact. A contagious process may then combine internal and external vectors of propagation (Prison, Revolution). One of the vectors may be the place or context of origin: internal dissensions within a community may transform a technical and localized controversy into a far-flung debate outside of the community (Controversy). Sometimes the contagion takes the form of population movements that can be visualized (Cartography, Migration, Suicide, Swamps, Transnationalism). Finally, propagation depends on the recipient, especially when contagion occurs by imitation, raising the question of whether the process is triggered by the person imitated or by the person performing the imitation by means of their imagination

(Consumption, Luxury, Spirituality, Yawning). Imitation appears to be a borderline case of contagion.

Contagion consists in a horizontal link that is by its very nature social. As a phenomenon of destabilization of the self by another person, it makes visible the lines that divide social groups (Aristocracy, Naming, Prison) or religious groups (Anti-Semitism, Belief, Judeity, Sanctity). In a society confronted by contagion, the challenges presented lead to new practices that offer concrete answers to the situation and to the constraints it engenders. The same is true of the remedies against contagion, which are of different sorts. Certain rituals are seen to have induced the population to come together and fight jointly against the evil's advance (Plague, Prophylaxis, Sanctity), while other measures promoted "distancing" (to use the term current in the coronavirus pandemic of 2020), restraining or accentuating a "dissolution of the social linkage" that followed many epidemics.[26] Hence distinguishing criteria were used to categorize suspects, separating contaminated from noncontaminated, or indeed to capture the influence of one social group upon another (Aristocracy, Clothing, Heresy, Prison).

By reducing social links and making them less flexible, the process of contagion also reveals the underlying power issues. It opens the way for certain groups to dominate others (Colonization, Red Guards, Tradition) and can reinforce distinctions among genres (Clothing, Dance). The process enable the spread of ideologies through invoking the metaphor of contamination (Judeity, Languages, Race) all while stimulating mechanisms of resistance. Strategies of propagation are opposed to those of restriction (Languages, Progress, Revolution). Political and economic issues get mixed up with scientific factors, as is shown by the history of technical or medical innovations (Epidemic, Innovation, Microbes, Progress, Smallpox) as well as that of environmental policies (Aluminum, Nuclear, Pollution, Swamps); Thomas Piketty shows as much regarding the 2020 COVID-19 pandemic in his afterword. The cultural productions of a particular period can appropriate medical concepts and rework them, thereby exemplifying hybrid interactions between areas of knowledge (Dance, Literature, Suicide, Theater). The interpretation of contagious phenomena calls upon the philosophical, scientific, and anthropological conceptions of a society; it tests its conception of the world, from mind-body relationship to interactions between human beings with their fellows and with the natural world (Analogy, Pollution, Yawning).

Contagion's horizontality also intersects with another dimension, which is vertical and transcendent, as contagion can develop in interaction with supraterrestrial entities, be they divine, demonic, or astral. Such interaction is notably evident in reactions of collective piety placing a community under divine protection (Plague, Prophylaxis, Sanctity) and in individual behaviors expressive of a personal and subjective relationship with God transmitted from one person to another by imitative contagion (Spirituality).

Examining these questions in this book provides many different angles of approach, and the perspective offered on contagion—or on demonstrations of contagion—is kaleidoscopic rather than unified. These instances also reveal the boundaries of using "contagion" as a tool and show what the concept cannot do. One of the problems exposed is a tendency to depoliticize described situations as instances of contagion, historical actors ceasing to be regarded as responsible agents when their behavior is depicted as inevitable (Anti-Semitism). In truth, the notion sometimes shows itself to be more useful in describing phenomena than in explaining or analyzing them, because it is more efficient at showing effects than underlying or explicit causes. It is an analytical framework that encounters difficulty in showing up the social connections, relationships of strength and power, and all of the interweaving factors at work behind the waves of propagation.

Moreover, the contagion metaphor sometimes leads to an excessively rigid view of a situation, setting it in concrete by privileging one form of interaction over all others. Showing that a particular phenomenon spreads inexorably can, for example, lead to homogenizing reality and failing to take account of its complexity (Aristocracy). When using models, historians run the risk of obscuring what is exceptional, ignoring circumstances, particular points, the behavior of historical actors, and surprises. This interpretative tool comes with a challenge, that of not forcing the sources, of not masking what does not fit the analytical framework.

How then should this book be read? The large number of contributions and the variety of their content may seem disconcerting. Nonetheless, each contribution is a singular entity that can be discovered and appreciated independently of the others. Each one combines three aspects: (1) it connects with the guiding principle of the volume and explores the notion of contagion as a process applicable to a historical context; (2) it is topped by a headword indicating the broad thematic area to which it belongs; and (3) it provides an individual title describing more narrowly the piece's specific subject. Readers wishing to select groups of contributions have several possibilities to choose from. They can follow lines of inquiry already suggested, or follow a route that looks at themes, namely: medicine,[27] politics,[28] and the environment[29] as related to contagious phenomena; social practices[30] and cultural practices[31] engendered by contagion; religious practices;[32] phenomena of exclusion arising from contagion;[33] mechanisms of transmission, creation, and copying activated in areas of artistic, literary, and intellectual endeavor.[34] Readers will find some historical answers here, and references are provided at the end of each piece to aid further inquiry. The book, which opens and closes with COVID-19, can also be read straight through, from cover to cover, allowing an effectively random overview dictated only by alphabetical order. This method of organization is deliberate, allowing for a mixing of ideas and avenues, and avoiding confinement within excessively restricted themes and meanings. It has already been pointed out that little is to be gained from dividing literal from metaphorical uses of the word "contagion." Similarly, thematic divisions ignore interactions between fields, the ebbs and flows between frontiers of knowledge and their historically constituted character. Alphabetical order is an alternative way of presenting knowledge, as it allows contagion to keep its polysemy and ambiguity and stops it from becoming frozen in one dimension. It also permits flexibility of thinking, enabling the volume to retain something of a partially untamed, labyrinthine character. Readers are therefore free to read this book empirically and to decide in what direction their reading should take them, and they will, we trust, find resources here to make it an agreeable journey.

NOTES

1. Jared Diamond, *Guns, Germs and Steel: The Fates of Human Societies* (New York: Norton, 1997); Mark Harrison, *Contagion: How Commerce Has Spread Disease* (New Haven: Yale University Press, 2012).

2. Frédéric Keck, *Un monde grippé* (Paris: Flammarion, 2010), especially conclusion.

3. Florent Coste, Adrien Minard, and Aurélien Robert, "Contagions: Histoire de la précarité humaine," *Tracés* 21 (2011): 8.

4. https://ahdictionary.com.

5. Bruno Latour, *Pasteur: Guerre et paix des microbes* (Paris: Éditions Anne-Marie Métailié, 1984); Peter Baldwin, *Contagion and the State in Europe, 1830–1930* (Cambridge: Cambridge University Press, 1999); Erwin H. Ackerknecht, "Anticontagionism between 1821 and 1867," *Bulletin of the History of Medicine* 22 (1948): 562–593.

6. Vivian Nutton, "Did the Greeks Have a Word for it? Contagion and Contagion Theory in Classical Antiquity," in *Contagion: Perspectives from Pre-Modern Societies*, ed. Lawrence I. Conrad and Dominik Wujastyk (Aldershot: Ashgate, 2000), 137–162; Vivian Nutton, "Seeds of Disease: An Explanation of Contagion and Infection from the Greeks to the Renaissance," *Medical History* 27, no. 1 (January 1983): 1–34; Mirko Grmek, "Les vicissitudes de la notion d'infection, de contagion et de germe dans la médecine antique," in *Textes médicaux latins antiques*, ed. Guy Sabbah (Saint-Étienne: Publications de l'Université de Saint-Étienne, 1984), 53–70; John Copeland Nagle, "The Idea of Pollution," *UC Davis Law Review* 43, no. 1 (November 2009): 1–78.

7. Owsei Temkin, "An Historical Analysis of the Concept of Infection," in *The Double Face of Janus and Other Essays in the History of Medicine* (Baltimore: Johns Hopkins University Press, 1977), 456–471; Lawrence I. Conrad and Dominik Wujastyk, "Introduction," in *Contagion: Perspectives from Pre-Modern Societies*, ix–xviii, x–xii; Justin K. Stearns, *Infectious Ideas: Contagion in Premodern Islamic and Christian Thought in the Western Mediterranean* (Baltimore: Johns Hopkins University Press, 2011), 91–105.

8. Jon Arrizabalaga, "Facing the Black Death: Perceptions and Reactions of University Medical Practitioners," in *Practical Medicine from Salerno to the Black Death*, ed. Luis Garcia-Ballester et al. (Cambridge: Cambridge University Press, 1994), 237–288.

9. François-Olivier Touati, "Contagion and Leprosy: Myth, Ideas and Evolution in Medieval Minds and Societies," in *Contagion: Perspectives from Pre-Modern Societies*, 179–201; "Historiciser la notion de contagion: L'exemple de la lèpre dans les sociétés médiévales," in *Air, miasmes et contagion: Les épidémies dans l'Antiquité et au Moyen Âge*, ed. Sylvie Bazin-Tacchella, Danielle Quéruel, and Evelyne Samama (Langres: Dominique Guéniot, 2001), 157–188.

10. Nutton, "Seeds of Disease"; Vivian Nutton, "The Reception of Fracastoro's Theory of Contagion: The Seed That Fell among Thorns?" *Osiris* 6 (1990): 196–234; Concetta Pennutto,

Simpatia, fantasia e contagio: Il pensiero medico e il pensiero filosofico di Girolamo Fracastoro (Rome: Edizioni di Storia e Letteratura, 2008), 381–453.

11. Gérard Fabre, *Épidémies et contagions: L'imaginaire du mal en Occident* (Paris: PUF, 1998), 118; Patrice Bourdelais, "La construction de la notion de contagion: entre médecine et société," *Communications* 66 (1998): 21–39; Erwin H. Ackerknecht, "Anticontagionism between 1820 and 1867"; Alain Corbin, *Le miasme et la jonquille: L'odorat et l'imaginaire social, XVIIᵉ–XIXᵉ siècles* (Paris: Aubier, 1982).

12. Béatrice Delaurenti, *La puissance des mots:* "Virtus verborum," in *Débats doctrinaux sur les incantations au Moyen Âge* (Paris: Cerf, 2007), 157–200.

13. Justin K. Stearns, *Infectious Ideas*, 99–105; Donald Beecher, "Windows of Contagion," in *Imagining Contagion in Early Modern Europe*, ed. Claire L. Carlin (New York: Palgrave Macmillan, 2005), 32–46; Aurélien Robert, "Fascinatio," in *Mots médiévaux offerts à Ruedi Imbach*, ed. Iñigo Atucha et al. (Turnhout: Brepols, 2011), 279–290.

14. Nutton, "Seeds of Disease," 29–30.

15. Nutton, "The Reception of Fracastoro's Theory of Contagion," 210.

16. Beecher, "Windows of Contagion," 32.

17. Arnaud Fossier, "La contagion des péchés (XIe–XIIIe siècle): Aux origines canoniques du biopouvoir," *Tracés* 21 (2011): 23–40, https://doi.org/10.4000/traces.5128.

18. Christian Borch, *Imitation, Contagion, Suggestion: On Mimesis and Society* (Abingdon: Routledge, 2019); Dan Sperber, *La contagion des idées: Théorie naturaliste de la culture* (Paris: Odile Jacob, 1996).

19. Beecher, "An Afterword on Contagion," in *Imagining Contagion*, 244.

20. In the sense of the title of the volume edited by Claire L. Carlin, *Imagining Contagion*. See also Beecher, "An Afterword on Contagion," 244, 254–259.

21. The current volume's confines are those of the Centre de Recherches Historiques (EHESS/CNRS, Paris), a research unit whose generalist remit covers historical periods and themes. All of the current volume's contributors are members in different capacities of the Centre de Recherches Historiques.

22. Conrad and Wujastyk, "Introduction," xv.

23. Jacques Cheyronnaud, Philippe Roussin, and Georges Vigarello, "Présentation," *Communications* 66 (1998): 5–7.

24. In his *Éloge de la variante: Histoire critique de la philologie* (Paris: Seuil, 1989), 10: "carcan de la fixité textuelle."

25. Cheyronnaud, Roussin, and Vigarello, "Presentation," 5: "donner une vie distincte, objectivable et circonstanciée à l'infravisible."

26. Gérard Fabre, *Épidémies et contagions*, 28.

27. Cartography, Epidemics, Microbes, Smallpox, Yawning.

28. Colonization, Progress, Red Guards, Revolution, Tradition.

29. Aluminum, Nuclear, Pollution, Swamps.

30. Aristocracy, Consumption, Crowd, Luxury, Migration, Solitude, Suicide, Transnationalism.

31. Dance, Languages, Literature, Theater, Vogue.

32. Belief, *Ex-voto*, Heresy, Plague, Prophylaxis, Relics, Sanctity, Spirituality.

33. Anti-Semitism, Judeity, Myth, Prison, Race.

34. Analogy, Calendar, Controversy, Iconography, Innovation, Manuscripts, Ritual, Writing.

SELECTED BIBLIOGRAPHY

Ackerknecht, Erwin. "Anticontagionism between 1821 and 1867." *Bulletin of the History of Medicine* 22 (1948): 562–593.

Arrizabalaga, Jon. "Facing the Black Death: Perceptions and Reactions of University Medical Practitioners." In *Practical Medicine from Salerno to the Black Death*, edited by Luis Garcia-Ballester, Robert French, Jon Arrizabalaga, and Andrew Cunningham, 237–288. Cambridge: Cambridge University Press, 1994.

Baldwin, Peter. *Contagion and the State in Europe, 1830–1930*. Cambridge: Cambridge University Press, 1999.

Bazin-Tacchella, Sylvie, Danielle Quéruel, and Évelyne Samama, eds. *Air, miasme et contagion: Les épidémies de l'Antiquité au Moyen Âge*. Langres: Dominique Guéniot, 2001.

Borch, Christian, ed. *Imitation, Contagion, Suggestion: On Mimesis and Society*. Abingdon: Routledge, 2019.

Carlin, Claire L., ed. *Imagining Contagion in Early Modern Europe*. New York: Palgrave Macmillan, 2005.

Cheyronnaud, Jacques, Philippe Roussin, and Georges Vigarello, eds. "La Contagion." Special issue, *Communications* 66 (1998).

Conrad, Lawrence I., and Dominik Wujastyk, eds. *Contagion: Perspectives from Pre-Modern Societies*. Aldershot: Ashgate, 2000.

Coste, Florent, Adrien Minard, and Aurélien Robert, eds. "Contagions: Histoires de la précarité humaine." Special issue, *Tracés* 21 (2011).

Diamond, Jared. *Guns, Germs and Steel: The Fates of Human Societies*. New York: Norton, 1997.

Fabre, Gérard. *Épidémies et contagions: L'imaginaire du mal en Occident*. Paris: PUF, 1998.

Grmek, Mirko. "Les vicissitudes de la notion d'infection, de contagion et de germe dans la médecine antique." In *Textes médicaux latins antiques*, edited by Guy Sabbah, 53–70. Saint-Étienne: Publications de l'Université de Saint-Étienne, 1984.

Harrison, Mark. *Contagion: How Commerce Has Spread Disease.* New Haven: Yale University Press, 2012.

Jarcho, Saul J. *The Concept of Contagion in Medicine, Literature, and Religion.* Malabar: Krieger Publishing, 2000.

Keck, Frédéric. *Un monde grippé.* Paris: Flammarion, 2010.

Latour, Bruno. *Pasteur: Guerre et paix des microbes.* Paris: Éditions Anne-Marie Métailié, 1984.

Nagle, John Copeland. "The Idea of Pollution." *UC Davis Law Review* 43, no. 1 (November 2009): 1–78.

Nutton, Vivian. "The Reception of Fracastoro's Theory of Contagion: The Seed That Fell among Thorns?" *Osiris* 6 (1990): 196–234.

Nutton, Vivian. "Seeds of Disease: An Explanation of Contagion and Infection from the Greeks to the Renaissance." *Medical History* 27, no. 1 (January 1983): 1–34.

Pelling, Margaret. "Contagion/Germ Theory/Specificity." In *Companion Encyclopedia of the History of Medicine*, vol. 1, edited by William F. Bynum and Roy Porter, 309–334. London: Routledge, 1993.

Pennuto, Concetta. *Simpatia, fantasia e contagio: Il pensiero medico e il pensiero filosofico di Girola mo Fracastoro.* Rome: Edizioni di Storia e Letteratura, 2008.

Snowden, Frank. *Epidemics and Society: From the Black Death to the Present.* New Haven: Yale University Press, 2019.

Sperber, Dan. *La contagion des idées: Théorie naturaliste de la culture.* Paris: Odile Jacob, 1996.

Stearns, Justin K. *Infectious Ideas: Contagion in Premodern Islamic and Christian Thought in the Western Mediterranean.* Baltimore: Johns Hopkins University Press, 2011.

Temkin, Owsei. "An Historical Analysis of the Concept of Infection." In *The Double Face of Janus and Other Essays in the History of Medicine*, 456–471. Baltimore: Johns Hopkins University Press, 1977.

ALUMINUM

The Hypothesis of an Alzheimer's Disease Epidemic?

Florence Hachez-Leroy

Aluminum is the third constituent element of the Earth's crust (8.1 percent), after oxygen and silicon and before iron (5 percent). Its affinity with oxygen rendered its extraction difficult, and it was not obtained in the form of metal mass until 1854. Aluminum oxide itself has been known since antiquity: alum is a hydrated double sulphate of aluminum used in tanneries and as a mordant in dyeing. Unlike other metals that are trace elements (copper, iron, zinc), aluminum is not necessary for the human metabolism. Beginning in the middle of the nineteenth century, its consumption in metallic form (kitchen utensils) and in the form of a food additive (baking powder), and then in the twentieth century in medications (acid reducers) and in cosmetics (deodorants), has raised concerns over its potential harmfulness via contamination of food and the body.

The history of aluminum and its safety involves the question of one or several pathologies linked to the absorption of the metal in different forms. Chronic fatigue syndrome and macrophagic myofasciitis are not, a priori, infectious diseases. However, the increase in cases of patients affected by Alzheimer's disease has made it possible for the term "contagion" to be used, and even more pertinently, work published in 2018 has argued that it could be transmitted between individuals, as with Creutzfeldt-Jakob disease. If contagion is defined as the transmission of a disease from one person to another, our point of view is that the generalized contamination of a population by a noninfectious agent, in this case aluminum, also participates in the phenomenon of contagion, with which specific pathologies are associated. We move from contamination to contagion.

There are many moments in the history of aluminum that raise the question of a contagion. At the end of the nineteenth century, two scientific polemics existed over the use of aluminum in food. The first, Franco-German, concerned the analysis of the material used for the equipment of French and German soldiers, their flasks in particular. Although no cases of intoxication were confirmed, three scientists challenged the safety of aluminum on the grounds that the liquids in the flasks corroded the metal. All three were quickly refuted by the rest of the scientific community, not unreasonably considering the nature of the material studied and the conditions of the analysis: the samples came from objects made of metal obtained from the early days of industrial production, when poorly controlled technical parameters would leave behind impurities. In addition, one of the scientists did even not carry out the analyses himself, effectively invalidating his conclusions.

The second, longer, scientific controversy was over food in the United States and set those in favor of baking powder containing aluminum salts against those who denounced it as toxic. The latter included producers of aluminum-free baking powder as well as independent researchers convinced of its toxicity. It is difficult to know whether any affected people were found, with the exception of a toxicologist from Yale University, who claimed to have identified casualties. For the first time, (brief) clinical trials were carried out on humans, but it was mainly dogs and rats that were sacrificed on the altar of aluminum. Increases in the dosage ingested systematically led to the deterioration of the animals' health or indeed to their death. These observations, although they did not prevent the use of aluminum in baking powder, nevertheless made it possible to record its neurotoxic effects when ingested in large doses as well as its presence in various organs such as the liver, spleen, and brain.

The first patients sick from aluminum were identified in the period between the First and Second World War, in the United Kingdom, thanks to the work of a general practitioner, Robert Montague Le Hunte Cooper, who observed among some of his patients major signs of chronic fatigue along with joint pain and dizziness. Proceeding empirically, he eliminated the possible causes of contamination one by one and observed that his patients' conditions would improve when they stopped using aluminum kitchen utensils. He delved into the scientific literature on the issue and discovered American studies on baking powder made from aluminum. He went on to perform laboratory experiments and confirmed his hypothesis: contamination by aluminum was the cause of an infection in a significant number of patients. The doctor did not, however, manage to assert his opinion successfully in the face of the opposition marshaled by the industrialists defending the metal's innocuousness.

In the 1960s, research nonetheless evolved in the direction of Cooper's conclusions. The role of aluminum in encephalopathies was a hypothesis raised in scientific publications worldwide. The case of dialysis in Denver, in 1975, would come to corroborate the doctor's suspicions, with a significant number of patients affected by senile dementia in the hospital that was caring for them. The use of a scanning electron microscope made it possible to confirm the presence of aluminum, associated with phosphorus, in the form of fine concretions in a deceased patient's brain. The intoxication was due to the absorption of aluminum salts by the digestive tract to combat phosphoremia. A decade later, the work of two British researchers identified "senile plaques" as characteristic of brains affected by Alzheimer, which comprised an identical distribution of aluminum and silicon. The year 1986 thus marked a turning point in the history of concerns over aluminum. Many mainstream newspapers, daily and weekly, took up the conclusions of this work and emphasized its sensationalism, declaring more or less peremptorily that aluminum was the cause of the Alzheimer's disease epidemic.

In 1998, a team led by professors Gherardi and Authier, at the Henri Mondor Hospital, described a novel histologic lesion among patients suffering from diffuse, debilitating myalgia, whose characteristics earned it the name "macrophagic myofasciitis." The investigations carried out showed the presence, in the histologic lesions' macrophages, of specular inclusions composed of aluminum hydroxide. The presence of the latter was due to its use as a vaccine adjuvant to improve the immune response of inactivated vaccines. As a result of its research, the team proposed the hypothesis that chronic fatigue syndrome could be caused by the presence of pathogenic agents or toxic compounds—aluminum in this case—that have immune stimulant effects, provoking an incessant stimulation of the immune system. According to their work, chronic fatigue syndrome is linked to aluminum salts. Macrophagic myofasciitis is therefore a chronic illness that, thus far, has not led to any deaths. Very disabling, it can persist, go into regression, or even disappear in a timeframe that varies greatly according to the patient, and the doctor's role is essentially to try to ease the patient's suffering.

From these works, a vast medical controversy has emerged, involving different groups of actors: the medical community, divided between those (the minority) willing to explore the potential harm of vaccine adjuvants and those (the majority) who refuse to do so; the association of patients with macrophagic myofasciitis who seek to bring attention to the developing research into adjuvants and who try to make their voices heard despite being numerically less important than other groups, such as those for autism or cancer; and institutions such as the Academy of Medicine that are hostile to these hypotheses. The debate is made very difficult by the fact that raising doubts about aluminum adjuvants is seen, or presented, as an attack against vaccination itself. Indeed, participants in the debate include antivaccine activists happy for an opportunity to reinforce their hostility.

Is it appropriate to speak of contagion here? Certain illnesses, despite being widespread, remain poorly understood by medical research. This is the case for autoimmune disorders and their trigger mechanisms or chronic diseases such as systemic exertion intolerance disease, still called chronic fatigue syndrome or myalgic encephalomyelitis, which is characterized by an inflammation of the spinal cord and brain with muscle pain. Researchers also suspect aluminum to be a cause for various other pathologies, such as Crohn's disease, breast cancer, or autism. Its very broad use in the food and agriculture, water purification, cosmetic, and pharmaceutical industries, as well as in transportation and in daily household objects, has over the course of a century multiplied the sources of exposure to it to the point that aluminum particles are now present in the air.

The significant increase in chronic and degenerative diseases, since the 1960s, would lead one to suppose that there are indeed some new factors of contagion, and some scientists even fear an epidemic. It remains to be understood what these factors are, especially the environmental ones. Faced with the proliferation of new substances after the Second World War and their possible interactions, the idea of "environmental contagion" has gained traction. Could it account for the scope as well as the complexity of a phenomenon now recognized by environmental medicine—the latest evolution, perhaps, of Neo-Hippocratic medicine?

translated by Jeffrey Burkholder

BIBLIOGRAPHY

Akrich, Madeleine, Yannick Barthe, and Catherine Rémy, eds. *Sur la piste environnementale: Menaces sanitaires et mobilisations profanes*. Paris: Presses des Mines, 2010.

Blanc, Paul B. *How Everyday Products Make People Sick: Toxins at Home and in the Workplace*. Berkeley: University of California Press, 2009.

Coste, Florent, Adrien Minard, and Aurélien Robert. "Contagions: Histoires de la précarité humaine." *Tracés: Revue de Sciences Humaines* [online] 21 (2011). http://journals.openedition.org/traces/5126.

Exley, Chris. "Human Exposure to Aluminium." *Environmental Science* 15 (August 2013): 1807–1816.

Gherardi, Romain. *Toxic Story*. Arles: Actes Sud, 2016.

Hachez-Leroy, Florence. *Menaces sur l'alimentation, Emballages, colorants et autres contaminants alimentaires, XIXe–XXIe siècles*. Tours: PUFR/PUR, 2019.

ANALOGY
Miniaturization, Multiplication, and Figuration in Medieval Christendom

Jean-Claude Schmitt

Insofar as the notion of contagion implies the reproduction and dissemination of a unitary entity (of a virus or microbe, for example), it necessarily links with that of analogy. By "analogy," we here use the term in the ontological sense assigned to it by the anthropologist Philippe Descola. "Analogism" in this sense—the tendency to resemble or multiply by analogy—is a feature of many cultures, including Christendom down to the eighteenth century.

Let us start with a concrete example. Around the year 1200, the Cistercian abbot Richalm von Schöntal (died 1219) declared in chapter 78 of his *Liber revelationum* (Book of revelations), "The image of our lady was often seen by me as she is painted in a picture, and no more, or rarely anything more, than from the chest and upward." His first reaction was to mistrust such an image; however,

> that very image began to multiply so that twenty or even thirty small images of the same form appeared to me on the same line. And moreover that image appeared to me like the one that pilgrims carry off with them from Saint Mary of Rocamadour, such that it was also completely the same image, to wit, it was like that leaden image that pilgrims have and which is of utterly the same form and size, and I was being told, "Dost thou now wish to believe?" As though she were saying, "I will make repeats and multiplications of my image so numerous for thee, that thou mayest be certain.[1]

This text, which is exceptional for more than one reason, appeals simultaneously to two of the senses in which the medieval Latin word *imago* was employed. Richalm uses the word to describe appearances to him of the Virgin Mary when he was awake (i.e., as *imagines spiritales*, to borrow Augustinian vocabulary). He then compares these appearances to material images, first to a painting (*pictura*: perhaps a mural) representing the Virgin and then to a small-scale model, multiplied twenty or thirty times, like the pilgrimage medals made of lead (*ymago plumbea*) distributed at Our Lady of Rocamadour, which figured the Virgin and Child in Majesty and in which the Virgin's right hand bore a scepter and her whole body was visible (see figure 1).

The abbot's testimony offers a series of analogies between the protypical Virgin who is in heaven—"spiritual images" of her or visionary appearances—and "image objects" modeled on the former and of differing sizes, be they paintings or small pilgrims' medals. In so doing, he points to a chain of relationships between the spiritual and material that belongs to what Anita Guerreau-Jalabert has termed the "generalized *spiritus-caro* (spirit-flesh) analogy." This analogy was characteristic of medieval Christian society's "implicit ideal": just as the flesh or body (*caro, corpus*) was ideally ruled by the spirit or soul, man was subject to God, the married layman to the celibate priest, the human female to the human male, the castle to the church, the material image to the spiritual image, and so on.

Such terms did not connote substances in themselves but relative polarities. For example, while man's body was made entirely of flesh, his head (the possible seat of the soul) was "spiritual" when viewed against the lower part of the body (which Richalm's vision censored in the case of the Virgin). The same went for social hierarchies and in spatial organization. However, every instance of ontology was special to its context. In Abbot Richalm's example, the relationship between the spiritual and material did not merely play on the different forms of the *imago*; it also turned on two transformations of the image, namely its miniaturization and its multiplication. In terms of today's world, do not such terms evoke microbes and contagion?

Within Christian culture, these terms referenced another paradigm— that of the eucharist. The eucharist, or more precisely the host consecrated

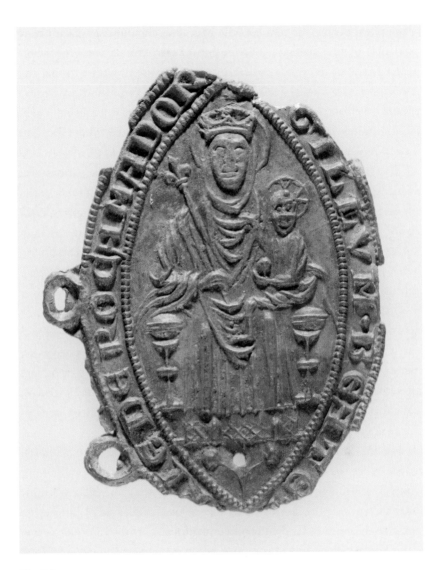

Figure 1

Pilgrimage medal from Notre-Dame at Rocamadour. *Source*: Musée National du Moyen Âge–Thermes de Cluny.

by the priest during the canon of the mass, was the most significant concretization of the analogical relationship of *spiritus* and *caro*. The sacramental words of the priest explicitly repeated those of Christ during the Last Supper; the consecrated host was the *Corpus Christi* (body of Christ) reduced in size to a mouthful of unleavened bread that could be reproduced infinitely and identically via a wafer mold to enable every Christian to communicate at least once a year, at Easter.

The same paradigm was at work in many other representations and practices typical of Christian culture, beginning with the cult of relics. The cult consisted of the dismemberment of the bodies of holy martyrs, confessors, and virgins and the dispersal of the same in fragments among a limitless number of Christendom's notable locations, such places becoming thereby so many magnetic poles of spatial social organization. Meanwhile, each small item, duly conserved in a reliquary, exercised the saint's power to work miracles as if he or she were fully alive and entire. Another example was the ex-voto, which, like a seal, was most often made of wax and represented materially—yet no less spiritually, since it was intended as an offering to a local saint or to the Virgin—the part of the body (arm, leg, breast, head, etc.) for which the pilgrim sought healing. In both instances, miniaturization and mass multiplication served the "generalized *spiritus-caro* analogy."

For the historian of medieval society, the miniaturization of hosts, images, relics, or seals, which was necessary to their mass reproduction, evokes a well-known notion—that of the microcosm. The full-page miniature shown in figure 2 reveals an awake Abbess Hildegard of Bingen listening to the word of God and contemplating an anthropomorphic image of the Trinity, which in its open arms holds the macrocosm (the circles of heaven, the stars, planets, and winds). In the center is the microcosm: a naked man, with chest full frontal, legs slightly turned toward his right, and arms outstretched to touch the inner circle of the clouds with his fingertips. Man is made "in the image of God" (*ad imaginem Dei*, Genesis 1:27); he is the microcosmic model of the Creation, a model that is incarnated in each individual man as generation succeeds to generation. The

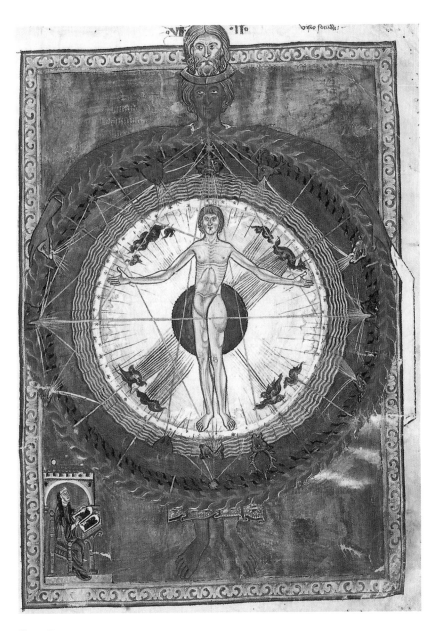

Figure 2

Hildegard of Bingen, *Liber operum divinorum*. *Source*: Lucca, Biblioteca Statale, lat. 1942, fol. 6, around 1230.

slight twist of the body indicates reveals the image to be not static but dynamic, ceaselessly replicated in every man as time goes on: the analogy reproduces itself without end.

The analogical interpretation of the world implied a further peculiarity of Christian ideology, namely the idea of universal time running from the Creation to the Last Judgment, in which the cardinal event (its *cardo* or "hinge") was the Incarnation. This event made analogy the key to Christian interpretation of the Bible, where the "types" of the Old Testament (its happenings and participants) prefigured the "antitypes" of the New (such as Christ, the Virgin Mary, and the Church). As Erich Auerbach (1892–1957) pointed out, what best characterized this Christian culture was not so much *mimesis* ("imitation," as in antiquity or the Renaissance) as the *figura* or, more precisely, as he defines it, "the figurative interpretation of reality." Such an interpretative method, which went back to Saint Paul, held, to take one example, that Joshua was a type or prefigurement of Christ and Christ was a fulfillment or definitive version of Joshua. The manuscripts of the *Bible Moralisée*, one of the most richly illuminated manuscripts of the thirteenth century, showed such typological relationships by systematically linking a medallion of a "type" (A) to its "antitype" (A′), reproducing this matrix four times on the same page throughout the manuscript (see figure 3a).

The pictorial representation of this "generalized analogy" is arresting, with its systematic relation of a more "physical" and "Judaic" "type" (e.g., in B, the creation of Adam and Eve) with a more "physical" and "Christian" "antitype" (in B′, the "birth" of the *Ecclesia* or Church from the wound in the side of the Crucified).

In sum, the plasticity of analogy allowed for a vast range of uses that worked throughout society. The miniaturization and multiplication of constitutive units permitted the *caro-spiritus* analogy to insinuate itself (not unlike a microbial infection) into all fields of representation and practice. All that was required, in each case, was for the functional legitimacy of the social order, its hierarchies, and powers to be thereby demonstrated.

translated by Graham Robert Edwards

(a) (b)

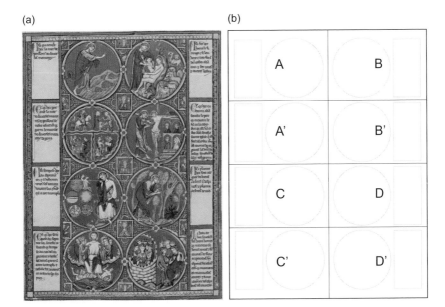

Figure 3

(a) *Bible Moralisée*. Source: Vienna, ÖNB, Codex Vindobonensis 25. (b) Pictorial representation of figure 3a.

NOTE

1. Richalm von Schöntal, *Liber revelationum*, in *Monumenta Germaniae Historica, Quellen zur Geistesgeschicht des Mittlealters*, vol. 24, ed. Paul G. Schmidt (Hannover, Hahnsche Buchhandlung, 2009), 97.

SELECTED BIBLIOGRAPHY

Auerbach, Erich. *Figura: La loi juive et la Promesse chrétienne*. Paris: Macula, 2003. First published in 1967.

Dahan, Gilbert. *L'exégèse chrétienne de la Bible dans l'Occident médiéval, XIIe–XIVe siècle*. Paris: Cerf, 1999.

Descola, Philippe. *Par-delà nature et culture*. Paris: Gallimard, 2005.

Guerreau-Jalabert, Anita. "Occident médiéval et pensée analogique: Le sens de *spiritus et caro.*" In *La légitimité implicite*, vol. 1, edited by Jean-Philippe Genet, 457–476. Paris and Rome: Publications de la Sorbonne-École française de Rome, 2015.

Kretschner, Marek Thue, ed. *La typologie biblique comme forme de pensée dans l'historiographie médiévale*. Fédération Internationale des Instituts d'Études Médiévales, Textes et Études du Moyen Âge 75. Turnhout: Brepols, 2014.

Lubac, Henri de. *Exégèse mediévale: Les quatre sens de l'écriture*, vol. 1–4. Paris: Cerf, 1959–1964.

Schmitt, Jean-Claude. *Les rythmes au Moyen Âge*. Paris: Gallimard, 2016.

Schmitt, Jean-Claude. *Penser par figures: Du compass divin aux diagrammes magiques*. Paris: Arkhé, 2019.

ANTI-SEMITISM

Anti-Semitism as a Disease: The History and Significance of a Metaphor

Olof Bortz

In October 2018, a white supremacist killed eleven Jewish worshippers at the Tree of Life Congregation in Pittsburgh. After the shooting, Deborah E. Lipstadt, a scholar of Holocaust memory and American-Jewish history, compared anti-Semitism to the contagious virus of herpes. She presumably employed this metaphor as a shorthand to convey her understanding of a phenomenon that is latent and not always visible and can spread imperceptibly. A few months later, in the spring of 2019, a case of measles spread within the Hasidic communities in the state of New York. The authorities quickly declared the outbreak a public health emergency due to the disease's extremely contagious nature. They then proceeded to shut down a number of Hasidic schools for failing to abide by vaccination regulations. This public health crisis created a link between Hasidic Jews and measles in the public mind, and a handful of incidents ensued in which Hasidic individuals were verbally and physically abused. Agudath Israel of America, a Hasidic umbrella organization, issued a warning against "infectious hatred" in an attempt to shield the Hasidic community from such attacks.

What is the significance of calling anti-Semitism infectious or contagious and depicting it as a form of disease or virus? Such language might be nothing more than rhetorical flourish to embellish dry academic jargon, but it has a specific resonance in the case of anti-Semitism. This text starts by examining criticism of these metaphors among scholars of anti-Semitism. It then proceeds to make the case for a different interpretation of them. In so doing, it makes two claims. First, it proposes that the persistence and the specific implications of disease metaphors for describing anti-Semitism need to be situated in relation to Jewish history. In more specific terms, it suggests seeing such metaphors as a result of a political transition in the way Western societies have perceived Jewish minorities. Second, it argues that every instance of anti-Semitism has a specific political context that metaphors of disease tend to obscure.

Metaphors of contagion and disease as a description of anti-Semitism are well known among scholars of anti-Semitism, and some have expressed criticism of them. Steven Beller tasks such metaphors with "reifying its subject as something with a will of its own, a contagious 'virus,' beyond the capacity of any individual to control or combat."[1] In Beller's view, metaphors related to disease relieve anti-Semites of responsibility for the disease with which they are afflicted. Instead of actors and purveyors of hatred, anti-Semites become passive recipients of disease.

Albert Lindemann and Richard Levy argue that metaphors of disease mimic the rhetoric employed against Jews throughout history.[2] In effect, Jews have been depicted as a contagious disease threatening Christianity and non-Jewish societies by their very presence. The imagery connecting Jews to disease dates back to the Middle Ages when Jews were forced to live in cramped conditions and in insalubrious areas of European cities. It gained renewed actuality during the late nineteenth century with the mass emigration of Jews from Eastern Europe. During the Holocaust, images of Jews as bacteria, disease, and vermin were the propagandistic equivalent of genocide. Historians such as Beller, Lindemann, and Levy thus point to problems of using disease metaphors concerning anti-Semitism. They present it as a way of recycling anti-Jewish imagery and absolving anti-Semites from responsibility.

There is, however, a political context at play that these historians fail to address, namely a reversal of perspectives concerning Jews and non-Jews in discourses on anti-Semitism during the twentieth century. What is the nature and cause of hatred against Jews? Historically, the answer to that question has to a large extent referred to Jews and their characteristics, even by those favoring the Jewish cause. In the eighteenth century, the German Christian Konrad Wilhelm von Dohm and the French Abbé Grégoire argued that a change of occupation, such as that from money lending to farming, and social integration would counteract anti-Jewish animosity. These ideas gained adherents in Prussia during the following century where Jews wanted to adapt to merit equal rights. Even after political emancipation and with the emergence of anti-Semitism as a political movement in the 1890s, both Jewish and non-Jewish observers regarded cultural and economic assimilation as a remedy.

Zionist thinkers of the late nineteenth century, such as the Russian physician Leon Pinsker, by contrast, presented anti-Semitism as a pathological phobia that Jews could do little about. Pinsker thus rejected the option of assimilation in favor of the creation of a Jewish state. Yet, Zionism as a political movement was also conceived as a normalization of Jewish existence by ending their constant minority status and providing them with a state of their own. In that regard, it was yet another way of changing Jews in response to anti-Semitism. From that perspective, Zionist youth organizations who taught their members how to till the land in preparation for their migration to Palestine were not all that different from earlier attempts at *Berufsumschichtung*. The belief in assimilation, however, was dented when the German Jews—the most assimilated of the European Jewish communities— were the target of the most violent onslaught in Jewish history.

Following the confrontation of the Allies with Nazi Germany, it made sense to present anti-Semites as a threat to democracy and world peace. In the spring of 1945, the American historian Koppel S. Pinson noted that the Second World War had "more clearly than ever before in the history of the Jewish problem identified the cause of anti-Semitism with the forces of political reaction, corruption and aggressive war."[3] Thus, a regime that saw the struggle against Jews as one of its most important objectives made it possible to argue that anti-Semitism represented a threat not only for Jews. Moreover, the condemnation of Nazism presented it as both a political extremism and a form of moral deviancy. Sociologists and psychologists published research presenting anti-Semitism as a social or mental pathology. They drew on an understanding of anti-Semitism that had been developed in the 1890s but seemed particularly apt because of the phantasmagoric nature of Nazi anti-Semitism.

In the decades following the Second World War, Jewish communities in Europe and North America became assimilated in a new and more fundamental way. Instead of being linked to a specific "Jewish problem," they now became one of several white religious or ethnic groups free from discrimination. Prejudice and stereotypes about Jews decreased, and the idea that they and their cultural or religious distinctiveness constituted a problem for society belonged henceforth to only the most extreme political fringe. Calling anti-Semitism a form of contagious disease reversed the perspective by arguing that non-Jews rather than Jews constituted a problem. This relieved Jews from the burden of accounting for the hatred directed at them.

Metaphors of contagion and disease can thus be taken as a sign of political progress in discourses about anti-Semitism. In scholarly terms, however, they might obscure more than they explain. First and foremost, claiming that anti-Semitism is a disease tells us little about the contexts in which it appears and is articulated. It intimates that the problem is always the same. Second, the move to biology marks a tendency to depoliticize, or even dehumanize, phenomena that are in fact political, cultural, and social. Metaphors need to be assessed for how efficiently they allow us to see things and aspects of reality that we would otherwise miss. Disease metaphors denote a transformation in how to approach anti-Semitism, from evaluating Jews to diagnosing anti-Semites. At the same time, they also point to a failure to address the threat against Jews in different times and places as distinct problems. Although anti-Jewish stereotypes certainly spread across countries and ages, as a form of contagion one might say, this does not mean that they represent the same phenomenon, either in social, political, or metaphorical terms.

NOTES

1. Steven Beller, *Antisemitism: A Very Short Introduction* (Oxford: Oxford University Press, 2015), 18.

2. Albert S. Lindemann and Richard S. Levy, "Introduction," in *Antisemitism: A History*, ed. Albert S. Lindemann and Richard S. Levy (Oxford: Oxford University Press, 2010), 7.

3. Koppel S. Pinson, "Antisemitism in the Post-War World," *Jewish Social Studies* 7, no. 2 (1945): 100.

BIBLIOGRAPHY

Ackerman, Nathan Ward, Marie Jahoda, and Carl Binger. *Anti-Semitism and Emotional Disorder: A Psychoanalytic Interpretation.* New York: Harper, 1950.

Beller, Steven. *Antisemitism: A Very Short Introduction.* Oxford: Oxford University Press, 2015.

Engel, David. "Away from a Definition of Antisemitism: An Essay in the Semantics of Historical Description." In *Rethinking European Jewish History*, edited by Jeremy Cohen and Moshe Rosman, 30–53. Oxford: Littman Library of Jewish Civilization, 2009.

Lindemann, Albert S., and Richard S. Levy, eds. *Antisemitism: A History.* Oxford: Oxford University Press, 2010.

Stimmel, Ernst, ed. *Anti-Semitism: A Social Disease.* New York: International University Press, 1946.

ARISTOCRACY
Tainted Blood and Aristocratic Values in Early Modern Spain

Sébastien Malaprade

For medieval and early modern people, epidemics, especially plagues, were among the worst scourges of the times along with war and starvation. Municipal archives bear witness to the preventive measures taken against epidemics; communities and their leaders were haunted by the fear that such scourges would return. They saw how drastic their effects could be in a world where population increase was seen as a sign of prosperity and divine blessing. But the dictionaries of the ancien régime attributed a second layer of meaning to contagion. They associated it with "vice" or "bad customs" or heresies acquired from communication with persons affected by them."[1]

It is the received historiographical view that the year 1492 saw the beginning of a new era, that of military and spiritual reconquest by Catholic forces over the Muslim and Jewish minorities in the Iberian Peninsula. The Catholic kings' decree that expelled the Jews three months after the kingdom of Grenada's surrender justified the measure in these terms: "that they who pervert the honest lives of the inhabitants of the cities and are likely to corrupt them by the contagion [of their customs] be expelled from the villages."[2] But paradoxically, in the decades that followed the restoration of religious unity and the discovery of the "New World," a developing literature within the confines of the Iberian frontiers pointed to the monarchy's degeneration. A group of reformist advisers known as *arbitristas* addressed the Spanish kings—from Philip II to Charles II—voicing their anxieties about the increasingly indolent mentality of the Spanish since the end of the Reconquest. They deplored their proclivity to abandon productive and commercial activities, leaving these to foreigners.

Such a diagnosis was often expressed through analogy with the spread of an epidemic. More generally, the discourse that included it made great use of a lexical field rooted in contagion. It was said that the values of the aristocratic elite had thoroughly contaminated society, even subverting the foundations of the third order, that of manual labor. In an opusculum published in 1600, the lawyer Martín González de Cellorigo discussed the causes of the Hispanic monarchy's decline. In that text, the depopulation of the peninsula was put down to the association of two contagionistic definitions, namely moral corruption and physical infection.[3] First, the rejection of labor was seen to have been nurtured by the financial windfall from the New World. This led to the Spanish becoming rentiers with expensive tastes and distracted them from the natural wealth that, in conformity to the canons of theology, was acquired by work and industry, hence the multiplied effects of the Castillians' "sloth," namely inflation, barren farmland, shortages, and migration to America in search of a better future. Second, the inadequate means allocated to fighting the plague—which struck between 1596 and 1602—and poor knowledge of the agents of infection had managed to "destroy the commonwealth." The two problems were of a piece: Cellorigo likened the rentier economy to a contagious ill, "a generalized plague that reduces these kingdoms to the greatest extremity, since all inhabitants, at least the majority, have been led to want to live off these means."[4] These views had an exceptional historiographical posterity. For all the dangers of essentialization, they contributed to the figure of a *homo hispanicus* frozen in time. Idle and indolent, he cultivated an exaggerated sense of honor, abhorred the mechanical and liberal arts, and aped the aristocracy with a contempt for hierarchies. Such were the characteristics that explained the economic inferiority of the Spanish in the eyes of early modern foreign observers. Travelers in the nineteenth century sometimes wrote of this resistance to labor in positive terms, as attesting a thirst for freedom. "In general, to the Spanish, work seems something humiliating and unworthy of a free man," penned Théophile Gautier.[5]

Such an interpretation, which presupposed the existence of anthropological invariants and interminable decadence, was reproduced by philologists and historians in the decades that followed the Second World War. It found expression in the polemic between Américo Castro and Claudio Sánchez Albornoz regarding Spanish identity and was in the ascendant when the French historiographical approach known as *histoire des mentalités* (history of attitudes) arrived in Spain from France. Though challenged by fresh approaches in social and economic history, this sort of interpretation has gone on feeding into numerous studies. An excellent early modernist scholar could still say in 2007 that "to live like aristocratics had become an ideal way of life for generations of Spaniards who identified with those values the honour and reputation to which they aspired."[6]

The solidification of such portrayals over the centuries helped them to appear natural and thus to deprive Spain of its proper historicity. Evoking the theme of the *trahison de la bourgeoisie* (betrayal of the bourgeoisie), Fernand Braudel popularized the notion that, from the end of the sixteenth century, the Mediterranean lands under Hispanic domination cut themselves off from capitalist networks—centered on northern Europe—and they entered a lethargic slumber that reflected an enduring crisis. The "contagion of *rente* (unearned income)," to use Bartolomé Bennassar's term, the quest for hypergamic marriages, and the diversion of capital to the land, led the bourgeoisie, according to Braudel, historian of the *Annales* school, to a form of self-renunciation.[7]

Moreover, the desire for security encouraged civil and religious elites to immobilize the market in land by means of legal instruments that alienated inheritances (entail, mortmain), while the burden of mortgage loans and perpetual rents paralyzed commercial life. If we may be permitted to caricaturize it a little, we might say that this notion of "the betrayal of the bourgeoisie" implied Spain, from the sixteenth century on, had become frozen in a historical epoch—that of aristocratic lineage—and that only a reintegration into capitalist dynamics could restore to it the historicity of which it had divested itself. Did not this idea already underlie what Gautier said, when he likened the Spanish to the sort of peoples who have no history and are ignorant of the social norms that are fundamental to advanced civilizations? "Like simple peoples close to the state of nature," Gautier says, "they have a rightness of judgment that causes them to despise the enjoyments of convention."[8]

While the analytical value of the contagion metaphor may be questionable in view of the principle of finality it induces—such a historiographical tradition suggesting that contagion spreads inexorably and homogenizes reality rather than makes it more complex—we still need to understand that term's spread from 1500. This entails examining the definition of a concept that has both physiological and cultural connotations. Denunciations of the introjection of aristocratic values into Spanish society were concomitant with policies of discrimination against *Judeo conversos* and *Moriscos*, that is, converts from Judaism and Islam, respectively. Pure blood laws, which excluded Christianized descendants of Jews and Muslims from religious institutions, the Inquisition, the universities, the aristocracy, and corporations, led to a hierarchy that distinguished between "new" and "old" Christians and prevailed throughout the ancien régime. By the action of bodily fluids (blood, semen, milk), any stigma was either effaced or reinforced through matrimonial alliances. Pure blood policies were thus a response to an obsession about the biological and moral contagion that converts would wreak on the rest of the population.

Regarding the expulsion of the Jews, another *arbitrista*, Pedro Fernández de Navarrete, observed that the kings of Spain had always preferred "to deprive themselves of an abundant population, rather than consent to the mystical body of the monarchy being subjected to ill humors whose contagious effects could corrupt the quality of the blood [of the kingdom's inhabitants]."[9] In a context in which new Christians were stigmatized, the adoption of aristocratic practices was seen as a defense against contamination and accusations of impurity. Such an attitude entailed not merely action of a racial nature by avoiding certain marriages but also the need to uphold cultural values that ran counter to those typically ascribed to Jews and Muslims. Despite their divergent opinions, Castro and Albornoz shared the view that Spanish contempt for labor was a reaction to the spirit of enterprise exhibited by the Jews or to the agricultural expertise that characterized the heirs of Al-Andalus.[10] Within this perspective, it was therefore not so much a question of a contagion of aristocratic values as of the construction of defensive strategies reckoned to obviate the assimilation of populations suspected of heresy.

translated by Graham Robert Edwards

NOTES

1. Antoine de Furetière's dictionary (1690) and the *Diccionario de la lengua castellana* (1726–1739).

2. *Real Provisión de los Reyes para la Corona de Castilla*, March 31, 1492.

3. Martín González de Cellorigo, *Memorial de la politica necesaria y util restauración à la república de España, y estados de ella, y del desempeño universal de estos reynos* (Valladolid: Juan de Bostillo, 1600).

4. De Cellorigo, *Memorial de la politica necesaria y util restauración à la república de España*, 4v.

5. Théophile Gautier, *Voyage en Espagne* (Paris: Charpentier, 1845), 269.

6. José Ignacio Fortea Pérez, "Les hiérarchies du privilège: Hidalgos, caballeros et aristocratas," in *Les sociétés au XVIIe siècle*, ed. Annie Antoine and Cédric Michon (Rennes: PUR, 2007), 424–432.

7. Bartolomé Bennassar, *Valladolid au Siècle d'or. Tome 1: Une ville de Castille et sa campagne au XVIe siècle* (Paris: Éditions de l'EHESS, 1999), 141–145 (first published, 1967); Fernand Braudel, *La Méditerranée et le monde méditerranéen à l'époque de Philippe II*, vol. 2, 2nd ed. (Paris: Armand Colin, 1966), 68 (first published 1949).

8. Théophile Gautier, *Voyage en Espagne* (Paris: Charpentier, 1845), 269.

9. Pedro Fernández de Navarrete, *Conservación de monarquías y discursos políticos*, 5th ed. (Madrid: Tomas Alban, 1806), 35 (first published in 1626 by Imprenta Real, Madrid).

10. Américo Castro, *La realidad histórica de España* (Mexico City: Porrúa, 1954); Claudio Sánchez Albornoz, *España: Un enigma histórico* (Buenos Aires: Editorial Sudamericana, 1956).

SELECTED BIBLIOGRAPHY

Bennassar, Bartolomé. *L'homme espagnol*. Paris: Complexes, 2003. First published in 1975 by Hachette (Paris).

Braudel, Fernand. *La Méditerranée et le monde méditerranéen à l'époque de Philippe II*, vol. 1–2. 2nd ed. Paris: Armand Colin, 1966. First published 1949 by Armand Colin (Paris).

Castro, Américo. *La realidad histórica de España*. Mexico City: Porrúa, 1954.

Sánchez Albornoz, Claudio. *España: Un enigma histórico*, vol 1–2. Buenos Aires: Editorial Sudamericana, 1956.

Sicroff, Albert A. *Los estatutos de limpieza de sangre: Controversias entre los siglos XV y XVII*. Madrid: Taurus, 1985.

BELIEF

Libertinism and Atheism (Sixteenth to Eighteenth Century)

Jean-Pierre Cavaillé

The denunciation of irreligiosity, impiety, libertinism, and atheism became one of the main rhetorical weapons in the religious and political controversies of the sixteenth century. It enabled multilevel attacks against an adversary, encompassing his modes of thought, opinions, morals, and behavior. In this regard, the denunciation was similar to the accusation of heresy; but it went even further than heresy at a time when that mode of stigmatization was weakening, particularly in places where the Reformation and religious pluralism had gained ground. The denunciation borrowed the metaphorical arsenal of heresiology inspired by medical discourse: notably, that irreligiosity, moral and religious licentiousness, and atheism were all contagious maladies, plagues, venoms, a poison.

This borrowing from medicine amounted to more than a question of lexical juxtaposition: the field of medicine at the time considered as contagious not only illnesses (plague and syphilis) but also poisoning by stinging or bites (scorpion, serpent) as well as poisoning by ingestion.[1] Hence, until the end of the eighteenth century, one can witness a flourishing of publications on the "antidotes" or "protectives" against "poison," "venom," or "plague" caused by heresy and also by "atheism." The relation established between the contagion of atheism and epidemics of maladies was no longer merely metaphorical. Indeed, for many authors including the most knowledgeable, it seemed evident that there must be an intrinsic, factual link between moral licentiousness and the contagion of syphilis. This was conceived as a divine sanction against "lasciviousness" that reached an unprecedented level. The proof of this was seen as the fact that the ancients had never known this evil.[2] The biggest anti-libertine offensive at the beginning of 1620s thus crystalized around the poet Théophile de Viau's obscene sonnet, which took the liberty of rhyming words to syphilis: "Phyllis, everything is all f—— up; I am dying of pox." This first verse sets the tone, but the last three were never forgiven:

> My God! I repent of having so badly lived
> If your anger does not kill me this time
> I swear from now on to f——only in the ass.[3]

The poet was not only exhibiting his pox—the fruit of his licentiousness—but also committing a "horrible blasphemy" in dreaming about sodomy, and blasphemy was usually considered as contagious as sodomy. It was the simultaneous combination of syphilis, licentiousness of morals and mind, atheism, and sodomy that represented the libertine contagion. In his *Apologie de Théophile*, Théophile denounces notably one of his accusers, the reverend priest Guérin who had cried out from his pulpit, "May God bless Mister first president and Mister public prosecutor who purged Paris from this plague! It's your [Théophile] fault that the plague is in Paris."[4]

Indeed, the plague was in Paris.

This type of accusation—suggesting that impiety, atheism, and the dissolution of morals were both causes and signs of the plague—was recurrent. In 1666, at the House of Commons, the *Leviathan* of Hobbes, regarded by his censors as the cesspit of atheism, was even cited as the possible cause for the devastating fire of London and the plague epidemics. In his *Discours très ample de la peste* (Very ample discourse on the plague), Nicolas de Nancel, a physician from the city of Tours in France, described for his readers the signs of imminent epidemics as follows: "[It looms] whenever you see that all divine and human justice is despised or abolished, service to God neglected, charity diminished, men swamped with all kinds of vices, fallen in atheism, impiety; blaspheming, swearing."[5] Furthermore, libertinism and atheism constituted in themselves a contagion with a diabolic origin and thus it was the will of God to punish them:

[. . .] the latter plague and poison so strange poured by him [the Devil] upon human species can never seize the heart of man unless there is God's supreme and just rage and judgement.[6]

In a more reasoned manner, atheism was perceived as a contagious malady whose diffusion would inevitably provoke the dissolution of society. In refusing God, atheists would destroy the foundation of all moral and human law:

> If this plague comes to spread within society, it only causes great miseries since it breaks the link between society and Republic, and wrecks the foundation that peoples' salvation and tranquility is based upon.[7]

This conviction was profoundly rooted, so it appeared logical to many. One can find it stated even in the texts of atheists such as *Theophrastus Redivivus* (1659), and this justified resorting to the most radical remedies including the capital punishment of the atheists (or those pretending to be so); the most severe laws against blasphemy; and the strictest control of books, a major agent of contamination. Nevertheless, the evil was transmitted first through direct contact, conversations, indecent bearings, and provocative discourses such as "witticism aiming to . . . discredit" religion to please a given assembly: "The contagion spreads as much as, and maybe even more rapidly! Is not a plague-ridden—I use this example consciously– much more dangerous when the plague is in his clothes than when it is just born without a body?"[8]

However, even if one can detect its provenance and places, the contagion is more often than not invisible. Michel Maudit, priest of the Oratoire congregation, distinguished three states of impiety: at one end there is the "secrete corruption" of minds; at the other an "open profession of impiety," exploding in the "public and universal depravity"; and in the middle an "internal annihilation of all religious sentiments that is communicated and spread in the minds through contagion. This state resembles to the first case in that it is secret, and to the second in that it commences to spread."[9]

How does evil pass from one mind to another? On this point, the analyses are quite sketchy. To find a theory on the contagion of erroneous opinions and deleterious conducts, one may turn to other authors such as

Montaigne or Pierre Charron. The latter identifies two obstacles to "wisdom": "one is external regarding with the opinions and popular vices, that is to say, the contagion of the world; the other is internal which concerns the passions." Self-contagion of passions produces the contagion of the other: "The passion conceived in our heart is immediately formed in our discourse, and through this discourse going out of us it enters into the other."[10] However, such a critical anthropology targets atheism less than it does other kinds of superstitions, absurdities, and aberrations that religions themselves contain in their irreducible diversity.

These analyses lead to an entirely philosophical religion, and hence a noncontagious one since it is based on reason; a deism that is not called so, and revisits the ancient theme of comparison between atheism and superstition. The latter is a "plague" much worse than atheism, according to Bayle, who ponders that atheism may be a contagious malady but one that is less deleterious for social life than superstition. He refers to the text of Paul Rycault (1666) that describes—in a quite ambiguous manner—an atheist sect's development at the very summit of the state in the Ottoman Empire: "Those who profess their faith for this sect love and protect each other; they are obliging and hospitable, and when they receive a like-minded guest in their home, they entertain him open-heartedly, and after offering a copious meal they provide him with a company for the night, a beautiful person in the sex of his preference."[11] Through the vocabulary of contagious evil, this hospitable sect, perceived through a proto-orientalist veil, became highly desirable.

Even though for a long time throughout the nineteenth century, and if one would like to scrutinize, until today, atheism (associated or not with moral licentiousness) has been presented by the confessional ideologues of all obedience as a terrible contagious malady threatening civilized life. From then on, the most radical minds of the Enlightenment were ready for the big turnaround through identifying superstition with religion. In his *Lettres à Eugénie; ou preservative contre les prejudges* (Letters to Eugenia; or Preservative against religious prejudices), Paul H. T. d'Holbach writes that "the devotion could be treated as vapors; superstition is an ingrained malady that one could heal through physical remedies."[12]

According to Nicolas Fréret, "religious fanaticism . . . is the most abundant source of evils inflicting human species."[13] However, it is not easy to submit oneself to the social constraints of religion without being contaminated, at least as long as those who carry such discourses remain as authority figures, and especially that of power: "There is a contagion that spreads in the minds and opinions of dominant figures in societies, and that can in fact persuade you to believe such maxims that had once utterly appalled us."[14] To be precise, Fréret's remarks go beyond denunciating religious fanaticism. Political interpretation of the epidemiological model of contagion becomes a powerful critical tool that works on the ravages caused in the minds and bodies by certain ideologies from the moment we give those supporting such ideologies access to power. Thus, the identified source of contagious evil is not religion, atheism, or any other belief system but the very structure of domination itself.

translated by Zehra Gulbahar Cunillera

NOTES

1. Jean Fernel, *De Abditis Rerum causis*, 1548, b 2, cap. 11.

2. David de Planis Campy, *La Verolle recogneue, combatue et abbatue* . . . (Paris: Nicolas Bourdin, 1623).

3. *Le Parnasse des poètes satyriques* (N.p., 1622), 1–2.

4. *Apologie de Théophile* (N.p., 1624), 36.

5. Nicolas de Nancel, *Discours très ample de la peste* [Very ample discourse on the plague], (Paris: Denys du Val, 1581), 77.

6. Philippe de Mornay, *Athéomachie* (Geneva: G. de Laimarie, 1582), 5.

7. Johann F. Buddeus, *Traité de l'athéisme et de la superstition* (Amsterdam: Pierre Mortier, 1756), 164.

8. Samuel Formey, *Le Philosophe Chrétien* . . . , vol. 1 (1750), 41.

9. Michel Mauduit, *Traité de religion contre les athées, les déistes et les nouveaux Pyrrhoniens* (Paris: Roulland, 1677), préface.

10. Pierre Charron, *De la sagesse* (Bordeaux: Simon Millanges, 1601), 250 and 643.

11. Paul Rycaut, *Histoire de l'état présent de l'Empire ottoman, contenant.* . . . (Paris: Mabre-Cramoisy, 1670).

12. Paul H. T. d'Holbach, *Lettres à Eugénie; ou preservative contre les prejudges* [Letters to Eugenia; or Preservative against religious prejudices] (N.p., 1768), 138.

13. Nicolas Fréret, *Lettre de Thrasybule à Leucippe* (1770); Nicolas Fréret, *Oeuvres philosophiques* (N.p., 1776), 196.

14. Fréret, *Lettre de Thrasybule à Leucippe* (1770); Fréret, *Oeuvres philosophiques* (N.p., 1776), 196, 288.

SELECTED BIBLIOGRAPHY

Cavaillé, Jean-Pierre. *Postures libertines: La Culture des esprits forts.* Toulouse: Anacharsis, 2011.

Charron, Pierre. *De la sagesse.* Edited by Barbara de Negroni. Paris: Fayard, 1986.

d'Holbach, Paul H. T. *Lettres à Eugénie; ou preservative contre les prejudges.* N.p., 1768.

Lachèvre, Frédéric. *Le libertinage au XVIIe siècle.* Paris: Champion, 1909–1928; reprint, Geneva: Slatkine, 1968.

Pintard, René. *Le libertinage érudit dans la première moitié du XVIIe siècle* [1943]. Geneva: Slatkine, 1983.

Postel, Claude. *Traité des invectives.* Paris: Les Belles Lettres, 2004.

CALENDAR
Circulation and Misuse of a Medieval Iconographical Model

Perrine Mane

Throughout the Middle Ages, the use of copies was a constant phenomenon of artistic production, whether of a large-scale sculpture or an illumination. The iconographical theme of calendars, lasting from the ninth to the sixteenth century, bears witness to these phenomena of contagion, by way of either the circulation of models or the spread of mistakes coming from the faulty copy of older images.

The artistic transcription of calendars had already been developed in ancient Greece where months were represented by religious festivals. Carolingian artists took up the theme, but it experienced its greatest popularity in the twelfth and thirteenth centuries. The months of the year illustrate manuscripts but are also found in churches, wall paintings, stained glass, and floor mosaics. Most often they are sculpted on church portals. France has eighty-nine large-scale sculpted calendars of this type. The majority of these calendar scenes relate directly to agriculture, grain, and wine growing as well as husbandry. Some, however, evoke other tasks, such as haymaking, woodcutting, fishing, or the fruit harvest. For the most part, peasants are absent from the months of April and May. Springtime scenes are filled with nobles celebrating this renewal of nature and bearing witness to their taste for refined pastimes. This distinct difference in the presentation of the annual cycle reflects medieval secular society's split into two groups.

The month of May is traditionally represented by a warrior, by horseback riding, or more often by a game-hawking horseman. The hunting theme was absent from calendars developed during the Carolingian period:

it appears in the twelfth century and spreads in the thirteenth, always with the aid of a falcon. Owning, training, and keeping such a bird of prey required a considerable fortune; hence the art of falconry was reserved for nobles. It glorified a taste for risk, required intense physical training, and constituted an excellent preparation for war. It was, in fact, part of knightly upbringing.

In most calendars, the horseman is pictured in profile, with his falcon perched on his gloved fist. And yet many painted or sculpted cycles innovate in both France and Italy. Such cycles illustrate the month of May with a horseman holding in one of his hands a sickle instead of a raptor. This is the scene painted in the twelfth-century cycle in Charly (Cher) as well as in several sculpted calendars. They can be found on the *voussoirs* of churches in the Saintonge region, such as Fenioux (1140) and Civray (1165) or again in Italy on the inner frieze of the Parma baptistery sculpted in 1196 (see figure 1) and on the porch of the west façade of the Cremona *duomo* circa 1225. These horseman are dressed like the peasants at various agricultural chores during the other months. In the two Italian calendars, the sickle is brandished with the arm forward, whereas in France it is toward the back.

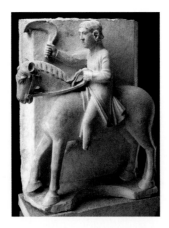

Figure 1

May, Baptistery of Parma, interior frieze of the loggia, 1196, sculpted by Benedetto Antelami.
Source: © P. Mane, courtesy of the author.

This unexpected scene has elicited numerous interpretations. It is unlikely that a simple peasant would be represented on horseback. And yet the tool could be a symbol of the upcoming harvest and the fast-growing wheat at that time of the year, unless the scene heralds the peasant's most important job, the harvest. Chiara Frugoni offers another interpretation: "In a miniature from the early fourteenth century, the *Sachsenspiegel,* an early thirteenth-century legal text in which the status of the peasant population is fixed for the first time, we find a horseman dismounting and harvesting a wheat field. The corresponding text explains that the traveler is authorized to harvest the grain of the field in order to feed his beast."[1] These figures could then be traveling horsemen. If such hypotheses cannot be categorically rejected, the anomaly might be otherwise explained. In 1927 Paul Brandt suggested a confusion between the terms for falcon (*falco-falconem*) and for sickle (*falx-falcem*).[2] Such an amalgam is further corroborated by the fact that in Old French, the term *faus,* close to *faucille* or "sickle," can mean "falcon."

This mistaken interpretation of handwritten or oral directions passed on to artists seems to originate in Poitou-Saintonge in the twelfth century. The sculpted cycles have such similarities that one must recognize the existence of a common model, distinct from the calendars in the rest of France containing only rare variants. Not only are there arches above the figures at the ends of the calendars of Fenious, Civray, and Cognac, but these figures, with their elongated proportions, are identically dressed in tight clothing, striated with strange horizontal wrinkles. Furthermore, these cycles are the only ones to integrate specific scenes, such as the month of November illustrated by two oxen before a trough. The cycles in Poitou were perhaps developed from a model circulating between different workshops, unless, given the short distances between the region's churches, the sculptors knew one of the cycles in the series and drew their inspiration from it. Or yet again, the different calendars could be the product of a single workshop moving from church to church. By contagion, this erroneous transformation of the traditional iconography of the month of May as sculpted by workshops of Poitou-Saintonge might have been passed on to Italian sculptors with whom they had close relations.

In another case, the spread of mistakes made while copying comes from the faulty interpretation of an earlier image within the context of one artistic technique, or also from one technique to another. In this way, in 17 percent of thirteenth-century illuminated calendars, the month of June is embodied by a walking peasant carrying a bundle of thin, green branches on his shoulder (see figure 2). But in the very middle of the period of the sap rising, it seems a curious date to picture woodcutting. This latter task is always pictured in sculpted or illuminated cycles for the winter months, in

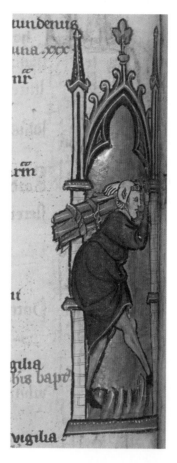

Figure 2
June, Psautier à l'usage de Thérouanne, illuminated in the late thirteenth century in Northern France. *Source*: Paris, Bibliothèque nationale de France, Smith Lesouëf 20, fol. 10v.

November or December, and sometimes but rarely in March. Doubtless, there must have been some confusion with the scene that originally showed the hay brought in for the month of June, such as on the north porch of Chartres Cathedral and on the Paris Cathedral between 1210 and 1230. The change was probably due to the faulty interpretation and circulation of a model that turned the haystack carried on the shoulder into a bundle of wood. Miniatures adopting the motif of wood bearing in June were moreover produced in the same region and at the same period, during the latter thirteenth century by workshops from Northern France[3] or Flanders.[4]

As Maurits Smeyers stresses, "The personal share of the illuminator in the decoration and especially in the illustration of manuscripts seems to have been rather limited, as much in the choice of subjects as in their elaboration. . . . In a given codex, to what extent can miniatures have been original creations or imitations of existing models? To what extent can we speak of invention or creativity in this discipline?" In fact, medieval iconographical tradition was forged by a mechanism of contagion and borrowings: "The repetitive character of religious art [satisfied] the obligation for an art aiming to be didactic, to be understood by the faithful by respecting the repertory of images that was familiar and intelligible to them."[5] The faulty copy of models is so patent that it even manifests a total misunderstanding of agrarian practices. This mechanism of the transmission of mistakes might thus be explained by a particular relationship with creating. Contagion and "precedent" were indispensable to medieval artists who were but little concerned with being original.

translated by Vicki-Marie Petrick

NOTES

1. Chiara Frugoni, "Chiesa e lavoro agricolo nei testi e nelle immagini dall' età tardo-antica all' età romanica," in *Medioevorurale: Sulle tracce della civiltà contadina*, ed. Vito Fumagalli and Gabriella Rossetti (Bologna: Il Mulino, 1980), 321–341.

2. Paul Brandt, *Schaffende Arbeit und bildende Kunst* (Leipzig: Kröner, 1927), 175.

3. Paris, Bibliothèque nationale de France, lat. 1076, fol. 3v and Smith Lesouëf 20, fol. 3v; Vesoul, Bibliothèque municipale, MS 6, fol. 4v; Saint-Petersburg, National Library of Russia, lat Q. v. I, 24, fol. 4v.

4. London, British Library, Royal 2 B III, fol. 3v; Oxford, Bodleian, Liturg. 396, fol. 3v; Saint-Omer, Bibliothèque municipale, MS 270, fol. Dv; Paris, Bibliothèque de l'Arsenal, MS 604, fol. 3v.

5. Maurits Smeyers, *La miniature* (Turnhout: Brepols, 1974), 59.

SELECTED BIBLIOGRAPHY

Brandt, Paul. *Schaffende Arbeit und bildende Kunst.* Leipzig: Kröner, 1927.

Comet, Georges. "Les calendriers médiévaux, une représentation du monde." *Journal des savants* 1 (1992): 35–98.

Frugoni, Chiara. "Chiesa e lavoro agricolo nei testi e nelle immagini dall'età tardo-antica all'età romanica." In *Medioevo rurale: Sulle tracce della civiltà contadina,* edited by Vito Fumagalli and Gabriella Rossetti, 321–341. Bologna: Il Mulino, 1980.

Mane, Perrine. *Calendriers et techniques agricoles (France-Italie, XIIe–XIIIe siècles).* Paris: Le Sycomore, 1983.

Mane, Perrine. "Comparaison des thèmes iconographiques des calendriers monumentaux et enluminés en France, aux XIIe et XIIIe siècles." *Cahiers de civilisation médiévale* 29, no. 115 (1986): 257–266.

Mane, Perrine. *Le travail à la campagne au Moyen Age. Étude iconographique.* Paris: Picard, 2006.

Smeyers, Maurits. *La miniature.* Turnhout: Brepols, 1974.

Toubert, Hélène. "Iconographie et histoire de la spiritualité médiévale." *Revue d'histoire de la spiritualité* 50 (1974): 265–284.

CARTOGRAPHY
John Snow and the Topography of Cholera

Sebastian V. Grevsmühl

The analysis of contagion through maps has a long tradition. The English-man John Snow (1813–1858) is a particularly renowned figure in this field. He is considered a pioneer of statistical mapping and one of the founding fathers of modern epidemiology. Although he published only two "epide-miological" maps during his career, he appears in all the major textbooks on the history of medicine, cartography, and, more recently, infographics. He is systematically cited for having contained a severe cholera epidemic in the mid-nineteenth century in the Soho district of London by using a powerful method of statistical visualization: the dot map. Dean of visual methods Edward Tufte writes that Snow's maps enabled him "to discover the cause of the epidemic and bring it to an end."[1] This compelling story is appealing in that it is short, dramatic, and heroic.[2] Many variations of Snow's maps have since been produced, some of which have become truly iconic, and continue to inspire practitioners of visualization methods from a variety of disciplines.

The problem, however, is that a number of historical studies have shown that Snow never actually claimed to have discovered the cause of the epidemic thanks to a map. In fact, he himself preferred to much more cau-tiously describe his map as a "diagram of the topography of the outbreak."[3] Moreover, despite their simplicity, Snow's two maps failed to convince the majority of his peers, who continued to advocate miasmatic theories, that is, contagion by airborne vapors. This has unfortunately escaped the major-ity of his commentators, who have not bothered to reconstruct his rigorous scientific approach. A number have attributed great power to Snow's maps, considering them to be the analytical tools of his thought, which is in fact quite debatable. Ultimately, such accounts say more about the intentions of their authors than the historical role of these famous maps.

What, then, was the function of Snow's maps, and what was his thought process? The best-known dot map in his work (figure 1) depicts the Soho district of London, modified by Snow to pinpoint cholera deaths that occurred over a six-week period between August and September 1854 by means of small black bars. He also used circles to indicate the location of thirteen public water pumps. But rather than being the source of a spectacular discovery, as has often been alleged, this map is a specific case study forming part of much broader fieldwork and intellectual research carried out by Snow over the course of many years at various sites.

Snow saw cholera firsthand on several occasions. In 1831, during the first of four major pandemics that ravaged England over the course of the nineteenth century, he was a medical assistant. At the time of the second epidemic, which occurred between 1848 and 1849, he worked as a doctor in London. It was then that he first theorized the transmission of cholera based on his clinical observations. He published this theory in 1849, without a supporting map, arguing that the key vector of cholera transmission was the contamination of drinking water by sewage. His theory openly opposed the dominant miasmatic theories, yet his argument raised a fundamental problem: as he himself remarked, "we are never informed in works on cholera what water the people drink."[4]

When a new epidemic struck England in 1853 and 1854, Snow decided to take advantage of the situation to fill in the data gap on water and to support his theory. To this end, he conducted two separate studies. One examined the links between cholera deaths and the practices of two water companies supplying water to the south end of London. The other, in a much more circumscribed way, concerns the Soho area. Published in 1855 as an expanded version of his *On the Modes of Communication of Cholera*, the results of these two projects also include the famous map of the Broad Street neighborhood (figure 1). The latter was meant to synthesize and illustrate his investigative work and to spatialize some of the

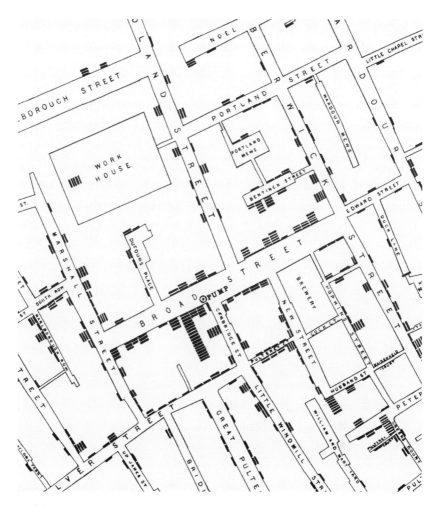

Figure 1

Detail of Snow's dot map showing cholera deaths in August and September 1854 in London around Broad Street (black bars) and water points (circles). *Source*: John Snow, *On the Mode of Communication of Cholera*, 2nd ed. (London: Churchill, 1855), 44–45.

epidemic's effects. In particular, it can be seen that the mortality rate is higher near the Broad Street water pump. But the cartographic reasoning stops there: the conclusion that the water from the Broad Street pump is the probable vector of the contagion, which prompted the authorities to remove the arm of this pump in September 1854, is based on the analysis of other elements.

The strength of the visual, but also its weakness, lies in the fact that each visualization process creates its own economy of visibilities and invisibilities. Everything that can be seen and everything absent from a map informs and potentially alters the narrative. In Snow's case, the invisibilities produced by the simple choice of map type weighs heavily on the development of the account. For example, one of the strong assumptions of the dot map is that it implies a more or less uniform distribution of people across the mapped space. If some houses do not have black bars, it is presumed that the inhabitants of these houses have successfully avoided contagion, whereas this may simply be due to the small number or even absence of people. In other words, mapping methods are never neutral, and biases also appear in alternative mapping techniques, such as the continuous tonal gradation method introduced by Quetelet to visualize variations in mortality as a function of population density.

In addition, Snow's map contains many anomalies, both visible and invisible, which require explanations only obtainable through a field survey. For example, the fact that some inhabitants are located close to the probable source of contagion does not necessarily lead to high mortality rates. Curiously, those who frequented the poor house on Poland Street and the workers of the Broad Street brewery remained largely untouched. It is only during his investigation that Snow learns these institutions have their own water sources—something the map does not show. In a similar vein, several deaths that occurred at a considerable distance from the source can be explained by regular use of the Broad Street pump.

A second map constructed by Snow also exists, published just six months later (figure 2), which is considerably less well known and rarely cited. However, it reflects Snow's desire to more precisely define a "cholera zone," particularly from a visual perspective. To this end, he added a dotted

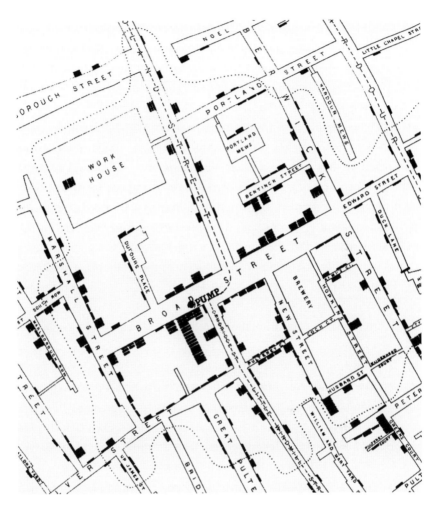

Figure 2

Detail from Snow's second dot-density map showing the addition of an equidistance line. *Source*: Cholera Inquiry Committee, *Report on the Cholera Outbreak in the Parish of St. James, Westminster during the Autumn of 1854* (London: Churchill, 1855), 106–107.

line to his original map that establishes the median pedestrian distance between the Broad Street pump and other nearby pumps. The highly irregular line was added to counter miasmatic theories that suggested a much more regular spatial contagion. Despite this effective visual novelty, Snow's opponents remained dubious, demonstrating that a map's interpretation can vary considerably depending on the authors and their intentions.

Indeed, Snow was not the only one to have published dot maps of this critical cholera episode. Others who came before (Edmund Cooper) and after (members of a scientific commission) produced maps that were often much more detailed, showing house numbers, a more comprehensive differentiation of deaths, and the sewer system superimposed on the neighborhood map. But the conclusions drawn from these maps all challenged Snow's theory. For example, members of the Committee for Scientific Inquiries of the General Board of Health strongly rejected his water transmission theory using the very same type of map, identifying instead an atmospheric influence of unknown origin, likely related to emanations from new sewers.

This much is clear: what is frequently presented as visual evidence is not actually so once we consider the context in which the cartographic object was made. Today, as infographics become omnipresent, there is a great temptation to transform historical cartographic objects into precursors of visual tools for "good" governance. In most cases, however, we depart considerably from historical realities to make this or that argument. In this way, when historians of cartography give a central place to Snow's map, they do so to support their own narrative of the centrality of visual thought in the sciences.

Today, mapping and contagion form an inseparable couple that often produces very useful public health results, especially when the mechanisms of contagion are known. The historical analysis of Snow's maps reminds us, however, that in the absence of a common paradigm of contagion, the visualization of spatial data relationships becomes a very complex analytical terrain, far from the simplistic explanations provided by heroic narratives. The latter, in fact, dangerously overestimate the power of the visual at the expense of more elaborate historical explanations. No one wins in this process, not historians, not visual culture specialists, nor political decision-makers.

translated by Maya Judd

NOTES

1. Edward Tufte, *Visual Explanations* (Cheshire: Graphics Press, 1997), 27.

2. Kari McLeod, "Our Sense of Snow: The Myth of John Snow in Medical Geography," *Social Science and Medicine* 50 (2000), 923–935.

3. John Snow, *On the Mode of Communication of Cholera* (London: Churchill, 1855), 45.

4. Cited by Tom Koch, "The Map as Intent: Variations on the Theme of John Snow," *Cartographica* 39, no. 4 (2004), 3.

SELECTED BIBLIOGRAPHY

Brody, Howard, Michael Russell Rip, Peter Vinten-Johansen, Nigel Paneth, and Stephen Rachman. "Map-Making and Myth-Making in Broad Street: The London Cholera Epidemic, 1854." *Lancet* 356 (2000): 64–68.

Cholera Inquiry Committee. *Report on the Cholera Outbreak in the Parish of St. James, Westminster during the Autumn of 1854.* London: Churchill, 1855.

Koch, Tom. "The Map as Intent: Variations on the Theme of John Snow." *Cartographica* 39, no. 4 (2004): 1–14.

MacLeod, Kari. "Our Sense of Snow: The Myth of John Snow in Medical Geography." *Social Science and Medicine* 50 (2000): 923–935.

Tufte, Edward. *Visual Explanations.* Cheshire: Graphics Press, 1997.

Vinten-Johansen, Peter, Howard Brody, Nigel Paneth, Stephen Rachman, and Michael Rip, with David Zuk. *Cholera, Chloroform, and the Science of Medicine: A Life of John Snow.* Oxford: Oxford University Press, 2003.

CLOTHING
Medieval Sumptuary Laws as Measures of Social Containment?

Mickaël Wilmart

One can easily combine the anthropology of clothing and the idea of contagion to analyze the processes through which fashion is spread. Given that, one might ask how the concept could also shed light on prohibitions that appear at different periods, especially at the end of the Middle Ages, under the generic term of sumptuary laws. Thoroughly examined for the Italian city-states, these regulations aimed first and foremost to limit luxury and conspicuous consumption. At the same time, they also attempted to match dress to social rank. While their economic and moral aspects have been discussed in depth, does the notion of contagion and its prophylactic counterpart, containment, allow us to explain these sometimes drastic measures as well as their evolution? With the towns of the Languedoc serving as an example in this text, we will show that such laws served not only to curb an epidemic of luxury at a time of strong economic growth but also to seal off certain groups into a particular vestimentary system, borrowing the terminology defined by Roland Barthes.

As Italian towns created one sumptuary law after another in the second half of the thirteenth century, the consulates of southern France put the same kinds of regulations into place with some local variations in their details. As examples, we can cite the texts that serve as the basis for our thoughts: Montpellier, 1273; Narbonne, 1274; and Montauban, 1275 and 1291. To the list we can also add Marseille, 1285.[1] With this, we have a first wave of prohibitions in dress concerning solely women, a phenomenon not exclusive to the region. In the long term it is symptomatic of a moralizing discourse about consumption, and its gendered character has often been noted. The legislative craze seems to be independent of the royal decrees of 1279, 1283, and 1292 limiting sumptuary practices of the nobility and the merchant sphere. A second wave of rulings came about in the middle of the fourteenth century, sometimes, though rarely, before the Black Plague, as happened at Rieux-Volvestre in 1343.[2] More generally, these laws were promulgated after the 1348 epidemic, such as that of Castres in 1357.[3] This time around it concerned both men and women, insisting specifically on respecting the social hierarchy, in imitation of the royal edicts.

In Languedoc, the thirteenth-century sumptuary laws strictly targeted women. They were enacted within the context of strong economic growth, after the first half of the century when the Albigensian Crusade undermined local structures. Economic growth manifested mainly in the role of exchange platform played by towns close to the Mediterranean coast, such as Montpellier and Narbonne. To a lesser extent, it also manifested in the successes of the Languedoc cloth trade. This growth allowed for the emergence of new fortunes and for the circulation of precious goods coming from all over Europe and the coast of the Mediterranean basin. More so than an attempt to control financial outflow by way of sumptuary expenditures, the urban regulations had a moral objective. Those of Montauban were formal: they were "for the honor of the ladies." The spread of metal trim and precious fabric was pointed out as an ill to be eradicated. Lust and luxury were not so far apart, as shown by the town's exceptions to the prohibitions. Prostitutes and female jugglers were authorized to adorn themselves in certain adornments or to take up certain cuts of dress that for other women were judged inappropriate.

Consequently, sumptuary laws concerned decency. Their purpose was to limit risk and restrain the spread of bad morals, thus saving the reputation of Montauban's ladies. To grasp the lengths to which these laws went to set up barriers, we must stress that dress restrictions went hand in hand with texts aiming to reduce opportunities for women to socialize by limiting the number of visits that they might receive on different occasions. Around 1270, the consulates, led by men, seem to have proceeded to a containment of women's sociability in supervising their appearances and their relations. They defined, de facto, the feminine collective as tied to sobriety and a restricted domestic universe, sheltered from the temptation and possible contagion of a new mode of consumption. As for men, they were free to wear the most precious metals and cloth and were restricted by the value of presents they could offer during their marriage proposals and engagements (Montpellier, Narbonne), distancing women from luxury.

The Narbonne regulations did not only limit the spread of women's luxury dress; they also restrained the importation of innovations in dress. Thus they specifically mentioned the prohibition of skirts made "in the Catalan style," although Catalonia is a region close to Narbonne. Here the law clearly proposes a practice of containment in the face of the contagion of a fashion coming from a neighboring region, from which Narbonne desired nonetheless to differentiate itself. The town's identity was thus defined by a vestimentary system that excluded Catalan influences, about fifteen years after the Treaty of Corbeil (1258) fixed the border between the Kingdom of France and Catalonia south of Corbières. Through exclusion or through measures of containment, sumptuary laws acted as identity markers for both gender and town. As for the second wave of regulations enacted in the middle of the fourteenth century, they highlight social identities intended to be insurmountable, thus restraining any possible porosity between groups.

The demographic crisis following the 1348 pandemic upset the social landscape, eroding its roots by the very dearth of population. The extreme mortality resulting from the plague made villages desolate and labor rare. At the same time, it opened up new economic opportunities. Decimated families of the elite seemed to fear competition with the parvenus and thus sought to limit pretensions toward social prestige by controlling appearances. Even little towns like Rieux-Volvestre or Castres, both new bishoprics created in 1317, set to work regulating the question of appearances, showing that this fear was widespread.

The two texts from Castres and Rieux-Volvestre differ in part of their terminology and in the details of their demands, but they adopt the same principle. The first articles took up the spirit of the thirteenth-century laws in targeting women, but the rest of the text also imposed important restrictions on men with regard to luxury. Above all, the two texts set down exceptions that no longer relate to those of thirteenth-century Montauban. Thus, in Castres, no woman could wear any decoration composed of gold, silver, or pearls on her head or gown, "unless she be wife of knight, of doctor of civil or canon law, of seneschal or of judge,"[4] that is to say the group that made up the social (nonmerchant) elite of small towns.

The same list is found at Rieux-Volvestre, including the prohibitions concerning men. This time, the legislative logic was not to restrain the contagion of luxury but rather to restrain the use of luxury to a certain category of person according to their social rank. The parvenus, coming from the sphere of merchants, were thus excluded as long as they had not acceded to the status or the functions listed. In this sense, the sumptuary laws can also be read as attempts at social containment but this time not to protect a group from temptation. Rather it was to keep the dominant group from being contaminated by those who have benefited from the demographic crisis to rise socially. In a society largely ruled by appearances, to keep someone from wearing the attributes of wealth comes down to a de facto restriction of social recognition. In opposition to that possibility, the established elite defined themselves as those allowed to luxuriously array themselves. And by these regulations, that elite intended to remind one and all of the boundary separating it from other groups so that there could be no confusion between them.

In looking at the experiences of the thirteenth and fourteenth centuries, sumptuary laws indeed appear as prescriptions for containment. From a moral standpoint, they were enacted to check luxury use at a period when modes of consumption were being disrupted. It is thus a question of avoiding the contagion of impropriety in all spheres of society, in particular the feminine. From a social standpoint, these regulations conveyed identity, as defined by the exclusion of certain practices judged contrary to a well-ordered society. At first the sole targets of these laws, women found themselves forbidden any luxury in appearance, conveying a sobriety thought to be redeeming. In addition, women's relations were reduced to a restricted circle, and consequently the definition of their identity resulted from a pronounced social containment. This arsenal of regulations took on another dimension in the fourteenth century when it restricted luxury to a particular social category. It was no longer a question of protecting the morals of a group considered weak but of putting a halt to any confusion in the social hierarchy, that is, to defend the dominant group by restraining the spread of its attributes to other categories.

translated by Vicki-Marie Petrick

NOTES

1. For Montpellier, Société archéologique de Montpellier, *Thalamus parvus: Le petit thalamus de Montpellier, publié pour la première fois d'après les manuscrits originaux* (Montpellier: J. Martel, 1840), 145–147; for Narbonne, Archives municipales de Narbonne: AA 103, fols. 47v–48 and AA 106, fols. 29v–30; for Montauban, Archives municipales de Montauban, AA 36v–37 and 74; for Marseille, Adolphe Crémieux, ed., *Le VIe livre des statuts de Marseille* (Marseille: F. Chauvet, 1917), 46–47.

2. The date, however, seems doubtful: there is but one late copy of the document surviving and seems rather to correspond to the 1350s.

3. For Rieux-Volvestre, Joseph Gleizes, "Notice sur la ville de Rieux (Haute-Garonne) et sur ses archives," *Mémoires de la Société archéologique du Midi de la France* 5 (1841–1847): 340–355, document published 349–351; for Castres, "Ordonnance somptuaire des consuls de Castres publiée en 1357," *Revue du Tarn* 1 (1877): 42–43.

4. Castes, "Ordonnance somputaire des consuls de Castres," 42.

SELECTED BIBLIOGRAPHY

Barthes, Roland. "Histoire et sociologie du vêtement: Quelques observations méthodologiques." *Annales ESC* 12, no. 3 (1957), 430–441.

de Grazia, Victoria, and Ellen Furlough, eds. *The Sex of Things: Gender and Consumption in Historical Perspective*. Berkeley: University of California Press, 1996.

Heller, Sarah-Grace. "Limiting Yardage and Changes of Clothes: Sumptuary Legislation in Thirteenth-Century France, Languedoc and Italy." In *Medieval Fabrications: Dress, Textiles, Cloth Work, and Other Cultural Imaginings*, edited by E. Jane Burns, 121–136. Blondes: Palgrave Macmillan, 2004.

Kovesi Killerby, Catherine. *Sumptuary Law in Italy, 1200–1500*. Oxford: Clarendon Press, 2001.

Riello, Giorgione, and Ulinka Rublack, eds. *The Right to Dress: Sumptuary Laws in a Global Perspectives, c. 1200–1800*. Cambridge: Cambridge University Press, 2019.

COLONIZATION
Social Contagion as a Civilizing Tool

Catarina Madeira-Santos

The ideology of the *civilizing mission* forged in France profoundly influenced the European colonial discourse of high-level administrators and experts in colonial sciences between the end of the nineteenth and the beginning of the twentieth century. In legislation and doctrinaire texts, the concept of "indigenous" had a more or less explicitly transitionary, mobile connotation. Indigenous people were those who, having not yet left behind their traditional and backward ways of life, were far removed from the civilized world. In the future, all would eventually cross the threshold of differentiation, with colonizers having the obligation to lead them to more advanced stages of civilization.

Imbued with evolutionary theories, the authors of the vast and eclectic colonial corpus debated at length the means to accomplish the work of civilizing the natives. Notable to this regard are the writings of Lopo Vaz de Sampayo e Mello (1883–1949), professor at the Escola Superior Colonial (High Colonial School) of Lisbon, who was well established in the international networks of colonialist sociability. Using results from the Congress on Colonial Sociology held in Paris (1900), he argued that each empire's adoption of the colonial system should be based on knowledge of their own sociological factors and not on colonial legislation with a supposedly universalist value. In his view, the law did not produce civilizing effects.

The main singularity of his work lies in the use of an epidemic *topos* to reflect on colonial politics. His book, *Questões Coloniais: Política Indígena*, begins with a lengthy discussion of Louis Pasteur's *La Théorie des Germes* (1878). He then develops the notion of *contágio social* (social contagion). By metaphorically mobilizing a contagion model, Sampayo e Mello explains social facts arising from colonization, in particular the spread of European civilization among African populations. His aim is to present social contagion as the tool of colonization par excellence, since it *naturally* triggers a process of sociocultural and ideological mutation or of civilization. The social level of colonized peoples would thus depend mainly on the degree of contagion exerted by the dominant civilization. This *social contagion*, put to good use by the law of imitation, common to the whole of humanity, is the most natural and perhaps strongest cause of the modification of legal institutions and political and administrative organizations.[1]

The social constitution of a "primitive" population would inevitably undergo slow but steady destruction at the hands of the advanced civilization; the transformative power of the social contagion would make the fragile and imperfect indigenous institutions disappear without violence. Although never directly quoting Gabriel Tarde (sociologist and rival of Émile Durkheim, much of whose work is based on the notion of "imitation," similar to that of "contagion"), the author gives *imitation* a central place in this contagionist model. The encounter between two different societies foments exchanges between individuals that lead to widespread mimicry. The social contagion thus results, sooner or later, in the end of otherness by overcoming the hierarchy between peoples.

Yet Sampayo e Mello also warns that social contagion does not automatically have a civilizing effect. While the civilized have the power to transform indigenous peoples, the reverse is also true. The transformation generated by the contagion is thus not necessarily ascending, linear, or irreversible, a view that went against the ideology of the civilizing mission. The European colonizer is both a contaminating agent (of civilization) and a target of contamination (of primitivization). To prove this, Sampayo e Mello takes up one of the oldest topoi of colonial literature: the *cafrealização*, that is, the white who "goes native" through isolated contact with Africans. In his view, the history of the colony of Angola provided a telling example. Over the centuries, the Portuguese colonists would have seen their way of life "degenerate," as they were largely a minority. Sampayo e Mello then finds a counterexample, with wonder and some naivety, in the United States. The grandchildren of African slaves, freed and educated in schools and universities, had become prominent American citizens and even intellectuals. The explanation was obvious: the white population, which was very large in America, had a powerful social contagion effect on Afro-descendants.

How, then, could social contagion be employed to colonize Africa, since Africans were the vast majority compared to Europeans? First, mestizo people had a role to play in resolving the colonial problem, as they were a contaminating vector, even a contagion agent par excellence. This perspective also differed from the dominant doctrine of the time, according to which miscegenation was a form of degeneration, resulting from unions between colonizers and African women. Instead, Sampayo e Mello took a positive view: "we cannot ignore this important sociological factor."[2] Starting from the first generation, mestizo individuals, having received by paternal inheritance an intellect already capable of scientific assimilation, were an intellectual element useful to colonial administration. Following this same argument, inexclusively adopting the customs and language of the dominant nation, mestizo people constituted "the most useful and suitable tool for the popularisation of these ethnic characteristics within the indigenous society, which they understand better than the Europeans."[3]

Consequently, it was in the interest of the colonial government to provide mestizos with equal social status and political privileges as the colonizers. Once they had the same rights as Europeans, they would qualify for administrative, religious, political, and military positions. Miscegenation would thus become the most powerful factor of the colonial system and political assimilation, that is, the exportation of all European laws and institutions to the colonies.

Second, exporting the contagion model to the colonies involved a political dimension. Since colonization is, by definition, an act of domination that entails a certain degree of physical and epistemological violence, it implies an *intentionality*. Social contagion is neither a (moral) stain nor a (medical) threat but a tool of governance and then of submission of the indigenous to a civilization model. Contagion thus had a positive connotation; its spread could and should be supported by administrative and institutional devices. It was with this reasoning that Sampayo e Mello proposed the establishment of missions and public schools as centers of instruction for indigenous people. Indigenous taxes were to be paid in colonial currency to create production and consumption needs that would gradually eradicate African ways of life. Free labor in turn would put an end to all forms of slavery. However, these measures were not to be used as a means of artificial, and therefore hasty, "inoculation." On the contrary, they were to be gradually imposed, supporting social contagion by respecting its natural dynamic of expansion.

In the long run, the social contagion would generate a society without otherness, where "temporary polygenism" would give way to monogenism. The attainment of this progression required a gradualist policy. In the granting of rights to African populations, Sampayo e Mello stated that "we must first make citizens and then give them full political rights, the true charter of social emancipation."[4]

However, the indigenous were not at the same evolutionary stage as Europeans, so they could not yet enjoy the same rights. An immediate granting of citizenship privileges to Africans would potentially prompt another contagion, this time insurrectionary. According to Sampayo e Mello, the history of the independence of the "black republics of Haiti (1804) and Liberia (1847)"[5] had proved that exaggerations of antislavery humanitarianism were a political error. Having just barely emerged from slavery and without having been educated to live in freedom, these peoples had misused their political and civil rights.

The denial of legal equality between colonizers and the indigenous was a critique of the Enlightenment doctrine and assimilationist policy toward colonized populations. Sampayo e Mello subscribed to the proposals of the 1900 Congress on Colonial Sociology: on the one hand, the negation of the universal value of the law as a tool of colonization, while on the other, the unreserved apologia of legal pluralism. The establishment of indigenous legal personality required exceptional moderation and caution, while the preservation of customary rights was indispensable "until the society

[had] acquired a high degree of civilization, which will, of course, prescribe these obsolete usages and these elementary and archaic forms of administration."[6] Hence there was a need to build up collections of customary law through ethnography. Later, once the indigenous were civilized, their institutions would disappear on their own, without shocks or social upheaval. Sampayo e Mello's conclusions regarding the need by the Portuguese to maintain legal pluralism until the evolution of Africans toward "civilization" would be completed were no different from those by other authors of the same period. The specificity of his proposal lies in the understanding that the "evolution" of Africans would need "social contagion." How did his theory impact Portuguese colonial policy?

Sampayo e Mello was an active and convinced colonialist who later strongly supported the dictatorship regime (established in 1926). His reflections on social contagion did not become the main colonial doctrine in Portugal; however, as a professor of colonial politics, ethnography, and ethnology at the High Colonial School, he trained many administrators who in turn took up the *topos* of contagion versus inoculation in discussions of colonial politics.

The consequences of gradualism are well known. The denial of citizenship to Africans led to the constitution of the legal status of "indigenous" in all European colonial empires, including the Portuguese empire in 1926. The process of social contagion and the very slow progression toward a society without otherness offered the colonial powers an immense pool of labor: the natives, the demographic majority of the colonial territories.

translated by Maya Judd

NOTES

1. Lopo Vaz de Sampayo e Mello, *Questões Coloniais: Política Indígena* (Porto: Magalhães e Moniz Editores, 1910), 530.

2. Sampayo e Mello, *Questões Coloniais*, 58.

3. Sampayo e Mello, *Questões Coloniais*, 340.

4. Sampayo e Mello, *Questões Coloniais*, 70.

5. Sampayo e Mello, *Questões Coloniais*, 70.

6. Sampayo e Mello, *Questões Coloniais*, 84.

SELECTED BIBLIOGRAPHY

Conklin, Alice. *A Mission to Civilize: The Republican Idea of Empire in France and West Africa, 1895–1930*. Stanford: Stanford University Press, 1997.

Madeira-Santos, Catarina. "L'esclavage en langues africaines." Université Paris Diderot, 2019.

Saada, Emmanuelle. "Penser le fait colonial à travers le droit en 1900." *Mil neuf cent: Revue d'histoire intellectuelle* 27, no. 1 (2009): 103–116.

CONSUMPTION
Addiction to Geophagy during the Golden Age of the Spanish Empire

Sofia Navarro Hernandez

Empty a vase that smells of wet earth after the rain, break off a piece and reduce to small fragments, and put them in your mouth to savor, soften, and finally swallow. The behavior may seem irrational, but it appears to have been contagious. At least that is what a variety of sources suggest about the consumption of clay jars—*búcaros* or *barros*—during the Golden Age of the Spanish Empire. These earthenware vessels, typically brick red in color, with an external luster obtained by hand polishing and a porous internal surface, were highly valued in aristocratic and religious circles in American and Iberian cities. Their uses were multiple and involved different senses: they cooled a room thanks to the steam they exuded upon contact with water, scented the liquids contained within them, and were also ingested, probably reduced to powder or dissolved in water. Inventories and correspondence of the time suggest their accorded value was a function of their origin and that the most successful lands, both in America and Europe, were those of Guadalajara (Mexico), Natá (Panama), Santiago (Chile), and Estremoz (Portugal). The notion of contagion, understood here as the transmission of a practice or behavior, provides a relevant window through which to assess the consumption of these objects, particularly their ingestion, given that this vice eventually necessitated control measures.

The consumption of *búcaros* was similar to that of a drug. It was addictive despite its well-known negative effects: in the language of the time, this form of geophagy led to "oppilations," or blocking of the flow in a body cavity, of the intestine or liver, for example, accompanied by severe pain. According to humoral medicine, earth is a cold and dry element, and therefore astringent, a quality also attributed to cocoa, and has been associated in medical discourse with oppilations. Physician Juan de Cárdenas, for example, held the "vice of eating earth, cocoa and similar filth"[1] responsible for these obstructions.

Yet is was these very oppilations that were sought by consumers, in particular the resulting production of a yellowish or pale complexion, which was very popular on the Iberian Peninsula. In her *Relation du voyage d'Espagne* (1679 and 1680), the Countess d'Aulnoy describes the situation as follows: "There were many who ate pieces of *terra sigillata*. I have told you that they have a great passion for this pottery, which usually causes an oppilation; their stomach and belly swell and become hard as a stone, and they are yellow as quinces."[2]

Pallor was not the only consequence of this practice, which could also lead to mental states close to hallucinations. This may explain its success among the religious, who would try by this means to get closer to God but risked finding themselves prisoners of the *búcaro* vice. This appears to have been the case for Sister Estefanía de la Encarnación, who had great difficulty recovering, holding the devil responsible for her addiction: "The Devil envious of my good wishes, since he could not be of my deeds, wished to slay them and distract me in inclining me to eat *bucaro*."[3] Thus, the consumption of *barros* was quickly identified by the Catholic Church as a threat to be brought under control to the point that, according to Countess d'Aulnoy, confessors of such consumption "were given no more penance than to be one day without eating them."[4]

Such regulation was all the more justified, as the vice is attributed, in most cases, to women. In literature, the theme of ingesting *barros* provides a pretext for constructing an image of woman that alternates between the pathetic and the erotic. Thus, the "oppilated" woman who has succumbed to the vice is the victim of a mockery that underlines the frivolous nature of her pallor and insists on her physical weakness. And yet the *barro* is simultaneously also a symbol of what is feminine and desirable, as shown in the lines of verse: "kiss me, young girl, kiss me with your *barro* mouth"[5] and "your mouth, *búcaro* of fragrances," the latter written by Sister Juana Inés de la Cruz and dedicated to the vice-queen of New Spain. In paintings, these objects mainly appear in still lifes, without human presence, although in Velázquez's *Las meninas* (1656), a small *búcaro* is offered by an infant-like maid of honor. The spread of this feminine infatuation is also described by the diplomat Lorenzo Magalotti in his correspondence with Marquise Strozzi: "Little by little, between curiosity, luxury and imagination, the desire, passion or frenzy for these vases has grown to such an extent, particularly among the ladies, that their production has risen in important workshops and the mastery of their manufacture refined, with great renown, such that they are on their way to appearing in almost every court in Europe."[6]

The authors of these writings and paintings acted as spreading agents of the contagion, constructing an imaginary that dramatized the ingestion of *búcaros* but also associated them with influential figures, such as the vice-queen or infanta. Images, whether they be literary or pictorial, play a role in the mimetic transmission of a behavior, especially when they portray models with whom their audience can identify. This suggests that the institutions of absolutist monarchical power did not necessarily seek to control the *barros* vice and may even have encouraged its contagion to restrain a target population—women—by making them ill.

However, it is also possible that the women themselves had their own reasons for pursuing this vice. To cure oppilations, doctors advised patients to drink water mixed with iron powders and then go for a walk. This remedy is, in fact, at the heart of the plot of the comedy *El acero de Madrid* (1618) by Lope de Vega, whose main character, Belisa, pretends to be ill after ingesting a *búcaro*. She is subsequently prescribed by an accomplice doctor a treatment of ferruginous water and, above all, the walks that will allow her to find the man she loves. We might thus imagine oppilations offered women an opportunity to leave the home and that the attraction of the *búcaros* may in fact have been linked to a desire for freedom.

Another hypothesis that would allow us to understand the enthusiasm for these clay vessels is that of their possible contraceptive power. Indeed, medical texts of the time insist on the gynecological disturbances caused by oppilations, including amenorrhea, which may in fact have been sought out by or for certain consumers, notably Infanta Marguerita, who is thought to have begun menstruating precociously. In any case, in a letter dated April 6, 1698 sent from Madrid to Mr. de Torcy, the Marquis d'Harcourt explains that his chaplain has prevented him from sending the "beautiful quantity of *búcaro*" that he had assembled for Mrs. de Torcy, "as it is forbidden for priests to give absolution to women who eat it, because it is contrary to creation." The Marquis adds that he will not be "so scrupulous" with his wife: "I will let her eat as much as she wants, for she will ruin me in the end by being too fertile."[7]

In *Craving Earth*, Sera Young proposes three reasons that push people and animals to consume earth: to stave off hunger, to compensate for a micronutrient deficiency, or to protect themselves from the effects of toxic substances. The first two hypotheses have been proven under certain circumstances: a context of food shortage regarding the former and higher consumption among iron-deficient populations concerning the latter. The third supposition has been put forth by various authors since antiquity, notably Pliny the Elder, who attributes to *terra sigillata* the property of being an antidote against snake bites and poisons.[8] The spread of geophagy might thus be thought of as a positive contagion, the diffusion of knowledge allowing one to face specific difficulties.

But what to make of those consumers for whom these explanations are not relevant? With regard to the *búcaros*, their contagious nature was perhaps linked to the rituals that surrounded their consumption—the effort to obtain them, the recipe followed to prepare them, the doubt and anticipation as to their effects, and the symbolic meaning of their ingestion: tasting earth from the four corners of the Empire as a way of overcoming distance.

translated by Maya Judd

NOTES

1. Juan de Cárdenas, *Primera parte de los problemas y secretos maravillosos de las Indias* (Mexico: Imp. National Museum of Archaeology, History and Ethnology, 1913), 192. First published in 1591.

2. Marie-Catherine d'Aulnoy, *Relation du voyage d'Espagne*, eighth letter (Paris: Plon, 1874), 288.

3. Sor Estefanía de La Encarnación, *La vida de Soror Estephanía de la Encarnación*, 1631, Madrid, Biblioteca Nacional, MS 7459, 16.

4. D'Aulnoy, *Relation du voyage d'Espagne*.

5. Francisca Perujo and Teresa Poggi Salani, "De los búcaros de las Indias Occidentales," *Boletín del Instituto de Investigaciones Bibliográficas (Mexico)* 8 (July–December 1972), 353.

6. Lorenzo Magalotti, *Lettere odorose (1693–1705)* (Rome: Liber Liber, 2007), 72, https://www.liberliber.it/mediateca/libri/m/magalotti/lettere_odorose/pdf/letter_p.pdf.

7. Cited by Alfred Morel-Fatio, "Comer Barro," in *Mélanges de philology romane dédiés à Carl Wahland* (Mâcon: Protat, 1896). Reissue in Geneva: Slatkine Reprint, 1972, 48–49.

8. Pliny, *Natural History*, vol. 9, book 35, translated by H. Rackham, Loeb Classical Library 394 (Cambridge, MA: Harvard University Press, 1952).

SELECTED BIBLIOGRAPHY

Morel-Fatio, Alfred. "Comer Barro." In *Mélanges de philology romane dédiés à Carl Wahland*. Geneva: Slatkine, 1972. First published 1896 by Protat (Mâcon).

Seseña, Natacha. *El vicio del Barro*. Madrid: Ediciones el Viso, 2009.

Young, Sera L. *Craving Earth: Understanding Pica—The Urge to Eat Clay, Starch, Ice, and Chalk*. New York: Columbia University Press, 2011.

CONTROVERSY

Propagation of the Quarrel between Rabbis Jacob Emden and Jonathan Eybeschutz

Jean Baumgarten

In 1751, a controversy erupted in northern Germany between two of the most eminent rabbinical authorities in the Ashkenazi community. The subject was an amulet believed to contain a hidden allusion to the false Messiah, Sabbatai Tsevi (1626–1676). Jonathan Eybeschutz (1690–1764), before being appointed to head the three Jewish communities of Hamburg, Altona, and Wandsbek, had been the rabbi of Metz. Members of the Jewish community often asked him to write amulets to protect women in childbirth, for example. His adversary, Jacob Emden (1697–1776), an eminent Talmudic scholar from Altona, was known for his virulent opposition to Jewish mysticism and the kabbala.

The force with which the controversy escalated was in part a reflection of the fierce internal conflicts tearing at the fabric of traditional Jewish society at a time when Judaism was entering the modern world. The quarrel could have remained a minor, local disagreement, but it became amplified and spread, as if by contagion, beyond the confines of the northern German communities. It involved the most diametrically opposed schools of thought and propagated itself in successive bursts into the principal centers of Ashkenazi Judaism. Judaism was splitting up into various antagonistic currents, ranging from rabbinical ultra-Orthodoxy to mysticism—including Hassidism—to the Haskalah of the Jewish Enlightenment. The quarrels between the proponents and opponents of the heretical movement surrounding Sabbatai Tsevi were having a profound impact on Jewish society. Small groups of followers continued to exist in Central and Eastern Europe, hoping for the return of the false Messiah and the advent of the Messianic era, and this constituted a threat to the unity of Jewish society.

The two main characters in the controversy were representatives of the most traditional rabbinical elite, but they embraced opposite views of Jewish tradition. Emden preached rigorous adherence to Jewish law while lending an ear, as a precursor of the Jewish Enlightenment, to secular voices and lauding Judeo-Christian dialogue. Eybeschutz, in addition to being one of the great rabbis of his era, was a kabbalist and healer who employed magical techniques. Their quarrel had begun several decades earlier. Already in 1725, Eybeschutz's adherence to the Sabbatian movement had raised eyebrows. The manuscript of a mystical treatise attributed to Eybeschutz, which revealed the existence of a clandestine network of heretics, was discovered in the baggage of an itinerant Sabbatian preacher. Eybeschutz, who was then a rabbi in Prague, denied any implication in the heterodox movement and signed a decree of excommunication against the sect.

But the word was out. The rumor only grew when Eybeschutz was appointed as the rabbi of the three north German communities in 1750. Members of the Altona community asked Emden to inspect an amulet that had been made by Eybeschutz. Emden held that it contained a hidden allusion to Sabbatai Tsevi and accused Eybeschutz of being a secret disciple of the false Messiah. Jewish leaders wondered if naming a rabbi who could be suspected of heresy and who could undermine the internal cohesion of the three communities was a good idea. Eybeschutz's hesitations and reversals only fed the fire of suspicion.

The rapid propagation of the controversy could be explained by the inflexible and uncompromising character of Emden, for whom combating Sabbatianism was a top priority throughout his life. But above all, the conflict should be seen as one of the many harbingers of the radical changes that were to shake up traditional Jewish society in the eighteenth century. Initially, the controversy between Emden and Eybeschutz remained within the three communities of Hamburg, Altona, and Wandsbek. Each camp sharpened its tools and put pressure on members of the community. The authorities took the side of Eybeschutz, the newly elected rabbi. The community council decreed that no one could communicate any information about the controversy. Anyone who visited Emden's private synagogue would be threatened with excommunication. Emden retorted that the prohibition had no legal value and anyone who signed an excommunication decree would in turn be excommunicated.

The controversy then overflowed its banks and engulfed the principal Jewish communities of Europe. At the time, the rabbinical authorities who dictated and discussed Jewish law formed a tight network of decision-makers. Legal questions were first examined at the local level. By the middle of the eighteenth century, however, rabbis were losing authority and were less and less able to resolve disputes that involved their whole community. In these cases, they called upon the preeminent rabbinical authorities in distant communities. It was in this way that Ezekiel Landau, the chief rabbi of Prague, came to be involved in the dispute. He published a missive that prohibited the use of amulets and public study of the kabbala, and he condemned any writings inspired by Sabbatai Tsevi. Nevertheless, wishing to avoid a direct confrontation with Eybeschutz, one of the foremost rabbinical authorities of the day, he sought a compromise.

Similarly, the rise of the printing press amplified the debate over Sabbatian heresy, fostering wide dissemination of the arguments. Answers to legal questions about the use of amulets could be published, copied, discussed, and circulated in the vast network of Ashkenazi communities. Excommunications and counterexcommunications were pronounced, and non-Jewish scholars and theologians were asked to arbitrate the debates. The north German Jewish communities were under the authority of the king of Denmark, who granted Jacob Emden a privilege authorizing him to open a print shop. This enabled Emden to greatly increase the volume of anti-Sabbatian pamphlets and diatribes against Eybeschutz as well as to publish a blacklist of books containing references to the "infamous sect," preceded by a warning: "The following books have absorbed, in some of their hidden parts, this snake's venom. . . . Impurity has thus spread through the people of Israel and lies in secret places."[1]

The rabbis of the three communities prohibited Emden from pursuing his work as a printer. Protected by a royal privilege, however, Emden was undaunted. The authorities then decided to expel Emden, who refused to leave and was put under house arrest in Altona. He hit back by activating networks of partisans to whom he sent missives, urging them to defend him in his battle against the heretical sect. Eybeschutz, wanting to counter these false accusations, also sent letters to rabbis, students, friends, and notable Christians, entreating them to support him in his struggle. He also drafted a plea in defense of himself and his followers, intended to silence Emden and his partisans.[2]

The two camps' unremitting attacks brought the conflict to the attention of the Jewish authorities at the European level. Reports thereof can be found in the proceedings of the Council of the Four Lands, an intercommunity body that oversaw the internal affairs of Jewish society in Eastern Europe. In 1753, the council outlawed writing—and disseminating any writing—about the controversy and excommunicated the Sabbatian sect. Rabbis from Lithuania, Moravia, Bohemia, and Italy entered the fray, which reverberated even as far as the Sephardic community in Constantinople, among other places. Eybeschutz, besieged by insults and threats, was ultimately forced to leave Hamburg.

When the controversy first began, discussion was confined mostly to the religious elite. But very quickly, it spread to the entire Jewish population and was a subject of debate in households, synagogues, and study and prayer groups. There was so much agitation that the dispute attracted the attention of Christian public opinion. It reached the ears of the authorities and of Catholic and Protestant scholars and theologians. It appeared in a multitude of writings, pamphlets, and invectives, in particular in the German and Polish press. The dispute even became a subject of discussion in literary circles.

When in 1751 clashes broke out in the Jewish quarters of Hamburg and Altona between partisans and adversaries of Eybeschutz, the civilian authorities took notice. Altona was under Danish rule; Hamburg was a Hanseatic city in which the Jewish population was governed by the Senate. Carl Anton, a converted Jew, professor of Hebrew, and former student of Eybeschutz, pleaded his teacher's cause before the Danish royal court, while Emden's partisans called upon the royal and municipal authorities.

The latter decided in favor of Eybeschutz, so as not to disavow their city's rabbi, but demanded clarification on the subject of the amulets. Meanwhile, Denmark's royal court of justice authorized Emden to return to Altona and resume his work as a printer. The court also punished those responsible for the turmoil in the city. The topic continued to inspire passionate debate, and it was not until the death of the two adversaries that it gradually subsided.

The controversy between Emden and Eybeschutz was propagated throughout Europe like a contagious disease. The slow disintegration of traditional Jewish society, its gradual secularization, and the effervescence that accompanied the advent of modern Judaism were all contributing factors. The community became a forum for combat between various conceptions of Jewish life at a time when the power and influence of rabbis was waning. The birth of modern Judaism came with religious convulsions, and the propagation of the controversy between these two rabbis was a precursor of them.

translated by Steven Sklar

NOTES

1. Jacob Emden, *Torat ha-kenaot* [The law of fanaticism] (Altona: N.p., 1752), fols. 71b–72a.

2. Jonathan Eybeschutz, *Sefer luhot edut* [The book of testimony] (Altona: N.p., 1755).

SELECTED BIBLIOGRAPHY

Carlebach, Elisheva. *The Pursuit of Heresy, Rabbi Moses Hagiz and the Sabbatian Controversies.* New York: Columbia University Press, 1990.

Katz, Jacob. *Hors du ghetto, l'émancipation des Juifs en Europe (1770–1870).* Translated by J.-F. Sené. Paris: Hachette, 1984. https://doi.org/10.1017/S0395264900074084.

Maciejko, Pawel. "The Eybeschutz Controversy." In *Sabbatian Heresy: Writings on Mysticism, Messianism, and the Origins of Jewish Modernity,* 115–139. Waltham: Brandeis University Press, 2017.

Maciejko, Pawel. *The Mixed Multitude Jacob Frank and the Frankist Movement 1755–1816.* Philadelphia: University of Pennsylvania Press, 2011.

CROWD

Gustave Le Bon, Sigmund Freud, Gabriel Tarde between Suggestion and Contagion

Yves Cohen

The discourse on crowds unfolded at the end of the nineteenth and early twentieth century under the influence of fear, and a dread of crowds was not new. Alarms from the French Revolution and uprisings that followed persistently fed such fright in Europe. At the end of the nineteenth century, these apprehensions were reinforced by the social protests of the Industrial Revolution and the growth of mass phenomena in all sectors, in industry certainly, but also in politics, war, culture, and education.

As soon as it was published in 1895, *Psychologie des Foules* (published a year later in English as *The Crowd: A Study of the Popular Mind*) by Gustave Le Bon was an international bestseller and was translated into some fifteen languages.[1] "Men forming a crowd cannot do without a master," proclaims the author in many variations (218). Left alone, crowds can only go wrong: "In consequence of the purely destructive nature of their power crowds act like those microbes which hasten the dissolution of enfeebled or dead bodies" (19). This medical metaphor blends crowds, germs, and contagion.[2] Le Bon's truths became those of several generations of political and social thinkers and doers, right or left; the book was read and used by all. Its impact was immense, no less in the social sciences of the twentieth century.

The notion of contagion is essential to Le Bon's approach to explaining crowds. It functions as a pair with that of "suggestion," which was at the heart of all debates in psychiatry and psychology at the time. At the end of the First World War, Sigmund Freud felt a need for a social psychology he lacked and borrowed that of Le Bon. In fact, he made Le Bon his first interlocutor in his 1921 book, *Massenpsychologie und Ich-Analyse* (*Group Psychology and the Analysis of the Ego*), where he incorporated the notion of contagion.[3] Five years before Le Bon, Gabriel Tarde had written *Les Lois de l'Imitation* (published in English in 1903 as *The Laws of Imitation*).[4] We find there the notion of "contagion of imitation" (98), raising the interesting question as to whether Le Bon would not have borrowed some nuance from him, or more. Contagion is central to the discourse on crowds and not incidental nor anecdotal, and not rhetorical either.

None of these three authors mention either any firsthand investigation of a crowd or even an in-depth study of one. This chapter, in turn, sticks to the point and even to the letter of their written work. Indeed, the historical evocation made here does not aim to test the effectiveness of the notion of contagion but rather to understand how it was used in service of the widely shared goal of crowd control.

Contagion appears in two ways in Le Bon's interpretative framework. First, three "causes" contribute to creating the "special characteristics" (26) that make up crowds. The first is sheer number, the second contagion, and the third suggestibility: "Contagion . . . is a phenomenon of which it is easy to establish the presence, but that it is not easy to explain. It must be classed among those phenomena of a hypnotic order. . . . In a crowd every sentiment and act is contagious, and contagious to such a degree that an individual readily sacrifices his personal interest to the collective interest" (34). Contagion in numbers comes from "suggestibility of which, moreover, the contagion . . . is neither more nor less than an effect" (34). Here, we see the extent to which Le Bon's remarks follow in the aftermath of disputes over Jean-Martin Charcot's work, led by the likes of Hippolyte Bernheim, Pierre Janet, and Alfred Binet, among others. Contagion allows the suggestion to go from one to multiple.

Second, contagion is one of the three "processes" of crowd control, which are affirmation, repetition, and contagion: "When an affirmation has been sufficiently repeated and there is unanimity in this repetition . . . what is called a current of opinion is formed and the powerful mechanism of contagion intervenes" (143). The medical metaphor reappears because "ideas, sentiments, emotions, and beliefs possess in crowds a contagious power as intense as that of microbes" (143).

In *Massenpsychologie und Ich-Analyse*, Freud turns to Le Bon's analyses to define the crowd, clearly agreeing with the latter despite some objections. Yet, on more than one occasion a surprising phenomenon occurs: these objections are little founded and serve more simply as a means of inserting a psychoanalysis perspective. Some of these points relate to contagion, and long passages of *Psychologie des Foules* are cited. Among these, we find the following remarks on the conscious and the unconscious: "We see, then, that the disappearance of the conscious personality, the predominance of the unconscious personality, the turning by means of suggestion and contagion of feelings and ideas in an identical direction, the tendency to immediately transform the suggested ideas into acts; these, we see, are the principal characteristics of the individual forming part of a crowd."[5] This conception of "the disappearance of the conscious personality (and) the predominance of the unconscious personality" in nearly term to term adopted by Freud (12).

This passage is followed by a long commentary by Freud: "We wish only to emphasize the fact that the two last causes of an individual becoming altered in a group (the contagion and the heightened suggestibility) are evidently not on a par, since the contagion seems actually to be a manifestation of the suggestibility. Moreover the effects of the two factors do not seem to be sharply differentiated in the text of Le Bon's remarks" (13). Yet this is precisely what Le Bon does in a passage quoted just before by Freud himself: "I allude to that suggestibility of which, moreover, the contagion . . . is only an effect."[6] Freud's objection is an artifice, and in fact his agreement with Le Bon is complete.

Another Freudian objection to Le Bon confirms it: "We may perhaps best interpret his statement if we connect the contagion with the effects of the individual members of the group on one another, while we point to another source for those manifestations of suggestion in the group which he regards as similar to the phenomena of hypnotic influence. But to what source? We cannot avoid being struck with a sense of deficiency when we notice that one of the chief elements of the comparison, namely the person who is to replace the hypnotist in the case of the group, is not mentioned in Le Bon's exposition" (13). Who else but the leader (*le meneur*) emerges from the Le Bon's crowd and endeavors to suggest it? Le Bon spends a significant amount of time on the latter, with numerous mentions of his suggestions. To this regard, in writing of parliamentary groups, he observes that "parliamentary crowds are very open to suggestion; and, *as in the case of all crowds*, the suggestion comes from leaders possessing prestige" (217; my emphasis).

At the very place where Freud sees no one in Le Bon, he introduces the libido and the father of the primitive horde, demonstrating for many and for long the advantage of thinking with psychoanalysis: "The leader of the crowd always incarnates the dreaded primal father" (99). Indeed, the word contagion (*Ansteckung*) appears in the German version of the text only in this Freud's discussion of Le Bon and of another author, William McDougall, and then again in just one other place in his 1921 book. Thus although Freud wrote of the "emotional contagion" with which "we are already familiar" (27), the expression is absent from the rest of the corpus of his writings. His reservations with regard to Le Bon nonetheless appear not only to be a way to introduce his own conceptions but also a posture so as not to show his unity with him.

Notwithstanding, it echoes Tarde's "imitative contagion" (218). There is, in fact, somewhat of a competition between Le Bon and Tarde. The latter presents a powerful interpretation of the world as imitation. He writes, for example, of what we call the circulation of technology as an imitation that "must have spread like a contagion . . . in the beginning of societies" (17). No invention without borrowing, as Leroi-Gourhan would say.[7] The conversion of peoples to this or that religion or social thought is a "political or religious contagion" (30) that can be compared to "a cyclone, an epidemic, an insurrection": "An epidemic . . . rages in a zig-zag line; it may spare one house or village among many. . . . An insurrection will spread still more freely from workshop to workshop, or from capital to capital. It may start from a telegraphic announcement" (35).

The "radiant contagion of civilization" derives from the continual action of one on the other in a generalized reciprocal copy (49). These "imitative contagions" form groups, communities, peoples, and civilizations.

Institutional forms similarly imitate one another and spread across borders. In the process, they are transformed. Tarde describes exactly what today we call "circulation"—here simply a question of contagion: "The parliamentary constitution of England began to be copied before its general diffusion in the nineteenth century, under two original forms, first by the United States . . . and then by revolutionary France, which hastened to drive parliamentarism into Rousseau-inspired radicalism. Contagious in turn, this last transformation . . . called forth I do not know how many ephemeral republics in South America" (293).

We have here what Tarde calls "contagious innovations" (*contagion novatrice*)[8] and no longer an exact reflection (as the mere term "imitation" implies)—that is, we have a circulation.[9] If the crowd is in no way a theme of consideration for Tarde, Le Bon was able to borrow from him the strength of the notion of contagion. Yet he is not ready to acknowledge what he owes to the latter and rejects the parallel drawn by Tarde between imitation and contagion. Allusion to Tarde is clear when Le Bon writes that "imitation, to which so much influence is attributed in social phenomena, is in reality a mere effect of contagion" (144), thus putting Tarde and his imitation in their place.

This vision of pathological and contagious crowds lasted the century. Crowds are "like women," says Le Bon (56). They need leaders and their contagious suggestions. One never finds in them exchange, objection, reflection, argumentation, or deliberation, and crowds have an incapacity to reason. Any linking action is either vertical from above and called suggestion or is reciprocal and called contagion. But have we not now left Le Bon's century behind? Is not the deliberative capacity of crowds better recognized? Can we still tell them that they need a master? Whatever the answers, are we done with the notion of contagion? Nothing is less certain.

translated by Maya Judd

NOTES

1.   Gustave Le Bon, *Psychologie des foules* (Paris: F. Alcan, 1895); translated as *Crowd: A Study of the Popular Mind* (London: T. Fisher Unwin, 1920). Citations refer to the 1920 translation.

2. Le Bon was far from being the first to speak of contagion as a mental and crowd phenomenon: see the bibliography of Scipio Sighele, *La Folla delinquente* (Turin: Bocca, 1891).

3. Sigmund Freud, *Massenpsychologie und Ich-Analyse* (Vienna: Internationaler psychoanalytischer Verlag, 1921); translated as *Group Psychology and the Analysis of the Ego* (London: Hogarth Press, 1949). Citations refer to the 1949 translation.

4. Gabriel Tarde, *Les lois de l'imitation: Étude sociologique* (Paris: F. Alcan, 1890); translated as *The Laws of Imitation* (New York: Henry Holt, 1903). Citations refer to the 1903 translation.

5. Freud, *Group Psychology*, 12.

6. Freud, *Group Psychology*, 11.

7. André Leroi-Gourhan, *Évolution et technique: Milieu et techniques* (Paris: Albin Michel, 1973), 392–395.

8. Tarde, *The Laws of Imitation*, 313; *Les lois de l'imitation*, ed. of 1895 (Classiques des sciences sociales), vol. 2, 93.

9. Yves Cohen, "Circulatory Localities: The Example of Stalinism in the 1930s," *Kritika: Explorations in Russian and Eurasian History* 11, no. 1 (2010): 11–45.

SELECTED BIBLIOGRAPHY

Barrows, Susanna. *Distorting Mirrors: Visions of the Crowd in Late Nineteenth-Century France*. New Haven: Yale University Press, 1981.

Cohen, Yves. *Le siècle des chefs: Une histoire transnationale du commandement et de l'autorité (1891–1940)*. Paris: Éditions Amsterdam, 2013.

Geiger, Roger L. "Democracy and the Crowd: The Social History of an Idea in France and in Italy, 1890–1914." *Societas* 7-1 (1977): 47–71.

Kelsen, Hans. "The Conception of the State and Social Psychology, with Special Reference to Freud's Group Theory." *International Journal of Psycho-Analysis* 5 (1924): 1–38. First published in *Imago* 8 (1922).

Moscovici, Serge. *The Age of the Crowd: A Historical Treatise on Mass Psychology*. Cambridge and New York: Cambridge University Press; Paris: Editions de la Maison des Sciences de l'Homme, 1985.

Schnapp, Jeffrey T., and Matthew Tiews, eds. *Crowds*. Stanford: Stanford University Press, 2006.

DANCE
Waltzmania in the Paris Pleasure Gardens
Elizabeth Claire

After the violence of the Terror that had marked the French Revolution, when Parisian pleasure gardens multiplied to offer new places of expression for the "frenzy to celebrate" that characterized the "madness of Thermidor," balls took center stage in the new nocturnal culture transforming Paris.[1] Louis-Sébastien Mercier described dancing as a "universal fury" that had everyone "from rich to poor" twisting about.[2] This culture of dancing madness would continue to develop until the Restoration and coincided with the emergence of a (first) romanticism and a new way of imagining the figure of the couple in Europe.

As the eighteenth-century salon culture of *bon mots* gave way to the passionate experience of the new social dances, their contagious vertigo became polemical. Under the reign of the Directory, during the winter season of Republican Year VII (1798–1799), the fashionable German "walsces" were all the rage. The first dance with a closed-couple hold to be adopted by an elite society in Europe, waltzing had already created trouble in certain German-speaking regions where it was promptly banned. The acceptance of the waltz in France merely increased concerns. The German poet Ernst Moritz Arndt described the French "nationalization of this German dance" in moralizing terms: the closed-couple hold, he said, allowed the male dancers to squeeze "the lady dancers as close as possible against themselves" while placing their hands "firmly on the breasts" of their partners.[3]

In this turning dance, the familiar *Contredanse* figures disappeared as the couple advanced with simple, repetitive steps, improvising their path across the dance floor while negotiating a shared center of gravity. Partners experimented with a vertigo whose centrifugal force and intoxication "exhausted" their bodies and "heated" their imaginations.[4] Through touch, the exchange of perspiration, and a rapidity that solicited the imaginations of the dancers embracing one another, the dazzling intimacy of the waltz was said to produce a ravishment that—according to the doctors who described it—menaced the health of an entire generation of youth.[5]

This "universal fury" of dancing was described according to several medico-philosophical notions: enthusiasm, passion, desire (*envie*), madness, and a whole ensemble of phenomena connecting body and soul, in which the mental faculty of the imagination played a pivotal role. Mental health medicine (*médecine morale*) at the time considered that the impressions of the imagination gave way to physical expressions called "nervous sympathies" (*sympathies nerveuses*) and that these could be transmitted from one individual to another.[6] Doctors wrote about the force of the imagination to explain the collective contagion of revolutionary violence: a mental contamination linked to a deviant behavior produced involuntary imitation. Following the same logic, *waltzmania* was understood as an epidemic of deviant dancing transmitted via the imagination.

The arrival of the German waltz in France coincided with the first publications of the new "Psychological and Political Sciences Class" of the National Institute of France as well as the 1802 creation by the Prefecture of Police of a Council of Hygiene in Paris. In the context of this political dynamic of early hygienism under the French Consulate, *waltzmania* came to be understood within a genealogy of European *choreaic* contagions: the eleventh-century legend of the Dancers of Kölbigk, Tarantism in Mediterranean Europe, the *Veitztanz* maligned by Martin Luther and cases of the *Danse de St. Guy* in Alsace and Rhineland during the Wars of Religion, the Convulsionaries of Saint-Médard in the early seventeenth century, or even the ecstatic Quaker dances taking place in the North American frontier (figure 1).

Under the auspices of the new hygienism, the posthumous publication of the heterodox physician Paracelsus, *Les causes des maladies invisible* (1565), had a particular impact on the interpretation of *waltzmania*.

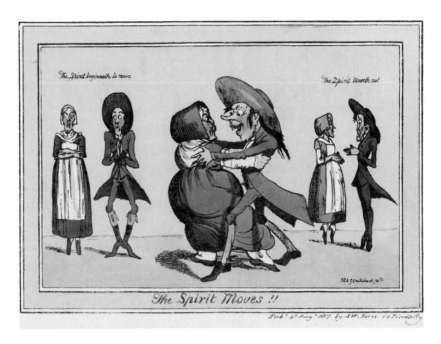

Figure 1

The iconography of the period also links ecstatic or "enthusiastic" dancing with the new *walse*. *Source*: Isaac R. Cruikshank and George Cruikshank, *The Spirit Moves!!*, British Museum, v. 9, no. 13098.

Paracelsus wrote about the 1518 dance epidemic in Strasbourg, reworking his 1537 theory of the cause of dance mania as published in "The Seven Defenses":[7] in sum, the imagination strikes the heart and tickles the nerves, and it provokes a turbulent joy and contracts the muscles, inducing the dance. Paracelsus also invented the figure of Frau Troffea, described as having set off the epidemic with her conjugal anger. The phenomenon according to Paracelsus, thus becomes a gendered one, since we are to understand that the *chorea lasciva* of the Strasbourg epidemic was born from the female imagination. In the eighteenth century, a renewed interest for Paracelsian theories of the imagination followed the very mediatized scandal concerning the medical practices of the Viennese physician Anton Mesmer, who cured Parisian women by touching them in very theatricalized ways (as reported by the Royal Commission in 1784).[8] The scandal of Mesmer's "animal magnetism" reinforced the idea, thereafter widely accepted, that the female imagination was particularly susceptible to contagion provoked by touch and theatrical gesture, that is to say, "nervous sympathies."

In 1804, P. J. Marie de Saint-Ursin, one of the most prolific physicians to treat the dangers of the new closed-couple dances, published his *L'ami des femmes: Du luxe privé. De la walse* (*A Friend to Women: On Private Luxury. On Waltzing*), a medical text dedicated to Madame Bonaparte and written in a literary prose destined for a female readership. He cites the harmful effects of Johann Wolfgang von Goethe's novel, *The Sorrows of Young Werther*, which begins with a sumptuous waltz shared between Werther and Lotte, and the events of the Revolution that "deformed" young women's morals in France. Marie de Saint-Ursin describes the waltz as a "battle" of the sexes that, through "the confusion of the senses" and the "degradation of love," upsets "women's desires" and destroys the bonds of marriage. As the male dancer embraces the waist of his partner "with a nervous arm," the couple pivots, "gazes merged, wholly absorbed in one another, they trace a multitude of circles in a state of delirium." This practice, according to the physician, was responsible for a "general contagion" of dance mania in France.[9] Other doctors considered that simply by observing a waltz, the "nervous sympathies" of a young woman could be activated, placing her in a state of contagious mania in which she risked sacrificing her mental health.

In this political period marked by speculation and the emergence of a new elite, the imperial aristocracy, the academic medical world took a keen interest in health problems stemming from social practices linked to the accumulation of private wealth ("luxe privé"). Urban illnesses like those of the women cured by Mesmer were categorized as nervous diseases specific to the female body. Faced with the excessively passionate dancing fashionable in the Parisian pleasure gardens, the medical establishment, in the interest of public health, alerted families about the potential contagion of the "perpetual" spinning dances that could strike their daughter's imaginations and induce madness. Doctors and moralists feared the new form of the closed-couple dancing but also the liberalization of the public balls that allowed for unprecedented social diversity within high society exactly at a moment when tensions concerning women's place in the imperial regime were unresolved.

In this way, the waltz participated in a sociomedical and philosophical debate centered on the powers of the female imagination and the question of republican motherhood, and these tensions were echoed in the specialized press. In the medical lexicon, a connection was established between the vertigo of the waltz and the "exaltation" or "striking" of the female imagination; the contagious character of the dance was correlated to "enthusiasm" or a form of physical and emotional "excess."[10]

In the French dance mania, physicians observed the distressed passions of women waltzers and considered this responsible for a "reversal of the natural order of things" and the manufacture of "mannish women" attracted by masculine ambitions.[11] They denounced the "very-vexing consequences" brought on by the "exciting and magnetic contact" of waltzing: vertigo, premature menstruation, syncope, spasms, miscarriage, the spitting of blood, tuberculosis, sudden death, *clitorimania*, and other "false pleasures."[12] These ills contradicted the "pleasures of maternity" that Louis-Jacques Moreau de la Sarthe and other physicians posited as a natural phenomenon.[13] If marriage were to serve as a foundational element of modern society, as suggested by the 1804 Civil Code, the exaggerated pleasures of the waltz ran contrary to this recommendation.

In the wake of the Revolution and its fervor, the proper channeling of the collective imagination appeared vital for the successful orchestration and governing of a new imperial "social body." The public balls remained an ambivalent space in this regard: on the one hand, they were controlled spaces and were monitored by municipal and military forces, yet they also legitimized a framework for the transmission of passionate practices that were susceptible to trouble the social order, especially when it came to gender relations. The circulation of medical discourse on *waltzmania* had the effect of rendering urgent, in the name of public health, the problem of the involuntary transmission of waltzing and its particular *jouissance*. The objective was to avoid a moral contagion of the "perpetual dances" that might lead to a collective female mania imprinted with revolutionary republican ideas, that is to say, a *chorea lasciva* that, by keeping female citizens away from the state-condoned imperative to reproduce, might destabilize the imperial project itself.

NOTES

1. Antoine de Baecque, *Les nuits parisiennes, XVIIIe–XXIe siècle* (Paris: Seuil, 2015), 52–53.

2. Louis-S. Mercier, "Les bals d'hyver," in *Le nouveau Paris* (Gènes, 1795).

3. Ernst M. Arndt, *Reisen durch einen Theil Teutschlands, Ungarns, Italiens und Frankreichs in den Jahren 1798 und 1799* (Leipzig: N.p., 1804).

4. Christoph W. F. Hufeland, *L'Art de prolonger la vie humaine* (Lausanne: Hignou en Company, 1809), 217–218 and 320; Samuel A. Tissot, "Des causes morales des maux de nerfs," *Traité des nerfs et de leurs maladies*, in *Encyclopédie des sciences médicales*, vol. 10; *Œuvres de Tissot* (Paris: N.p., 1840).

5. Salomon J. Wolf, *Beweis daß das Walzen eine Hauptquelle der Schwäche des Körpers und des Geistes unserer Generation sey* (Halle: Johann Christian Hendel, 1799). First published in 1797.

6. Pierre J. G. Cabanis, *Rapports du physique et du moral de l'homme* (Paris: De Crapelet, 1805). First published in 1802.

7. Paracelse, *Œuvres médicales*, éd. Bernard Gorceix (Paris: PUF, 1968).

8. *The Reports of the Royal Commission of 1784 to Examine on Mesmer's System of Animal Magnetism and Other Contemporary Documents*, new English translation and an introduction by I. M. L. Donaldson, 2014, http://www.rcpe.ac.uk/sites/default/files/files/the_royal _commission_on_animal_-_translated_by_iml_donaldson_1.pdf.

9. P. J. Marie de Saint-Ursin, *L'ami des femmes: Du luxe privé. De la walse* (Paris: Barba, 1804), xiii, 49 and 58–68.

10. Samuel A. Tissot, "Des causes morales des maux de nerfs," in *Œuvres de Tissot*, 126, 130–132, and 367; "Tanzmoden in Breslau, Aus einem Briefe," *Journal des Luxus und der Moden* 6 (June 1797): 289–292; Christoph Wilhelm Friederich Hufeland, *L'Art de prolonger la vie humaine* (Lausanne: Hignou, 1809), 320.

11. Jean Etienne Dance, *De l'influence des passions sur la santé des femmes* (Paris: Didot Jeune, 1811), 15.

12. E. Pariset and A. C. L. Villeneuve, "Danse," in *Dictionnaire des sciences médicales*, vol. 8 (Paris: Panckoucke, 1814), 1–8; G. J. Raparlier, *Dissertation sur le vertige* (Paris: Didot Jeune, 1815), 10; Louis-Jacques Moreau de la Sarthe, *Histoire naturelle de la femme*, vol. 2 (Paris: Duprat and Letellier, 1803), 393–395; Dance, *De l'influence des passions*, 9; Jean-Joseph de Brieude, *Traité de la Phthisie Pulmonaire, par Brieude, Membre de la Société de Médecine de Paris, Membre de la ci-devant Société Royale de Médecine, de l'Académie Royale*

de Médecine-Pratique de Barcelonne; l'un des Auteurs de la partie médicale de la nouvelle *Encyclopédie*, book 1 (Paris, Chez Levrault frères, 1803), 32–33; Jean-Joseph de Brieude, "Imagination (Pathologie)," Louis-Charles-Henri Macquart, "Imagination (Hygiène)," in *Encyclopédie méthodique. Médecine, contenant: 1° l'hygiène, 2° la pathologie, 3° la séméiotique et la nosologie, 4° la thérapeutique ou matière médicale, 5° la médecine militaire, 6° la médecine vétérinaire, 7° la médecine légale, 8° la jurisprudence de la médecine et de la pharmacie, 9° la biographie médicale, c'est-à-dire, les vies des Médecins célèbres, avec des notices de leurs Ouvrages*, book 7, ed. Félix Vicq-d'Azyr (Paris, Vve Agasse, 1798), 465–491, at 471 and 489.

13. Moreau de la Sarthe, *Histoire naturelle de la femme*.

SELECTED BIBLIOGRAPHY

Claire, Elizabeth. "Inscrire le corps révolutionnaire dans la pathologie morale: la valse, le vertige, et l'imagination des femmes." In *Orages: Littérature et culture 1760–1830*, no. 12: "Sexes en Révolution" (March 2013): 87–109. http://orages.eu/wp-content/uploads/2017/05/inscrire.pdf.

Claire, Elizabeth. "Monstrous Choreographies: Waltzing, Madness and Miscarriage." *Studies in Eighteenth Century Culture* 38 (2009): 199–235.

Goldstein, Jan. "Enthusiasm or Imagination? Eighteenth-Century Smear Words in Comparative National Context." In *Enthusiasm and Enlightenment in Europe, 1650–1850*, 29–49. San Marino, CA: Huntington Library, 1998.

Hess, Remi. *La Valse, un romantisme révolutionnaire*. Paris: Métailié, 2003.

Lécuyer, Bernard P. "L'hygiène en France avant Pasteur 1750–1850." In *Pasteur et la révolution pastorienne*, edited by Claire Salomon, 65–139. Paris: Payot, 1986.

Poma, Roberto. "Paracelse et la danse de Saint-Guy." In *1518, La fièvre de la danse*, edited by Cécile Dupeux, 95–114. Strasbourg: Éditions des Musées de Strasbourg, 2018.

Rohmann, Gregor. "Veitstanzähnliche Bewegungen. Dimensionen eines Deutungsmusters zwischen Martin Luther und Ozzy Osbourne." In *Mythen der Vergangenheit. Realität und Fiktion in der Geschichte*, edited by Ortwin Pelc, 111–158. Göttingen: V and R Unipress, 2012.

Vermeir, Koen. "Guérir ceux qui croient: Le mesmérisme et l'imagination historique." In *Mesmer et Mesmérismes: Le magnétisme animal en context*, edited by Bruno Belhoste and Nicole Edelman, 119–146. Paris: OmniScience, 2015.

EPIDEMIC

Bovine Tuberculosis in France and the United Kingdom (Nineteenth Century): From the Miasma to the Microbe

Alessandro Stanziani

While animal epizootics and their transmissibility to humans are a contemporary problem (mad cow disease, foot-and-mouth disease, avian influenza), they have, in fact, been an issue since the boom in meat consumption in the Middle Ages and even more so since the eighteenth century, with the expansion of consumption and scientific knowledge. In France, several rulings of the Parliament of Paris, from 1714 to 1784, forbade "corrupted" meat as well as that from "sick" animals. After the Revolution, these two categories persisted, as did the problems they posed. Meat can indeed be unfit for consumption because it has spoiled due to heat, the presence of bacteria, and so forth. But meat may also come from an animal with a contagious disease. In the latter case, should its sale be banned?

In the nineteenth century, "local practices" prevailed, the disadvantage being that a disease considered in one locality as a critical flaw (and therefore prohibiting the sale of the animal or its parts) might not be considered as such in another. Given these uncertainties, a new law established a list of diseases that imposed a ban on the sale of affected animals and their parts: rinderpest, contagious pleuropneumonia, sheep pox and scabies, foot-and-mouth disease, glanders, farcin, dourine, rabies, and anthrax. However, as new diseases emerged, a debate quickly arose over the logic of the nomenclature: should the lists be closed or, on the contrary, extended to include new scourges, particularly tuberculosis?

A true plague of the nineteenth century, tuberculosis fueled all sorts of fears and forms of social exclusion. It also called into question biological order at a time when, with Darwinism, the boundary between man and animal was once again under discussion. Tuberculosis proved to be a privileged field for this frontier due to queries over the disease's transmissibility. On the one hand, the majority of hygienists insisted on the transmissibility of this disease and the need to exclude all affected animals from consumption. On the other hand, breeders' associations, with the support of other hygienists, thought the animal disease to not be transmissible to humans and that, regardless, even in an affected animal, some parts of its body remain "healthy."

However, in practice tuberculosis, while important, was not actually the most widespread epizootic. In 1893, in the French department of Seine, the most significant contagious animal disease was pleuropneumonia, which affected 107 feeding establishments, comprising 2,247 animals. In comparison, tuberculosis touched 73 barnyards in Paris and its surroundings, with 78 animals affected and losses estimated at 30,945 francs. The attention paid to tuberculosis was therefore partly a media effect. Scientific uncertainty further fed the situation, led by two competing explanations for the transmission of germs. There were, on the one hand, supporters of the theory of "miasmas," thought to be responsible for the contagion; on the other hand, the Pasteurians emphasized bacteriological elements. The majority of veterinarians in the late 1870s favored the first interpretation but then switched to the other side over the next two decades.

The gradual shift from a miasma theory to epidemiology stemmed from an increased emphasis on observation. Any legal or health dispute, any real or actual epidemic, any death (and autopsy) suspected of being linked to the ingestion of contaminated meat was an opportunity to test one or the other theory. This approach dealt a definitive blow to organoleptic analysis and called into question the practices of former inspectors and veterinarians. The new expert now had to have skills in microscopy, physiology, and epidemiology. Observation of the case became fundamental; the narrative being part medical diagnosis, part judicial investigation, and part journalistic reporting.

A later consequence of this epidemiological shift was a renewal of debate over the distinction between "ordinary meats" and "luxury meats."

A number of hygienists thought the "poor" might largely be the recipients of meat from sick animals and that the latter should thus be banned from sale. Others, however, argued that the poor had better immune defenses and were consequently less likely to be victims of contagious diseases transmitted through meat consumption. Excessive bans would therefore have the sole effect of depriving the very poorest of meat consumption, which would otherwise be too expensive. This issue has continued to be a source of dispute with each food security crisis. Whether it be the contaminated chickens of the 1960s and 1970s, "mad cow disease," or raw milk cheeses, the use of bans continues to provoke fierce discussions between "hygienists," who today adhere to the precautionary principle, and those who see in these bans (or their removal) a way to revive a market in crisis at the expense of the most disadvantaged social groups. In this context, in the eyes of administrative officials, protecting health and supporting the economy are not always compatible objectives. Can we both avoid consumer panic and support French livestock farming?

With regard to bovine tuberculosis, certain politicians and experts feared that the spread of scientific theories could cause consumer panic. It then became a matter of understanding when the disease is "advanced enough" in the animal to be transmittable to humans. Depending on the answer, the ban on infected meat will be more or less extensive (i.e., the entire animal or only certain pieces). However, on this subject, the main scientific societies, such as the Belgian Royal Academy of Medicine or the Central Society for Veterinary Medicine in Paris, were divided. In parliamentary committees and debates, these doubts were amplified by pressure from various lobbies. In reality, the solution lay not only in the science but in the ties between epizootics, animal husbandry, consumption, and insurance. The greater the number of legal seizures and the higher the food safety, the more the question of compensation became important. In the event of mass seizures, everyone accepted the idea of compensating the owners of animals and meat, but to what extent and, above all, with what resources?

Unlike the present day, state support at the turn of the nineteenth and twentieth centuries was nonexistent. Instead, the government encouraged livestock farmers to take out insurance. Farmers' mutual savings and loans societies consequently began to offer this service. Yet this solution raised an additional question: to compensate owners of slaughtered animals, it must first be established that the necessary measures to avoid contagion have been taken. But what are these measures?

Here opinions diverged. On the one hand, those in favor of hygienic measures advocated a range of measures to be adopted not only in the acquisition and feeding of animals but also in the barnyard. Pasteurians, on the other hand, thought vaccines to be the only remedy. After much discussion, and with scientists remaining divided, the French authorities opted for the vaccine solution. Insurance companies followed suit and concluded that only owners who have vaccinated their livestock can claim compensation. If failing to resolve the scientific questions, this institutional solution gave life to a flourishing insurance and vaccine market. Moreover, as a result of these measures, tuberculosis cases dropped significantly at the beginning of the twentieth century, both in animals and humans: Pasteurians cried success.

A quite similar outcome was, however, achieved in the United Kingdom before the compulsory vaccination was introduced in 1939. The majority of scientists and politicians across the Channel were instead convinced of the effectiveness of hygiene measures and skeptical of Pasteur's theories and vaccines. This feud continues to this day: during the mad cow and avian flu epidemics, French scientists and authorities immediately imposed an obligatory vaccination, while on the British side, hygiene measures were preferred. Once again, the results obtained in both cases did not allow the question to be settled.

translated by Maya Judd

BIBLIOGRAPHY

Atkins, Peter. *Liquid Materialities: A History of Milk, Science and the Law*. Farnham: Ashgate, 2010.

Stanziani, Alessandro. *Histoire de la qualité alimentaire*. Paris: Le Seuil, 2005.

EX-VOTO
Votive and Political Accumulations in the Public Space

Pierre-Olivier Dittmar

Thousands of coins in the basin of the Trevi Fountain, hundreds of wishes hanging upon the branches of a tree, dozens of marble plaques near a statue of the Virgin. The votive phenomenon appears as a provocation for historians to the extent that its deployment in time and space, from sanctuaries of antiquity to churches of contemporary Brazil, defies ordinary frameworks of analysis. The collective, and apparently spontaneous, dimension of these deposits intrigues us, suggesting spaces intermittently contaminated with suffering and desire.

During the twentieth century, researchers widely commented upon the nature of the contract constituted by any votive deposit, the famous *do ut des*[1] linking offerer and deity in a dialogue structured by the deposited object: I offer an object to an invisible power in thanks for an exceptional intervention or to provoke one. In fact, the bibliography has focused on a *vertical axis* passing through notions of materialization and transcendence. In doing so, a *horizontal axis* of the ex-voto phenomenon has been largely overlooked. However, for those who frequent these objects inserted in their ritual contrivances, the collective dimension imposes itself powerfully. An ex-voto rarely exists alone; it is almost always surrounded by offerings in the same format. To create commensurable objects, we have collectively produced a definition articulating the following two axes: "A votive offering is a physical gift to an active force supposedly acting in a specific place and the expression of a formulated or satisfied desire. This gift is the act of an individual or group, always surrounded by other gifts of the same type."[2]

How should the dimension of community be considered? At any rate, it cannot be interpreted as a survival of a lost holistic world, the last echo of a tradition that would have ignored individualism. Far from dwindling, votive deposits have multiplied since the 1990s and are part of a revival of what Jack Santino and Ceri Houlbrook call *folk assemblage*. The proliferation of gum walls, roadside shoe trees, placement of memorial objects after a terrorist attack, cairns along hiking trails, and other contemporary phenomena develop without ties to traditional religious framework. They require us to think of ex-votos not only as a contract with the invisible but also, above all, as collective accumulations in public spaces.

What happens when a tourist places, at the base of a replica of the Statue of Liberty's torch on the *Pont de l'Alma* in Paris, a thank you note to Princess Diana for helping him to find a "little apartment"? Why, a few years later, does the same site attract love padlocks? Today the wall of Juliet's House in Verona, Italy is covered with a strange collective composition of Post-it Notes, love letters, requests, and thanks, affixed to the venerable stones of the supposed home of Shakespeare's heroine (figure 1). By what means do a princess who died in a traffic collision and a literary heroine who committed suicide become solicited intercessors in fields as diverse as finding a soulmate or an apartment?

These practices may be seen as the consequence of a transfer of sanctity from saints to celebrities. At the same time, we may consider that it would be naive to imagine that tourists in Verona really believe that Juliet will bring them love. Undoubtedly, we benefit from thinking that these media figures participate in a process of "I know very well, but even so,"[3] as operators of collectives, pretexts making it possible to gather significantly (figure 1).

Let's take a step further. The love padlocks analyzed by Ceri Houlbrook testify to an even more radical situation, since here the wish is not accompanied by any transcendental entity. Even more, the remarkable coin wish trees of the British Isles offer a wealth of learning opportunities, since what was once the attested votive practice of inserting coins into the bark of a tree does not stop augmenting, even when none of the participants encountered in her study claim to have expressed a wish.

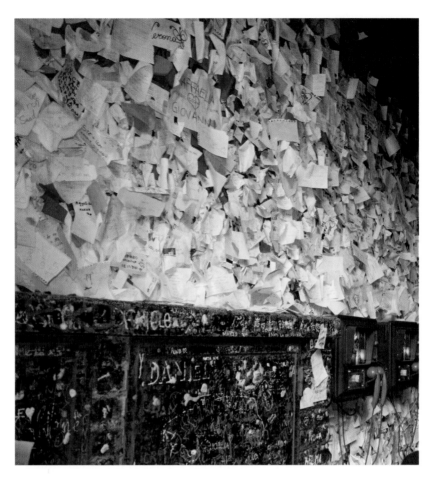

Figure 1
Love letters on the wall of Juliet's House in Verona, May 11, 2020. *Source*: Luu (wikimedia).

Without deities or vows, these dispositions oblige us to weigh a common and collective desire by unidentified people with the complicity of a largely reinvented material world. By physically occupying public places in an unplanned way, these objects validate and perpetuate a sensitive and political geography.

Clearly, there is a horizontal diffusion of desires by "things" that no longer respond to any pattern of transcendence. If we attach a padlock to another padlock or slip a letter of request behind an old votive offering, rather than in front of an image of worship, these techniques of diversion and reuse contribute to make each individual into a stakeholder and therefore, in a sense, an intercessor. If an invisible entity exists in this apparatus, it is no longer a deity but instead all of our contemporaries—the people?—whom we never seem to entirely perceive.

How should we think about these horizontal mobilizations? One might be tempted to use Tarde's model based upon imitation and contagion, or better yet, its rereading by Gilles Deleuze and Félix Guattari that would make these folk assemblies an appropriate process of subjectivation. Yet however relevant these approaches may be, they do not allow direct thinking about the trace or object in its very materiality within the transmission process. Perhaps the concept of *stigmergy* may help in this conceptual approach.

The concept of stigmergy, defined in 1959 by Pierre-Paul Grassé, combines the Greek terms *stigma* (sign) and *ergon* (work). In its initial context, the concept was used to describe spectacular constructions such as termite mounds by social insects. Since then, the concept has been transformed and its use extended to other avian, and subsequently mammalian, organizations. Since the 2000s, the concept has been applied to humans in a wide variety of fields, from the theorization of social movements such as Occupy Wall Street to management techniques in large companies, including the analysis of illegal garbage dumps.

Today it is important to take this concept as a new creation, without reference to its context when it was originally created, thereby avoiding any naturalizing appeal that might assimilate anonymous crowds with termites or ants operating on an extremely basic stimuli/response mode. In fact, the concept has been taken up more inventively, notably by Lachlan MacDowall, to conceptualize certain features of spontaneous occupation of public space. Following this precedent, I propose to redefine stigmergy as follows: A mechanism of indirect coordination between agents. The principle is that any trace left in the environment by the initial action invites a new action of the same order, by the agent who will encounter this trace. In this way, successive actions tend to strengthen and thereby lead to a spontaneous emergence of coherent activity.

Taken as such, the concept makes it possible to think of indirect complicities, based not upon the meeting of bodies, or even the contagion of ideas, but rather upon physical traces as the result of work upon matter. Therefore, encounters may occur in unusual historical sequences, such as when an individual arrives to scrawl a miraculous story as graffiti on an ex-voto painted fifty years previously by someone unknown to the graffitist. More generally, stigmergy helps us to think not only of collective *action* but also of collective *productions* without coordination, representation, or foreshadowing.

If the revival of this concept goes hand in hand with the proliferation of streetside folk assemblies, it is perhaps because both respond in their own way to the crisis of representation, both aesthetic and political, which has characterized the past two decades (figure 2).

From this perspective, it must be considered that today, stigmergic objects such as ex-votos are more political than ever. Submitting an ex-voto

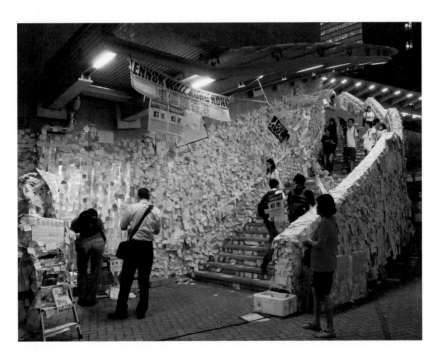

Figure 2
Lennon Wall in Hong Kong, October 21, 2014. *Source*: Underbar dk (wikimedia).

is not merely a donation but especially a testimonial to a situation and call to witness. Hence the message, often formulaic and repetitive, is less of a dissension than the practice itself, which establishes a balance of power, sometimes beyond the framework accepted by the public powers. In many cases, this placement amounts to the *occupation* of sites of worship in general, pilgrimage sites, current touristic sites, and sites of visibility in general.

Public accumulations of objects conveying wishes, desires, and sufferings *demonstrate* individual needs but also allow individuals to demonstrate *themselves* around rallying points. The political dimension of these popular arrangements was present in their structure and has been emerging openly over the past few years. During the umbrella revolt of 2014 in Hong Kong, then in 2019 in Algiers and again in Hong Kong, entire walls were covered with Post-it Notes expressing desires and demands and opposing the political regime (figure 2). Strikingly, these share a format with the Post-it Notes on Juliet's house in Verona containing love requests, although altered to a political medium. Regardless of the genealogy of this globalized phenomenon, it is important to consider the nature of these mobilizations, consisting in leaving a trace, not only bearing an individual message but also encouraging passersby to reproduce the gesture and continue a collective work.

The concept of stigmergy is not intended to exhaust the meaning of the ex-voto phenomenon but to instead enable us to specify how it works. In fact, *do ut des*, originally used to describe votive deposits, must be understood as conveying an ambiguous message: *I do so that you may do*, where the "you" simultaneously addresses both an abstract entity, a deity, or government as well as passersby who discover the object.

translated by Benjamin Ivry

NOTES

1. [A Latin formula in the civil law, meaning "I give that you may give."—Trans.]

2. Pierre-Olivier Dittmar et al., "Un matérialisme affectif," *Techniques and Culture* 70, no. 2 (2018): 12–41.

3. [A chapter in Octave Mannoni's *Clefs pour l'imaginaire ou l'Autre scène* (Paris: Éditions du Seuil, 1969) is titled "Je sais bien mais quand même," discussing denial and semi-belief. Frédéric Lambert's *Je sais bien mais quand même: Essai pour une sémiotique* (Le Havre: Éditions non Standard, 2013) further investigates the subject.—Trans.]

SELECTED BIBLIOGRAPHY

Deleuze, Gilles, and Félix Guattari. *A Thousand Plateaus: Capitalism and Schizophrenia*. Trans. Brian Massumi. Minneapolis: University of Minnesota Press, 1987.

Dittmar, Pierre-Olivier, Pierre-Antoine Fabre, Thomas Golsenne, and Caroline Perrée. "Un matérialisme affectif." *Techniques and Culture* 70, no. 2 (2018): 12–41.

Elliott, Mark Allan. "Stigmergic Collaboration: A Theoretical Framework for Mass Collaboration." PhD dissertation, Centre for Ideas, Victorian College of the Arts, University of Melbourne, Melbourne, 2007

Grassé, Pierre-Paul. "La reconstruction du nid et les coordinations inter-individuelles chez Bellicositermes natalensis et Cubitermes Sp. La théorie de la stigmergie: Essai d'interprétation du comportement des termites constructeur." In *Insectes Sociaux*, vol. 6. Paris: Masson, 1959.

Houlbrook, Ceri. *The Magic of Coin-Trees from Religion to Recreation: The Roots of a Ritual*. Cham: Palgrave Macmillan, 2018.

Lambert, Frédéric. *Je sais bien mais quand même: Essai pour une sémiotique*. Le Havre: Éditions non Standard, 2013.

MacDowall, Lachlan J. "Graffiti, Street Art and Theories of Stigmergy." In *The Uses of Art in Public Space*, edited by Julia Lossau and Quentin Stevens, 33–48. London: Routledge, 2015.

Santino, Jack. "Performative Commemoratives, the Personal, and the Public: Spontaneous Shrines, Emergent Ritual, and the Field of Folklore." *Journal of American Folklore* 117, no. 466 (2004): 363–372.

HERESY

Fighting the Crypto-Protestant "Infestation" under the Habsburg Monarchy

Marie-Élizabeth Ducreux

In the first third of the eighteenth century, the Archbishopric of Prague produced a nondated normative memorandum on the difficulty of recognizing heretics. It was perhaps written at the end of Emperor Charles VI's reign (1711–1740) or at the beginning of Maria Theresa's (1740–1780).[1] It came after the rescript emitted in 1726 by Emperor Charles VI in Bohemia that codifies the punishments to inflict on heretics and "seducers" (*Verführer* in German). To consider what in other local and contemporary ecclesiastical documents is called the *pravitas haeretica* (deformity, vice), the vocabulary has recourse to the semantic field of dissemination, contamination, plague, or contagious illness (*lues haeretica*), and remedy (*medela*, *remedium*).

To understand the lexical choices of the memorandum and its reference to the notion of contagion, one must go back a century earlier to the situation of the kingdoms and lands of the House of Habsburg with regard to heresy. After his victory at the Battle of White Mountain on November 8, 1620, Emperor Ferdinand II (1619–1637) reimposed Catholicism in the Archduchy of Austria and Czech lands. The political measures taken by Ferdinand II and his son Ferdinand III (1637–1657) to convert their Austrian and Bohemian subjects were parallel and comparable. Due to the long-term effects in Bohemia of the religious and political movement arising in the early fifteenth century by Jan Hus and his disciples, however, the definition and boundaries of heterodoxy with regard to Catholicism proved to be different.

In the duchies of Inner Austria, this religious imposition had begun twenty years earlier. There, as in Lower Austria and Upper Austria, "heresy" was clearly identified by civil and ecclesiastic authorities. The nobility, the inhabitants of the cities, and peasants had often become Lutheran as well, sometimes Calvinist, during the sixteenth century. In Bohemia, on the other hand, Hussitism and its different branches had grown deep roots in the fifteenth and sixteenth centuries among Czech-speaking people. It preceded the appearance of Lutheranism, which became very present afterward in the German-speaking cities and regions of North and East Bohemia. There were few native Calvinists, in local competition with the Czech (or Moravian) Unity of the Brethren, a minority offshoot within Hussitism that appeared in 1457.

In 1487 a religious peace settlement legalized the coexistence of Catholics and Hussite Utraquists in the Kingdom of Bohemia and rejected the Unity of the Brethren as heretics. In this way, the Utraquists could no longer be considered as heretics within the country. Put another way, until the 1609 Letter of Majesty recognized the free exercise of the non-Catholic, evangelical faiths in Bohemia, the exact content of religious beliefs and affiliations of the populace was unclear, outside of ritual characteristics based on doctrinal understanding of the Eucharist as distinct from that of the Catholic Church. For the Utraquists, eternal salvation depended upon lay communion under both kinds. Unlike nobles and urban elites who could emigrate if they refused to convert, non-free peasants and inhabitants of seigniorial towns had no recognized right to emigrate in the Treaty of Westphalia. This is another difference from non-serf Austrian peasants persecuted for their religious beliefs at the same time as the writing of the normative memorandum of the first third of the eighteenth century.

In the eighteenth century, when Austria's civil and religious authorities discovered the persistence of Lutheran practices among the people in some regions of Carinthia, around Vienna and at the frontier of the ecclesiastical principality of Salzburg, they were seen as crypto-Protestants and were deported within the Habsburg Monarchy to Transylvania, where Lutheranism and Calvinism were still allowed. Others were later transported to repopulate and develop the Banat along with prostitutes, beggars, and delinquents. Yet, in the two Bohemian or Czech lands, Bohemia and Moravia, they were not deported and were spoken of as "suspected" of heresy and not as crypto-Protestants. But where does heresy come from? From the outside? From the depths of the countryside as a sign of the failure of a century of efforts to reconvert people to Catholicism? This is where the documentation of the Archbishopric of Prague comes in.

This memorandum was written to give a *modus operandi* directly to the local vicars forane (*Vicarii foranei*), substitutes of the Prague Official, who oversaw about fifteen parish priests within each circle, or province, of the kingdom. It was also meant for parish priests and permanent missionaries who had been in place since the 1730s. These were the ecclesiastics who in fact led the first interrogations and were tasked with establishing, in connection with the officiality of the archbishopric, whether a suspected person might be called a heretic. The memorandum indeed specifies why one must not call "heretics" those who are nonetheless extremely (*vehementissime*) suspect in this matter.[2]

Other sources, such as the annual reports on the state of religion in the Archdiocese of Prague, establish statistics of all acts pertaining to the "heretical scourge" that "prowls" in the many places where it "roams" (*grassabatur*).[3] The vocabulary used goes beyond the semantic field of contagion and sickness. In these sources, one finds the number of suspects denounced at the Royal Appeals Court of Bohemia (458 in 1735, 105 in 1751, for example). They are called "heretical emissaries" and "seducers," leading the inhabitants of the realm into their errors. The latter are designated as "born of Catholic parents" or even sometimes as *catholici ficti*. These same people, suspect and even "infested with their principles," "can only barely be distinguished from true Catholics."[4] One can therefore note an ambiguity in defining the origin and kind of heresy, even in the sources devoted to counting the offenders of the Catholic unanimity of the Kingdom of Bohemia.

In this context, the memorandum produced by the Archbishopric of Prague examines the difficulty in determining the criteria that can, with certainty, distinguish a proven heretic from a simple suspect who was perhaps "seduced" by an emissary of error. To do this, it uses the vocabulary of illness. Where do we situate the origin of heresy? The "seducers" come from abroad, but what should be done with the fugitives from Bohemia found among them, who have returned to "disseminate" books and errors? From there, its author reviews all the signs that are not to be interpreted as proof of a true heretical attitude. Moving to foreign lands like Saxony and even Hungary—land of the emperor, like Bohemia—which, writes the author, "one might say that it is part of heretic lands," to have planned one's departure, sold one's furniture and agricultural tools, taken one's niece, nephew, or own father abroad before returning home, none of this would necessarily be enough to establish the reality of one's heterodoxy. Prudence is required.

The inquisitor, parish priest, missionary, or vicar forane is under an obligation to "mitigate the rigor" of his conclusions in most cases. If these people, coming and going as they please, who do not denounce the "emissaries" of heresy that they may even have sheltered and who are strongly suspected of deception and dissimulation, still might have left their original home for reasons other than religion. This leads to an imagined sickness that one must nurse: one must give medicine and spiritual remedies, avoid excommunicating them all, and not make them sign under oath too many letters of reversal. Finally one must not turn to the seigniorial authorities for all of them and even less so give them over to the secular arm. An excellent medication to apply to those who have been contaminated by the error of others is to have them pray for the conversion of the unfaithful, over and above the recitation of the Acts of Faith, Hope, and Charity. This painstaking work of distinction between the contaminants and the contaminated is led by doubt, for "it is nearly impossible to tell the intentions of such men, and it is not easy to believe those who would exile themselves."[5]

It is the prescriber's doubt that categorizes the suspects, for all are suspect before being declared "sick." If they are sick but not declared heretics, the hope for healing must be encouraged. In this document meant to be normative, the imaginary of contagion is thus put into the service of an elusive concept of heresy and its propagation.

translated by Vicki-Marie Petrick

NOTES

1. National Archives of Prague (Národní archiv, abbr. NA), Archives of the Archbishopric of Prague (abbr. APA), call numers B 30/5 and B 30/6.

2. NA Prague, APA, B 30/5.

3. NA Prague, APA, B 30/5. The term is often used in the description of epidemics.

4. NA Prague, APA, box H 2/5 4293, *De Statu religionis*, 1751e (leaflet 5e).

5. NA Prague, APA, B 30/5: *Verum quia de intentionibus talium hominum constare minime potest, nec profugituris facile credendum est.* One can also find in this document a mention of the prayer for the conversion of infidel heretics and the recitation of the theological acts.

SELECTED BIBLIOGRAPHY

Ducreux, Marie-Élizabeth. "Reading unto Death: Books and Readers in Eighteenth-Century Bohemia." In *The Culture of Print: Power and the Use of Print in Early Modern Europe*, edited by Roger Chartier et al., 191–230. Princeton: Princeton University Press, 1989.

Ducreux, Marie-Élizabeth. "Le livre et l'hérésie, modes de lecture et politique du livre en Bohême au 18e siècle." In *Le livre religieux et ses pratiques: Der Umgang mit dem religiösen Buch*, edited by Hans-Erich Bödeker, Gérald Chaix, and Patrice Veit, 131–155. Göttingen: Vandenhoeck and Ruprecht, 1991.

Leeb, Rudolf, Martin Scheutz, and Dietmar Weikl, eds. *Geheimprotestantismus und evangelische Kirchen in der Habsburgermonarchie und im Erzstift Salzburg (17./18. Jahrhundert)*. Vienna: Böhlau/Munich: Oldenbourg Verlag, 2009.

Pörtner, Regina. "Policing the Subject: Confessional Absolutism and Communal Autonomy in Eighteenth-Century Austria." *Austrian History Yearbook* 40 (April 2009): 71–84. https://doi.org/10.1017/S006723780900006X.

Steiner, Stefan. *Rückkehr unerwünscht: Deportationen in der Habsburgermonarchie der Frühen Neuzeit und ihr europäischer Kontext*. Vienna: Böhlau Verlag, 2014.

Steiner, Stefan. *Reisen ohne Wiederkehr: Die Deportation von Protestanten aus Kärnten 1734–1736*. Vienna and Munich: Oldenbourg Verlag, 2007.

ICONOGRAPHY

Dynamics of Innovation at Work in the Representation of the Hellmouth

Élise Haddad

In the past, medieval iconography has occasionally been described as a code, the elements of which were fixed and known quantities, allowing for certainty of interpretation. Today, that idea is largely criticized. In fact, infinite variations can be observed in the documents, variations that question the dynamics of innovation at work in the images, in particular the mutation of motifs and codes. Some creations remain a *hapax*, meaning that they remain one of a kind. But a certain number of them meet with a wider audience, integrating iconographical tradition. Can the notion of contagion aptly characterize the way in which these motifs spread when they flourish?

The use of the Hellmouth in some episodes of Revelation will serve as a case study in which to address the question. This motif, well known in the context of the Last Judgment, shows a monstrous head, its maw open wide upon the zone of the underworld, where we often see the damned. The contexts of the use of the Hellmouth are, however, larger and more diverse than those this definition has delimited, and furthermore they evolve with time. The Hellmouth is first the representation of the underworld and an attribute of the apocalyptic horseman who corresponds to Death and then becomes this horseman's point of origin. Later, it becomes a more widely spread element spouting various evil creatures, particularly locusts, those monstrous creatures sent by God to earth to torture men. This mutation happens through successive and independent micro-innovations, each being sufficiently limited so that the motif of the Hellmouth remains recognizable and comprehensible.

The Four Horsemen of the Apocalypse illustrating the manuscripts of the central Middle Ages are variously identified. There is consensus concerning three of them: Death, Famine, and War. The fourth, who leads them, is often identified as Conquest but also sometimes as Christ or the Antichrist. These horsemen are represented with attributes that allow us to recognize them. Famine, for example, holds a scale. Death, who rides a pale horse, sometimes has a Hellmouth as attribute, knotted to the tail of his mount and opening onto the souls of the dead. This is the case in a manuscript in the British Library[1] that was surely produced around 1260. We can also find an example in 1265 in the so-called *Douce Apocalypse*.[2] In both cases, the mouth is wide open behind the fourth horseman shown at the moment he rides forth from it. In the first of these two manuscripts, the Hellmouth is double, opening upward and downward. In the second, the mouth opens only upward but has feet allowing it to follow the horseman without being tied to the horse's tail. A devil is visible in the two images above the crowd of the damned in the infernal maw. In certain rarer cases, the attribute could be Satan following the horseman alone, as in the 1220 *Beatus* of Las Huelgas,[3] thus filling the same role. But these occurrences are minor, and the Hellmouth is the motif that more habitually characterizes this horseman.

Several shifts happen after this point. By the mid-thirteenth century, other images make the Hellmouth the point of origin for this apocalyptic horseman. This is the case, for example, in an Oxonian manuscript in which we see the rump of the horse freeing itself from the interior of the immense Hellmouth open at a right angle on the lower left edge of the image.[4] Inscriptions (*Infernus* and *equus pallidus*) confirm these identifications and describe the actions. In the manuscript the Hellmouth is not only used as a standard attribute allowing for identification, as this would be redundant given the inscriptions naming each horseman. Rather, it is also used as a characterization, that is, in this case, the horseman's place of origin. The same iconography is replicated in many manuscripts of the Anglo-French Apocalypse tradition.[5]

A further step is taken by the illuminator of the Lambeth Palace Library manuscript 75,[6] dating to 1238, which illustrates a gloss of Revelation by

Gilbert of Poitiers. This apocalyptic horseman surges forth from a supposed Hellmouth, although it is no longer explicitly such since it does not contain the souls of the dead. It has become a motif characterizing the frightening place whence emerge destructive figures, such as the Four Horsemen of the Apocalypse. This change does not happen at once; it is slow and complex, and the innovation is not generalized. Thus in the fourteenth century, the Cambridge manuscript kept at Trinity College[7] still pictures a mouth attached to a horseman. The different formulas are used concurrently by the illuminators.

Beyond the change of status of the Hellmouth attached to the Horsemen of the Apocalypse, the successive shifts continue and the motif is

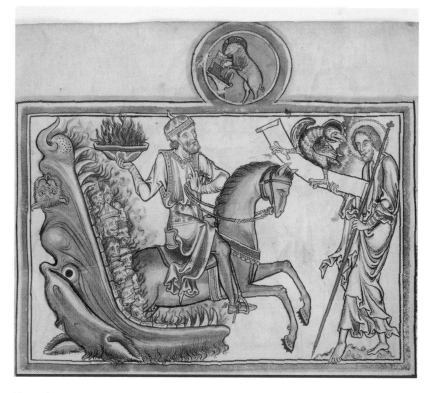

Figure 1

Horseman of the Apocalypse emerging from a Hellmouth, mid-thirteenth century. *Source:*
Apocalypse, Paris, Bibliothèque nationale de France, 403, fol. 9r.

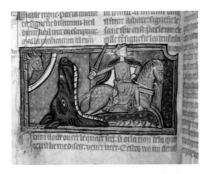

Figure 2

Horseman emerging from a Hellmouth, thirteenth century. *Source*: *Apocalypse* gloss by Gilbert de la Porrée, Lambeth Palace Library, MS 75, fol. 12v.

applied to other apocalyptic creatures. The tradition of images included in the manuscripts of Revelation or its commentaries include, in fact, many monsters, locusts among them, from chapter nine. They appear shortly after the horsemen in the order of both text and image. Older representations contained in the *Beatus* manuscripts do not picture the place of origin of these creatures and neither does the Trier Apocalypse.

Then, toward the year 1000, and the Bamberg Apocalypse,[8] locusts emerge from a seemingly octagonal well. It is likely the representation of the "bottomless pit" mentioned in the text of Revelation. This formula, which hews close to the text, pictures a well or a hole in the ground and has a certain popularity. It is taken up again in the first half of the twelfth century in a manuscript from Oxford[9] but also in 1175 in the *Beatus* of Rylands Library.[10] In the fourteenth century, by 1320–1330, a new motif comes into play: in the manuscript of the Apocalypse kept at Lincoln College,[11] the locusts explicitly come from what we will call a chthonian mouth. The latter has all the hallmarks of a Hellmouth, except it does not contain the souls of the dead. Rather, it serves simply as a point of origin for apocalyptic creatures.

The notion of contagion is rich for describing these successive micro-innovations. If it does not account for the often deliberate character of each individual innovation, the notion allows us nevertheless to grasp an effect of critical mass. The higher the number of images and producers of

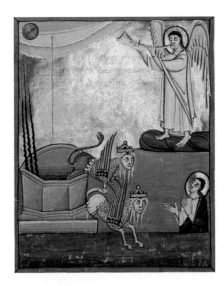

Figure 3

Locusts emerging from an octogonal well. *Source: Bamberg Apocalypse*, Bamberg, Staatsbibliothek Bamberg, MS A ii 42, fol. 23r.

images that adopt an innovation, the more this innovation has a chance of integrating the common language. After a certain threshold it becomes key. But, as with viruses, it can also mutate. The word "contagion" also throws light on the spontaneous nature of the process. None of the actors planned for the emergence of a new iconographical motif, but each consented to adopt an element of it and thus to transmit it. Finally, the notion of contagion allows us to characterize certain anomalies otherwise difficult to explain, unless we suppose long lines of lost images. In the examples given, one exceptional case has been left aside. It is a sculpture that dates to about 1130, thus well within our chronology, on the tympanum of Beaulieu-sur-Dordogne, which presents probably one of the first images of locusts emerging specifically from a chthonian mouth. This extremely early occurrence upsets the orderly chronological narrative and recalls that a motif can emerge and have little posterity at a given moment and then, later, proliferate epidemically once all the conditions for success are in place.

In summary, the notion of contagion allows for a description of the dialectic between innovation and tradition. Within this dynamic can be

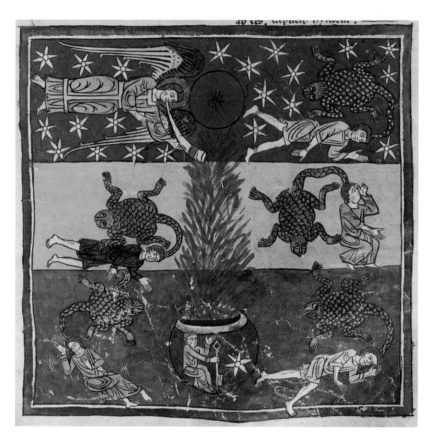

Figure 4

Locusts emerging from a circular pit, circa 1175. *Source*: Beatus's commentary on the Apocalypse, Manchester, Rylands Library, MS lat. 8, fol. 130r. © The University of Manchester.

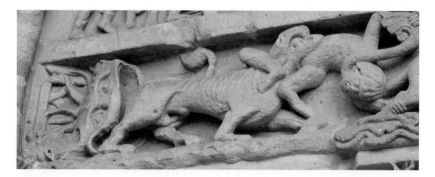

Figure 5

Locust emerging from a Hellmouth, circa 1130. *Source*: Beaulieu-sur-Dordogne, Corrèze, France. © E. Haddad, courtesy of the author.

found the nature of the system of signs at work in medieval iconography. This system gathers many elements reproduced as is and whose meaning is stable, but it also makes mutability and inventiveness possible, in the form of transmission from one to another. It constitutes an example of collective action without consultation, without command and without plan.

translated by Vicki-Marie Petrick

NOTES

1. London, British Library, MS 35166, fol. 8 v.

2. Oxford, Bodleian Library, MS 180, p. 16.

3. New York, Morgan Library and Museum, MS 429.

4. Bodleian Library, MS Auct.D.4.17.

5. See Bibliothèque national de France, Fr. 403, f. 9r.

6. London, Lambeth Palace Library, MS 75, f.12v.

7. Cambridge, Library of Trinity College, B-10-2.

8. Cote: Bamberg, Staatsbibliothek Bamberg, MS A ii 42, fol. 23r.

9. Bodleian Library 352, fol. 7v.

10. Manchester, Rylands Library, MS lat. 8, fol. 130.

11. Lincoln College, MS lat. 16, fol. 154.

SELECTED BIBLIOGRAPHY

Baschet, Jérôme. "Inventivité et sérialité des images médiévales: Pour une approche iconographique élargie." *Annales: Histoire, Sciences Sociales* 51, no. 1 (1996): 93–133. https://doi.org /10.3406/ahess.1996.410835.

Bord, Lucien-Jean and Piotr Skubiszewski. "De l'homme-scorpion mésopotamien à la 'sauterelle' apocalyptique: À propos des illustrations d'Ap 9, 1–12 aux IXe–XIe siècles." *Cahiers de civilisation médiévale* 177 (January–March, 2002): 5–24.

Emmerson, Richard Kenneth, and Suzanne Lewis. "Census and Bibliography of Medieval Manuscripts Containing Apocalypse Illustrations, ca. 800–1500." *Traditio* 40 (1984): 337–379; 41 (1985): 367–409; 42 (1986): 443–472.

INNOVATION
Organ Building and Diplomatic Exchanges in the Renaissance

Hugo Perina

In 1471, Alfonso of Aragon, Duke of Calabria and son of King Ferdinand, commissioned an organ from Lorenzo di Giacomo da Prato for the Castel Nuovo in Naples. Beyond the construction of a new instrument and the transfer of Tuscan (so-called modern) techniques to Campania, this is significant in that it also highlights a rapprochement in relations between the Aragon and the Medici dynasties. Certainly the interplay of alliances sometimes put Naples and Florence in enemy camps. In spite of it all, however, personal relationships did develop, as shown by the exchange of letters between the two reigning families and supported as well by exchanges in the cultural domain. In their diplomatic dealings with the Medici, Aragon's cultural policy gave a large role to the organ. This was not new. Even as early as 1450, the highly celebrated organist of Florence's cathedral, Antonio Squarcialupi, had sojourned at the Neapolitan court. If musical interpretation is a source of interest, a totally new way of organ building revolutionized soundscapes.

The case of Lorenzo da Prato (1417–1492) is particularly interesting since he is of the exact period of Lorenzo the Magnificent, of Ferdinand I, King of Naples and of his son Alfonso. Furthermore, he also connects distinct cultural regions. His career developed around two geographical poles. Although anchored in central and northern Italy, it was interspersed with two stays in the Kingdom of Naples, giving him a very particular status in the history of Italian organ building. In central Italy between 1459 and 1473, we see Da Prato's production punctuated by prestigious commissions for the cathedrals of Siena, Arezzo, Perugia, Pistoia, and for San Petronio in Bologna. Thus, until around 1475, his activity is centered around Tuscany, Emila-Romagna, Umbria, and the Veneto before shifting to the Kingdom of Naples. There the master also trained several students who in turn diffused Tuscan-style organ building. Given that, two questions come to the fore. What are the technical elements allowing us to establish contagion between relatively distant, and indeed rival, regions? Furthermore, to what extent are the builders and the patrons the agents of this contagion?

Lorenzo da Prato's first trip to Naples occurred in June of 1470. At that time, the Duke of Calabria was allied with the Florentines against Venice. Even then, the organ formed a link between Lorenzo the Magnificent and Ferdinand I. The latter writes Lorenzo de' Medici in 1473 asking him to allow a young man named Angelo to study with the organist of Santa Maria del Fiore, that is, the selfsame Squarcialupi who had gone to Naples in 1450. The King of Naples seems to have weighted his musical requests with a strong diplomatic connotation. Da Prato was certainly sent by Medici, and there is no doubt that this gift was particularly appreciated by the Neapolitan sovereign.

The Tuscan organ builder's first stay cannot have lasted more than a year given that he was present in Bologna between 1471 and 1475 to build the organ of San Petronio (and between 1473 and 1476 in Pistoia for their *duomo* San Zeno). Still, Da Prato returned to Naples during his years in Bologna. He was in Campania again in 1477.[1] In fact, only two organ projects can be placed in the years following the Tuscan organ builder's stay in Naples, and both went unfinished. There was the organ of San Agostino of Padua and that of the abbey church of San Fedele in Poppi, which was completed by Aretino di Jacopo da Città di Castello. Thus the hypothesis of a longstanding sojourn by Lorenzo di Giacomo in Campania becomes plausible.

At the same period, Lorenzo da Prato took on Stefano Pavoni and Giovanni Mormando as students, two founding figures of the Neapolitan School. This lineage from master to student helped to transmit Lorenzo's Tuscan manner to a few students who formed a veritable school. Once trained, Mormando took on a great number of apprentices in his work-shop: Gaspare de Sessa, Fra Tommaso de Angelis, Maestro Baccino (Da Prato's future heir), Giovanni Matteo di Niccolò, and Jacopo, son of mae-stro Da Prato. For this reason, Mormando can be considered the father of the Neapolitan School. Comparing his activity with that of his master we can see how a local school formed from a few instruments manufactured in a region that was underdeveloped in this domain. Furthermore, if it is rare to be able to measure a master's influence on his pupil this clearly, Pavoni's introduction in 1474 of flute stops is directly linked to Lorenzo's teaching. He had elaborated this innovation a few years earlier for San Petronio in Bologna. If certain modern traits were spread by the requests of the patrons, we can note in this case that the network of organ builders was a means of diffusion at least as important as that of the patrons.

The contagion of the Tuscan conception of the organ "alla moderna" in southern Italy can be measured along two criteria: the fixture of the organ to the wall and the presence of flute stops in the composition of the acous-tic apparatus. The first southern organ adjoined to the wall and hoisted onto the tribune is documented in 1483 in the Carmine of Naples, forty-five years after the prototype elaborated by Brunelleschi in the cathedral of Florence. This architectural innovation marks a watershed of the first order in the history of both the organ and liturgical space. In the 1470s the flute stops were the first set of pipes developed in Italy that sought to imitate and an existing instrument because of a widespread taste for the recorder. Attempts at imitation spread to practically all instruments in the Baroque period, but because of its popularity, and doubtless too its technical limita-tions, the flute was likely the first stop integrated into Italian organs, either at building or after the fact.[2] To obtain a "fluted" sound, pipes must have large diameter but a small mouth. This did not seem to pose any particular technical challenges to the builders once the diffusion of this innovation was well underway.

In fact, compared to the reed pipe stops, the flute stops were not far removed from a *ripieno* pipe, that is, the type of sound body dominant in Renaissance Italian organ building. The first Italian organ to be given a flute stop was built by Da Prato in 1471–1475 for San Petronio in Bologna.

After Bologna and Lucca, between 1490 and 1496, flute stops came to Milan, Florence, Padua, Pisa, Bergamo, Gemona, and Sacile. With a first specimen in 1474, Campania was paradoxically ahead of Tuscany thanks to Lorenzo da Prato and his student Stefano, cited above. By 1474, the latter had added a flute stop to his master's 1471 organ for the Castel Nuovo of Naples. These technical criteria are objective evidence of the contribution and strength of the exchanges between the courts of Naples and Florence.

The second phase of Da Prato's production in Campania allows us to study the interpenetration of diplomatic relations by way of the organ. One year after the Pazzi conspiracy (1478) and the war between Florence and the papal troops, the Medici leader declared a truce. Alfonso directed Medici to Naples, where he spent nearly three months at court (December 1479–March 1480). The renewed peace led to Da Prato's return to Naples in 1481 to build organs for the monastery of San Severino, the *duomo* of Amalfi, Santa Maria del Carmine, and San Eligio of Capua.

A short time later, in 1483, Ferdinand named Lorenzo the Magnificent *camerario del Regno*. In this way, the transfer operated by an organ builder was tasked with expressing or reinforcing the friendship between the princes. Joampiero Leostello's chronicle on the life of the Duke of Calabria confirms the friendship that his lord felt for Medici who in return accorded him all honor during his visit to Florence in 1484. The chronicler mentions all the masses the duke attended, at Santa Maria Novella and elsewhere in the city. On October 4, he heard the Saint Petronius Mass sung in Bologna in the *ecclesia major* (in fact, more likely the basilica of San Petronio, whose organ is the work of Da Prato). Potential patrons listened to (as well as looked at) prototypes, and thus models were circulated. The Duke of Calabria, for instance, compared the organs of his kingdom to those of Bologna in Florence at every ceremony. Works as well as men gave rise to an emulation between the princes, who competed in the generosity of their artistic and musical patronage.

In this way, Da Prato made a solid reputation for himself in Tuscany and played his part in making it a center of the production of organs in Italy. From his technical innovations such as fixture to the wall, the elevation to the tribune, and the addition of the flute stops, the Tuscan organ builder gained a prestige that covered the whole of Italy. The importance of the instrument in the construction of political power led the princes of the Medici and Aragon houses to lay hold of it, personally, to the point that they made the organ a point of connection in their diplomatic relations. A man we might perceive a simple "artisan" in fact crafted the cultural and diplomatic rapprochements of Naples and Florence. This was due to his skill in organ building, recognized as exceptional. Further to that, teaching exponentially spread the influence that the Tuscan master had acquired from his production of instruments in Campania. The organs, builders, and organists must hereafter be perceived as agents of a contamination stimulated by the patron princes, who invested so much more than gold in this project. In sum, technical innovation is at once a criterion allowing us to measure the contagion of an instrumental concept and the dynamics of exchanges within a given framework in space and time.

translated by Vicki-Marie Petrick

NOTES

1. Pier Paolo Donati, "Corpus dei documenti sulla manifattura degli organi in Italia dal XIV al XVII secolo. Vol. II: Documenti dal 1451 al 1480," *Informazione organistica, Nuova serie* 34 (2013): doc. 297.

2. Pier Paolo Donati, "L'arte degli organi nell'Italia del Quattrocento. Vol. II: La comparsa dei registri, Informazione organistica," *Nuova serie* 14 (2006): 125.

SELECTED BIBLIOGRAPHY

Bentley, Jerry H. *Politics and Culture in Renaissance Naples*. Princeton: Princeton University Press, 1987.

Fantappiè, Renzo. *Organari, organisti e organi a Prato. XIV–XX secolo*. Prato: Società pratese di Storia patria, 2012.

Filangieri, Gaetano, ed. *Documenti per la storia le arti e le industrie delle provincie napoletane*. 6 Vols. Naples: Tipografia dell'Accademia reale delle scienze, 1883–1891.

Pontieri, Ernesto. "La dinastia aragonese di Napoli e la casa de' Medici di Firenze (dal carteggio familiare)." *Archivio storico per le provincie napoletane* 65 (1940): 279–280.

JUDEITY
Identity and Otherness: Jews in France circa 1900

Catherine Fhima

The Jews of France in 1900 were the product of the emancipation process that had begun in 1791. Their search for social standing as legitimated by civil equality and the creation of a French identity led them to enter into a new relationship of otherness with the Christian majority. This initiated a process of acculturation to the national community as it was being formed. Unprecedented kinds of interactions resulted, as can be seen in uses of the French language that became common. Thus, throughout the nineteenth century, the modes of expression of the Jews were contaminated in a new way, consciously or unconsciously, by the dominant Christian culture. These modes of expression were contaminated as well by the centuries-old representations of Jews that the larger Christian society reflected back to the Jews themselves. In return, these interactions modified their relationship with society as well as with their image and presentation of self.

Basing our argument on a corpus of private and public writings produced by Jewish writers between 1890 and 1930—personal correspondence and literary texts—we will examine the phenomena of contamination via language, meaning the voice of the other that one appropriates as one's own.[1] We can distinguish three discursive registers where this contamination takes effect: a lexical register borrowed from the Christian religious vocabulary, a register related to anti-Semitic discourse, and a register inspired by thought of "race."

The religious register shows the pervasiveness of Catholic culture, but in this case the borrowed vocabulary does not refer to Jews as people. The contamination here is expressed in the naming of time according to the calendar and in the organization of daily time. Thus, in family letters, certain writers sometimes joined their heading dates with names drawn from Catholicism, for example, Palm Sunday, All Souls' Day, and Easter Monday. These calendar references intersect with terminology used in essays: "Old Testament" and "sainthood" were commonly employed when the authors were (nevertheless) writing about Judaism.[2]

With this qualifying vocabulary, there are also expressions admiring Catholic religious images. We have letters in which, whoever the correspondent may be, the writers confidentially articulate their fascination with Christian spirituality. Edmong Fleg admitted to kneeling before "Cimabue's great Christ" in Florence. Jean-Richard Bloch evoked his ideal of a monkish life in thinking of Albrecht Dürer's Saint Jerome.[3] In contrast, Max Jacob's discourse held no admiring element when he converted. He declared to his cousin, Bloch, "I'm not renouncing anything. I had no religion. I'm choosing one."[4] From the vocabulary used in ordinary life to the expression of an aesthetic admiration, these cases show the need the writers felt to demonstrate that they had mastered the cultural codes, codes that were moreover supposedly shared ones. Writers wished to show this mastery both to the majority "other," the non-Jewish, and to the minority "other," the Jews themselves. The contamination reveals the depth of the desire to incorporate the majority culture in which Catholicism embodies the religion par excellence.

In the case of the anti-Semitic register, circulating polysemous phrases centered Jews. Take the designation of "the Jew." Its definite article "the" singularizes at the same time that it creates a stereotype of an overarching unitary category. It often introduces a stigmatizing description. Many Jewish writers used this kind of stereotyping.[5] But the meaning of the contamination varied according to whether these writers adhered to the conceptions of the world typical of the social and political environments in which anti-Semitic discourse was expressed, be it in socialist or far-right contexts. When they were socialists, Jewish writers excoriate "Jewish finance," for example, or "the Rothschild bank." The reason for this was that the very use of these syntagmas seemed to mean less an attack against Jews than against capitalism. Because it was important for these writers to show their "group alignment"[6] to the majority other, in this case socialist, this kind of contamination at its base functioned in such a way as to erase Jewish difference in the name of a universalism of social justice. It forbade, for example, questioning the stigmatizing association of Jews with money. And yet, paradoxically, they rejected these same stereotypes, clearly felt as anti-Semitic, when used by the followers of Edouard Drumont or the Action Française, and the nationalist right.

The contamination of the anti-Semitic lexicon can be seen yet again in the realm of novels with the physical and moral description of Jews. An analogous descriptive rhetoric can be noticed among very different authors. Bloch evoked "red eye brows" and an "oily nose";[7] Fleg observed "kinky-haired children";[8] and Irène Némirovsky described a "greasy, redheaded, pink Jew" with "his murderer's hands."[9] When a few Jewish critics, hesitating to detect any anti-Semitism, nevertheless pointed out the harshness of these stereotypes, the writers responded that, faithful to the French literary tradition, they were describing an objective truth. The intersecting perspectives of these different "othernesses" obviously influences the writings. Yet this literary realism bore most particularly upon characters of foreign Jews, most often Russian. The stereotyped descriptions of these fictional immigrants were perceived as what one might call "the interior other." Jewish writers attempted to use them to distinguish between these "foreigners" and themselves, that is, between the "excluded" or the "outsiders" and the "established."[10] The contamination is apparent then, according to a chain of interlocking representations of a similar nature.

In the third register of discourse, that of the thought on race, Jewish writers in turn inverted meaning. The race was "good"; one had "the courage of one's race." Stigma became a source of pride and was joined by a thematic of blood. André Spire described the talent of Marcel Proust as that of a "half-Jew,"[11] according to a concept reflecting modes of classification that were becoming common usage by the 1920s. In drawing on Proust's portion of "Jewish blood," Spire shows to what degree scientific and parascientific discourses concerning biological heredity were internalized. Proust himself had recourse to the notion of "race" to turn the heavy stigma of Judeity on its head. This is also what he did with homosexuality and with Judeity, associating both identities with a "cursed race."[12] Here, the operation of contamination produced a dissonant discourse. It turned the negative value of "race" into a positive. Taking hold of the vocabulary of scientific doxa on race, Jewish writers acted on two interdependent planes. First they showed that they were imbued with the framework of thought of their time. Second, they created a language validating their difference of identity through a reversal of meaning that lessened the effects of subordination intrinsic to the notion of race.

The notion of contamination allows us, then, to account for cognitive operations performed by Jews around 1900, during the entire process of their integration into French society. Writers in particular, by their uses of the language, bear witness to these borrowings and appropriations from the words of the majority, including those who designate themselves as Jews and assign to them a negative status. By the contaminated forms of their expression, Jewish writers aimed to share in common aspects of the whole of French society. They also sought out modes of presentation of their difference. The notion of contamination therefore, through several registers of discourse, offers us the possibility of understanding the order of interactions and thus to evaluate the power differentials between various groups involved. It restores the collective and historical tendency of Jews to absorb the culture in which they are immersed. At the same time, it also throws light on that which, in the Judeity of those concerned, either finds itself altered or undergoes a recomposition as an effect of interactions with the majority other, including during periods of rejection. Finally, as it shifts the usual historiographic ideas about the assimilation of Jews into French society, the notion of contamination makes for one of the most appropriate analytical tools in attempting to grasp how individual and collective identities are created while measuring, in a system of open modernity, the degree of porosity between the groups involved.

translated by Vicki-Marie Petrick

NOTES

1. Mikhail Bakhtin, *Problems of Dostoevsky's Poetics*, ed. and trans. by Caryl Emerson (Minnesota: University of Minnesota Press, 1984), 202.

2. One example is enough: James Darmesteter, *Les prophètes d'Israël* (Paris: Calmann-Lévy, 1892).

3. André É. Elbaz, ed., *Correspondance d'Edmond Fleg pendant l'affaire Dreyfus* (Paris: A.-G. Nizet, 1976); Edmond Fleg to Lucien Moreau, May 12, 1897, 56; Bibliothèque nationale de France (Paris), Manuscripts Department, NAF 28222; Jean-Richard Bloch Collection, Bloch to Marcel Cohen (copy), August 15, 1919, *Cahier no. 9*, 71–72.

4. Catherine Fhima, "Max Jacob ou la symbiose des identités paradoxales," *Archives juives, Revue d'histoire des Juifs en France* 35 (2002): 77–101.

5. We will only cite Bernard Lazare, *L'antisémitisme, son histoire et ses causes* (Paris: Léon Chailley, 1894).

6. Erving Goffman, *Stigma: Notes on the Management of Spoiled Identity* (Englewood Cliffs-New Jersey: Prentice Hall, 1963), chapter 3, "Group Alignment and Ego Identity."

7. Jean-Richard Bloch, *Lévy, premier livre de contes* (Paris: NRF, 1912), 23.

8. Edmond Fleg, *L'enfant prophète* (Paris: NRF, 1926), 151.

9. Irène Némirovsky, *David Golder* (Paris: Grasset, 1929), 43.

10. Norbert Elias and John L. Scotson, *The Established and the Outsiders: A Sociological Enquiry into Community Problems*, 2nd ed. (London: Sage Publications, 1994). First edition 1965.

11. André Spire, *Quelques Juifs et demi-Juifs*, 2 vols. (Paris: Grasset, 1928).

12. Marcel Proust, *Contre Sainte-Beuve* (Paris: Gallimard, 1987), 250.

SELECTED BIBLIOGRAPHY

Elias, Norbert, and John L. Scotson. *The Established and the Outsiders: A Sociological Enquiry into Community Problems*. 2nd ed. London: Sage Publications, 1994.

Goffman, Erving. *Stigma: Notes on the Management of Spoiled Identity*. Englewood Cliffs, NJ: Prentice Hall, 1963.

Yuval, Israel Jacob. *Two Nations in Your Womb: Perceptions of Jews and Christians in Late Antiquity and the Middle Ages*. Translated by Barbara Harshav and Jonathan Chipman from Hebrew. Berkeley: University of California Press, 2006.

LANGUAGES

Hybrid Languages or "Impure" Languages? From Hisperic Latin to Arabo-Latin (Sixth to Fifteenth Century)

Benoît Grévin

Language historians know that no language has been preserved from "contaminations." They know that contagions are an integral part of linguistic ecology. Without even mentioning the cases of creolization or grammatical hybridization, the integration of a lexicon that comes from other languages, close or far from the host language, has always been part of the life of language. From the rise of linguistic nationalisms onward (nineteenth century), the idea of language purity has taken a specific dimension (the Magyarization campaign of Hungarian vocabulary, the Slavization campaign of the Czech language), but the question of the link between the parts of society that were supposedly in charge of language and the words that were felt as foreign, even "contaminating," may also be considered in the long duration of traditional cultures.

With regard to that, medieval Latin is an especially relevant instance given that its lexical "contamination" has had very diverse aspects. Moreover, there has always existed a structural tension between lettered people who endeavored to practice a language that was close to classical norms and technicians who developed "alter-Latins" that were more open to innovation according to specific needs. Latin vocabulary could be enriched (positive vision) or altered (negative vision) according to at least three guiding principles:

the integration of words coming from countless vernacular languages spoken by Latin Christian people;

the integration of words coming from Greek and Hebrew, the two other sacred Christian languages of reference as the bearers of the biblical text; and

the integration, both for prestige and scientific convenience reasons, of a specialized vocabulary coming from classical Arabic (and technical Arabic languages depending on classical Arabic), a cultural language partly unconnected to Latin Christianism but having a very eminent status compared to other vernacular languages.

Considering the contamination phenomena of medieval Latin according to that triple perspective may enable one to decenter an analysis often limited to the study of the contaminations of Latin by "modern" European languages and of classicizing Latin reactions like humanism, the most famous one. Studying the contamination phenomena of medieval Latin by Greek and Hebrew and considering the punctual contamination of Latin by Arabic can show that "linguistic contagions" debated by contemporaries responded to specific sociolinguistic reasons and that the debates about language "contamination" used to be richer than what the cliché of the struggle between "medievals" and "humanists" may suggest. Medieval and Renaissance arguments standing in favor or against the Greekization, Hebrewization, and Arabicization of Latin did exist, but they have not been compared yet.

In sociolinguistics, some hostile reactions allow us to prove the existence of tensions that are not always mentioned in ordinary documentation. A famous testimony regarding the reluctance toward medieval Latin contamination belongs to that type of source. It is a passage from an important treaty written in 870 by Archbishop Hincmar of Reims (d. 878), an important politician and thinker in Charles II the Bald's reign. In that treaty, Hincmar of Reims reproaches his nephew Hincmar of Laon for liking the use of Greek and barbaric terms in Latin.[1] There are enough "Latin words you could have used in the lines where you used Greek words, inserted by force, and even Irish words, as well as other barbarisms *ubi graeca et obstrusa et interdum scottica et alia barbara . . . posuisti.*"

The decoding of that passage (from which only an excerpt is quoted here) refers to the last step of a long linguistic story: the invention by Irish clerks (the "Scots") from the sixth to the ninth century of plays on words and neologisms—full of Greek-originated lexical constructions—based on Greek, Hebrew, and even Irish roots, whose most spectacular examples are the mysterious poetical games called *Hisperica famina* (Ireland, seventh century?). Hincmar of Laon's Latin was certainly not up to the inventiveness of those riddles, and his uncle's attacks may have been about the use of a form of Hellenized Latin according to the great contemporary philosopher John Scotus Eriugena, one of the last representatives of Irish intellectual traditions on the continent.

That controversial passage nevertheless allows us to guess the logic of a confrontation between, on the one hand, a linguistic opening strategy that accepted, as part of the language, a series of foreign terms not belonging to classical Latin and, on the other hand, a a show of ostentation of a simpler style preserving a "maternal" form of Latin. "*Lingua . . . in qua natus es*," said Hincmar of Reims: Latin still seems to be indivisible from the emerging Romance language, even if the existence of the latter was more and more perceived during this century, which saw the redaction of the partly Romance Oaths of Strasbourg in 843. Hincmar associates "violently contaminated" Latin *verba obstrusa* (words inserted by force) with an exogenous world, the world of Irish clerks whose influence was targeted for two centuries on the continent (see the proverb *ut Escotus mentit* [*sic*] in the correspondence between Frodebertus and Importunus around 665). Read literally, Hincmar of Reims seems to criticize maximal contamination, referring back to Greek, Barbaric, and Irish terms, like in *Hisperica famina*. Read figuratively, he undoubtedly refers to lettered games that were closer to his time as the clergy's linguistic *habitus*. The *verba scottica* might have been, rather than Celtic words, "Hellenisms in the Irish style."

In practice, Carolingian clerks had to use Latinized Greek terms in their theological discussions. The polemic about contagion primarily reveals several loopholes among the court and the Carolingian clergy concerning the resistance to influences that were felt as foreign and the more or less pronounced engagement in a certain type of conceptual game, all that translated into stylistic choices. The linguistic tensions linked to the restauration of imperial Latin, to its remoteness from Proto-Roman dialects and to confrontations within the high clergy who were the depositaries of normative uses, appeared unexpectedly on the occasion of a rather political quarrel.

A quite unknown testimony from the very end of the fifteenth century showed that linguistic contamination, on the contrary, might have been subjected to apologetic discourse for reasons far more complex than mere stylistic sensitivity. In a letter sent to Count Belisario Acquaviva in 1500,[2] the humanist Antonio de Ferrariis, called Galateo, took the opposing view of his day's doctrine that aimed to expunge a language that was more and more classicizing of exogenous influences, by defending philosophy's and medicine's interests to keep Arabic words in the Latin language. In his surprisingly relativist argumentation, he underlined the fact that if Arabic words seemed barbaric to Latin ears, the reciprocity was certainly true: "*arabica . . . vere barbara et latinis auribus, ut et nostra illis gentibus, horrenda vocabula.*" He also emphasized that because vocabulary continuously renews, it was pointless to restrict ourselves to antiquity.

That "defense and illustration" of Arabic contamination in Latin had socioprofessional reasons. Antonio de Ferrariis was a doctor and had humanist knowledge highly (but not only) conditioned by Greco-Latin tropism. Since the twelfth to thirteenth centuries, Arabisms were particularly represented in Latin in the medical field, as Avicenna's translations and other classics had integrated a number of Arabic or Arabo-Persian terms without translating them. Moreover, the most successful attempts to appropriate the Arabic language were made by doctors and were documented in Italy in the fifteenth century with Andrea Alpago's and Girolamo Ramusio's works.

Nevertheless, as it was the case with "Irish Latin," the 1500s discussion about Arabisms in Latin depended on a quarrel that lasted more than a century. In 1370, in a letter to the doctor and astronomer Giovanni Dondi dall'Orologio, Petrarch violently took to task the admirers of Arabic sciences and triggered a polemic that combined stylistic considerations (Latin culture had to, according to him, get rid of "debilitating and feminine influences") and social promotion strategies (it was in humanists' interests to combat doctors and jurists' technical jargon to better reinforce their ascendance over Renaissance courts). Antonio's defense of the contamination of Latin by Arabic shows that 130 years after Petrarch, and despite the triumph of Greco-Latin humanism, the hard line did not manage to achieve their ends. The "contagion by Arabic" had new supporters and new arguments because it met socioprofessional needs and satisfied cultural appetites that counterbalanced the purist temptation.

Open-mindedness, narrow-mindedness: in those medieval and Renaissance cultures, the reactions of lettered people in charge of normed languages facing "linguistic contagions" show to what extent it would be prejudicial to analyze this dialectic, inextricably linked to the lives of languages, solely from a linguistic or literary perspective. In traditional societies, dealing with linguistic contaminations has taken various aspects (literary, normative, emotional). It has always been linked to sociolinguistic stakes that must be studied in a historical perspective as well. Petrarch's and Antonio's choices, and long before, Hincmar of Laon's and Hincmar of Reims's, choices were as linked to political and/or socioprofessional assertiveness as to stylistic consideration. It is our role to identify the logic of those confrontations to write the history of a language in perpetual debate.

translated by Anne Claire Levy

NOTES

1. See Hincmarus Remensis, "Opusculum et epistola in causa Hincmari Laudunensis," in *Patrologie Latine*, vol. 126 (Paris: Garnier, 1879), 448.

2. See "Antonii Galatei viri doctissimi epistolae selectae ex codice vaticano, ep. XVI," in *Spicilegium romanum*, vol. 8 (Rome: Typis Collegii Urbani, 1842), 579.

SELECTED BIBLIOGRAPHY

Berschin, Walter. *Griechisch-lateinisches Mittelalter: Von Hieronymus zu Nikolaus von Kues*. Berne: A. Francke, 1980. Italian edition, *Medioevo greco-latino da Gerolamo a Niccolò Cusano*. Edited by Enrico Livrea. Naples: Liguori, 1989.

Goullet, Monique. "Les gallicismes du latin." In *Gallicismes et théorie de l'emprunt linguistique*, edited by André Thibault, 17–44. Paris: L'Harmattan, 2010.

Grévin, Benoît. "De Damas à Urbino: Les savoirs linguistiques arabes dans l'Italie renaissante (1370–1520)." *Annales HSS* 70, no. 3 (2015): 607–635. https://doi.org/10.1535/ahs.2015.0140.

Grévin, Benoît. "Anamorphoses linguistiques: Le pentacle des langues référentielles dans l'Occident latin." In *Hiéroglossie I: Moyen Âge latin, Monde arabo-persan, Tibet, Inde*, edited by Jean-Noël Robert, 43–78. Paris: Collège de France, 2019.

LITERATURE
The Misdeeds of Reading upon Sensitive Imaginations

Judith Lyon-Caen

We could not here give the measure of all the religious, moral, or medical discourse that associates the reading of "bad books" with a poison dangerous to both the individual and social body. In the Catholic world, the Congregation of the Index, instituted during the run-up to the Council of Trent, produced until 1917 the catalog of prohibited books (*Index librorum prohibitorum*), before being merged with the Congregation of the Holy Office. For Catholics, the legal duty to comply with the decisions of the Index did not disappear until after the Second Vatican Council, in 1966. The metaphor of poison was accordingly quite commonplace in condemnations of bad books. As one example among many others, in 1736, Father Porée, regent of the school Louis-le-Grand, called for a ban on novels, writing that "the law forbids the sale of foodstuffs likely to introduce into the body the harmful germs of diseases (*noxia morborum semina*). Let it likewise forbid the sale of works that, by means of a food even more harmful, allow the heart to be infiltrated with the fatal poisons of love (*lethifera amorum venena*)."[1]

The moral noxiousness of reading—of the theater as well—more broadly reflects the obsessive fear of an overstimulated imagination, which pervades Western sexual morality. Of interest here is the translation of this fear into physiological terms, through a new medicalized understanding of reading: for example, Alexandre Wenger has studied how, in the second half of the eighteenth century, Western medical discourse attempted to establish and detail the psychosomatic effects of reading on various categories of readers (women especially but also men of letters). The idea was to describe and decry the harmful effects of bad reading while also exploring the effectiveness of medical books on a general readership far broader than that of doctors. The growth of the reading public, the flourishing of literature, and the medicalization of discourse on reading are thus closely linked. The "dangers of reading" concern a medical expertise that was attempting to understand the mechanisms of the imagination and to describe the pathologies of reading, all while being itself a successful literary motif, which can be found in libertine literature, in novels, and in the medical treatises themselves.

So if reading is indeed a pathogen, then for whom and in what way? The numerous discussions of bad reading, in the nineteenth century, focused on those readers deemed most vulnerable, owing to their physiological disposition or to their supposed moral weakness: women, the young, the masses. But this discourse also explored the genre and content of literary works and their manner of circulation. Beginning in the 1820s, the medical literature on female hysteria recommended moderation in the reading of novels, as it did with everything that could trigger nervous over-excitement, such as walks in town or visits to museums. The advent of the serial novel, at the end of the 1830s, renewed anxieties: the Catholic world in particular was very quick to be alarmed over the increased circulation of fictional content by the press. At the end of the 1840s, Alfred Nettement, the French Legitimist and Catholic literary critic, lamented that the "poison" of bad novels was circulating unconstrained and even affecting the very nature of the political press, as though the presence of novelistic fiction below the fold was weakening or contaminating the whole of journalistic discourse.

It was in this period that courts began to see cases of crimes attributed to the bad influence of literature. In France, the justice system involved itself, for example, in two cases of failed double suicide, the Bancal affair (1835) and the Ferrand affair (1837). Both concerned unhappy lovers: in each, a man killed a woman before unsuccessfully trying to kill himself, and in each, questions were raised before the court about the bad books that may have made the lovers want to disappear together. In 1840, Marie

Lafarge, née Cappelle, was accused of having poisoned her husband with arsenic. During the much covered and widely followed trial, the press blamed the malicious reading purportedly done by the accused, herself the author of the successful *Mémoires*. This poisoner was said to have herself been poisoned, corrupted by reading, in particular by the *Mémoires du Diable*, the long and often cynical novel of manners published serially by Frédéric Soulié in 1839.

In the second half of the nineteenth century, the vocabulary changed, moving from the register of corruption or poisoning to that of *contagion* or *suggestion*. In 1875, the alienist Paul Moreau de Tours presented in Paris a thesis entitled *La contagion du suicide: à propos de l'épidémie actuelle*. It argues that the publicity given by the press to many types of crime, including suicide, has deleterious consequences. While the "cause" of suicide lies in the particular character traits and history of the individual, the press plays the role of "propagation," of sparking and spreading the fire. "Pathological suicide thus finds its antidote: silence," he concludes.[2] In 1887, the doctor Paul Aubry published *La contagion du meurtre: Étude d'anthropologie criminelle* (*The Contagion of Murder: A Study of Criminal Anthropology*), in which he visits in detail the Bancal affair of 1835. The phenomenon of criminal suggestion was, at the time, a major subject of psychological thought, especially around the "École de Nancy," and occupied a central place in the constitution of this new discipline, which drew from law, psychology, anthropology, and medicine and became known as "criminology." By moving from contagion to suggestion, accounts of literature's effects seem to become less physiological and more psychological. But the terms remain uncertain.

On a Sunday in June 1881, in Tours, a young notary clerk named Lucien Morisset fired a revolver into a crowd, killing one person. The explanation for his action was to be found, according to the medical expert, Legrand du Saulle, in the "literary alcoholization" to which Morisset was devoted—a novel concept—recalling the heyday of literary poison. An avid reader of romantic literature and a great admirer of the famous murderer Pierre-François Lacenaire, the "alcoholized" Morisset was thus alleged to be another victim of the book. The court notably did not hear anything from

Morisset about his actual reading. In 1908, the Italian criminologist Scipio Sighele took another look at the cases discussed here, in a book entitled *Littérature et criminalité*.[3] There he considered the "frightening suggestion of literature" and used the term "literary crimes" to describe these homicides in which the influence of literature supposedly played a preponderant role.

Books and popular press, theater, photo comics, and then radio, cinema, television, series, and videogames: the fear of the harmful effects that the content, texts, and, above all, images of mass culture may have on readers' or viewers' sensitive imaginations fed into themes other than contagion. Between the moral concern and the scientific problem of locating, describing, and understanding the effects of narratives and images on readers or viewers, a vast, sometimes overlapping, range of discourse has been deployed. In 1982, the American sociologist David Philipps coined the term "Werther effect" to describe the correlation that he observed between media coverage of suicide cases and the increase in the number of suicides. He was also interested in the impact of fictional suicides (in television series) on real-life suicides.

Sighele likewise talked of "wertherites" in 1908, though without having recourse to statistical processing. In 1856, the doctor Alexandre Brierre de Boismont published a very lengthy study of *Suicide et la folie suicide, considérés dans leurs rapports avec la statistique, la médecine et la philosophie*, in which he pointed to the melancholic figure of young Werther alongside other characters from literary fiction, as well as some romantic authors, as a "microcosm of his time." Here literature was not being presented as a cause or an agent but rather as a symptom of the moral tendencies of the age. Literary studies, for their part, continued to brood upon the functions and effects of the fictional "character," occasionally attempting, in our time, to support their thinking with research from the cognitive sciences.

Insisting on the creative part of reading and on the diversity of appropriations to which all cultural productions are susceptible—within systems of social, cultural, mental, and material constraints that every reading brings into play, or perhaps reconfigures—the history of reading practices conducts its investigations independently of any uniform theory of contagion or imitation. On the other hand, this history invites us to consider representations of reading, including the image of the reader corruptly influenced to the point of becoming suicidal or a murderer, as cultural productions themselves, situated in their specific time and social space. It is a disturbing image, to which one might oppose a more optimistic figure: that of the emancipated reader, a poacher, the author of her own reading.

translated by Jeffrey Burkholder

NOTES

1. *De libris qui vulgo dicuntur romanes oratio . . .* , translation in *Mémoires de Trévoux* (July 1736): 1454.

2. Paul M. de Tours, *La contagion du suicide: À propos de l'épidémie actuelle* (Paris: A. Parent, 1875), 77.

3. Scipio Sighele, *Littérature et criminalité* (Paris: V. Giard and E. Brière, 1908).

SELECTED BIBLIOGRAPHY

Amadieu, Jean-Baptiste. *La littérature française du XIXe siècle mise à l'Index.* Paris: Éditions du Cerf, 2017.

Bosc, Olivier. *La foule criminelle: Politique et criminologie dans l'Europe du tournant du XIXe siècle.* Paris: Fayard, 2007.

Certeau, Michel de. *L'invention du quotidien*, vol. 1: *Arts de faire.* Paris: Gallimard, 1990.

Chartier, Roger, ed. *Pratiques de la lecture.* Paris-Marseille: Rivages, 1985.

Lyon-Caen, Judith. "Suggestion, alcoolisation littéraire, identification: Le crime romantique de Lucien Morisset (1881)." Fabula/Les colloques. March 1, 2018. http://www.fabula.org/colloques /document5088.php.

Proulx, François. *Victims of the Book: Reading and Masculinity in Fin-de-Siècle France.* Toronto: University of Toronto Press, 2019.

Wenger, Alexandre. *La fibre littéraire: Le discours médical sur la lecture au XVIIIe siècle.* Geneva: Droz, 2007.

LUXURY

"Holding India in Their Hands": Influx of Wealth into Republican and Imperial Rome

Maria Cecilia D'Ercole

In 146 BCE, on three occasions, majestic processions traveled down the *Via Sacra* in Rome: they celebrated the victory of Caecilius Metellus over Macedonia, Scipio Aemilianus over Carthage, and Lucius Mummius over Corinth. These performances of a power that now extended from one shore of the Mediterranean to the other effectively showcased the extraordinary influx of wealth pouring into the *Urbs* starting in the middle of the second century. Everything was on display: paintings, statues, valuable plates, silver and gold, exotic animals, prisoners, and slaves. In a matter of a few decades, this wealth had radically changed practices and lifestyles in Rome. Further to this, in the first-century BCE, trade opened up with the Far East. Ships now harnessed the strength of monsoons to make the journey to the Indian ports of Barygaza and Barbarikē in the space of a year; they brought back pepper, Indian precious stones and pearls, and silk from China. This massive diffusion of luxury goods, and the greed it generated, was akin to a true social epidemic. So much so, in fact, that even ancient authors perceived it as such. The desire to emulate became an absolute necessity, causing a contagion of practices, or as is sometimes described in the medical lexicon of contagion, a pathological anomaly.

As is often the case with epidemics, ancient historians sought the place and event that had triggered such an irruption: Polybius, Titus Livius, and Plutarch all point to the capture of Syracuse in 212 BCE, Salluste the defeat of Carthage in 146 BCE.[1] But the majority theory, perhaps already sketched out by Cato the Elder, asserted itself with Titus Livius:[2] the East is the origin (*origo*) of this foreign wealth (*luxuriae peregrinae*). Pliny, in retracing the different stages of the phenomenon, also points to this geographic area as the source of luxury.[3] He complains of the enormous flow of sesterces—no less than fifty million a year, he says—which leaves annually for India and the country of Seres, likely present-day China, emptying estates and causing a shortage of currencies, at the root of several financial crises in Rome.[4] Beyond Pliny's moralizing tone, which undoubtedly magnifies the actual scope of these commercial exchanges, we see here the beginning of a "hemorrhage," which would for centuries contribute to the pouring of precious metals from the Mediterranean into the East.

If the contagion thus originated from the distant countries of the East, a fairly long latency period seems to have preceded the high points of its outbreak. The case of Indian pearls provides a good example. These precious ornaments, *margaritai*, were known to the Greeks since the Indian voyage of Nearchus, admiral of Alexander the Great.[5] But it was not until the end of the first-century BCE, in Rome, that these exotic objects became so cherished that they gave rise to intense trade with the countries of the Far East. Material traces of the latter appear on coins from the first imperial period, such as the *aurei* and *denarii* of Augustus and Tiberius, which portray treasures found in southern India. At the beginning of the second century, such evidence increased. It then diminished, but did not disappear, toward the second half of the century. As with any contagion, these phenomena spread through contact, in this case both material and cultural.

Such practices were transmitted through a partly deliberate, partly uncontrolled process of emulation and imitation. The taste for luxury invaded all areas. The house of Lucullus in Rome and the "House of the Faun" in Pompeii were likely over three thousand square meters, larger than many public squares. In the Roman Republic shaken by violent crises, it was now customary to have a professional chef prepare refined and exotic dishes. To this regard, in a letter dating to 46 BCE, Cicero complains, with a touch of false modesty, of his cook who could not serve him a peacock, unlike that of Hirtius, consul of 43 BCE.[6] Pliny exclaims, "we drink in a heap of precious stones and lace our goblets in emeralds: to become intoxicated, we like to hold India in our hands."[7]

An infatuation with pearls and silks from the Far East caused excesses that largely defied good taste. Thus, the Emperor Elagabalus appears dressed entirely in transparent silk;[8] Caligula's wife, Lollia Paulina, attends a dinner party covered in emeralds and pearls worth some forty million sesterces, as she could prove on the spot with receipts.[9] The fabulous wealth of Crassus, who died in 53 BCE, is estimated to have been worth fifty million denarii, or forty times greater than that of Scipio Africanus, considered the richest Roman at the beginning of the second-century BCE.

Pearls, just like diseases, invited scientific description and classification. An echo of this attitude appears in Roman legal thinking: Sabinus, a jurist of the first-century CE, wondered about the nature of pearls, which belong neither to the category of gems nor to that of stones, as they originate and develop *apud Rubrum mare*, or in the present-day Red Sea.[10]

Parallels were drawn between this obsession with luxury and forms of physical or mental pathology. Sallust makes an explicit comparison in observing that "when the disease had spread like a deadly plague, the community was changed."[11] At the beginning of the Flavian period, in the tragedy *Octavia* attributed to the Pseudo-Seneca, *luxuria* is similarly compared to a seductive curse, a *pestis blanda*.[12] In a symmetrical fashion, Roman medical writers such as Celsus were concerned about the effects of extravagance (*luxuria*) and laziness (*desidia*) on health and lifespan: bad habits required recourse to complex medicine (*multiplex*), which the Romans had had little need of before.[13] Seneca pushes this analogy even further in describing the "vertigo that is sometimes of a man, sometimes of a century";[14] he uses the same word to describe women's obsession with pearls.[15] The passion for luxury seizes the body like a disease: indolence penetrates ever deeper into the marrow and muscles, provoking an inertia where the only consolation is the spectacle of others' debauchery.[16]

In other cases, the analogy evokes mental health: *luxuria* is qualified as *demens* in *Controverse* by Seneca the Elder.[17] It triggers uncontrolled forms of individual or collective dependence. For Pliny, luxury is an *insania*, an abnormal deviation of desire.[18] Another technical word is *furor*, a pathological state of the mind that, according to Seneca, even affects the movements of the body.[19] It was indeed a *furor*, according to Pliny, that drove a woman, a *mater familias* without great means, to spend some one hundred and fifty thousand sesterces for a rock crystal.[20] This language is all the more significant in that such curiosity about mental illness is also found in contemporary medical treatises, which distinguish three different types of *insania* and *furor*.

As for any disease, there are remedies and antidotes for *luxuria*. One such remedy appears in the rhetorical praise of poverty, considered a wrongly neglected good (*ignotum bonum*).[21] For Seneca the Younger, abstemious behavior, based on temperance (*frugalitas*), is an effective countermeasure.[22] Another remedy consists of taking appropriate legal measures in the form of sumptuary laws, already promulgated in Rome in mid-fifth-century BCE. The most enlightening remarks on this subject appear in a passage by Tacitus,[23] who describes a law presented to the Senate under the Principate of Tiberius, aiming to limit several forms of lavishness and ostentation: the use of silk garments for men, the number of slaves, the quantity of precious tableware, and many other things. The law was not adopted: Asinius Gallus prevailed with effectively subtle arguments, particularly their sway on an assembly that, writes Tacitus, shared the same weaknesses as the speaker. The *similitudo audientium*, the "audience of congenial spirits," led this austere remedy to be rejected. The contagion could freely continue its course.

Places of exotic origin, uncontrolled diffusion, analysis of symptoms, and search for remedies: all of these aspects allow us to compare the obsession with luxury in republican and imperial Rome to a truly epidemic phenomenon.

translated by Maya Judd

NOTES

1. Polybius, *The Histories*, volume 9, book 10, Loeb Classical Library 159 (Cambridge, MA: Harvard University Press, 2011); Livy, *History of Rome*, volume 25, book 40, trans. Frank Gardner Moore. Loeb Classical Library 355 (Cambridge, MA: Harvard University Press, 1940); Plutarch, *Lives*, volume 5: *Agesilaus and Pompey: Pelopidas and Marcellus*, Loeb Classical Library (Cambridge, MA: Harvard University Press, 1917); Sallust, *The War with*

Catiline, volume 10, Loeb Classical Library (Cambridge, MA: Harvard University Press, 2013).

2. Livy, *History of Rome*, volume 34, books 6–8, Loeb Classical Library 295 (Cambridge, MA: Harvard University Press, 2017).

3. Pliny, *Natural History*, volume 33, Loeb Classical Library (Cambridge, MA: Harvard University Press, 1952), 148–150.

4. Pliny, *Natural History*, volume 6, Loeb Classical Library 392 (Cambridge, MA: Harvard University Press, 1942), 26, 101; *Natural History*, volume 12, Loeb Classical Library (Cambridge, MA: Harvard University Press, 1945), 41, 84.

5. Arrian, *Indica*, volume 8, Loeb Classical Library 269 (Cambridge, MA: Harvard University Press, 1952), 5, 8.

6. Cicero, *Correspondances*, volume 7 (Paris: Belles Lettres, 1980); *Ad Familiares* IX, 16, 18, 20.

7. Pliny, *Natural History*, volume 33, Loeb Classical Library (Cambridge, MA: Harvard University Press, 1952), 5, 6–7.

8. *Historia Augusta*, trans. David Magie, Loeb Classical Library 140 (Cambridge, MA: Harvard University Press, 1924), 17; *Historia Augusta: Elagabalus*, trans. David Magie, Loeb Classical Library 140 (Cambridge, MA: Harvard University Press, 1924).

9. Pliny, *Natural History*, volume 9, Loeb Classical Library 394 (Cambridge, MA: Harvard University Press, 1940), 117.

10. Sabinus, *Digeste*, 2, 17–19, 34.

11. Sallust, *The War with Catiline*, ed. John T. Ramsey and trans. J. C. Rolfe, Loeb Classical Library 116 (Cambridge, MA: Harvard University Press), X, 34–37.

12. Seneca, *Tragedies II: Oedipus. Agamemnon. Thyestes. Hercules Oetaeus. Octavia*, Loeb Classical Library (Cambridge, MA: Harvard University Press, 1961), v. 428.

13. Celsus, *On Medicine, Prooemium*, book 5, trans. W. G. Spencer, Loeb Classical Library 304 (Cambridge, MA: Harvard University Press, 1935).

14. Seneca, *Epistles*, volume 3: *Epistles 93–124*, trans. Richard M. Gummere, Loeb Classical Library (Cambridge, MA: Harvard University Press, 1925), Epistle 114, 9, 306–307.

15. Seneca, *De beneficiis*, volume 7, trans. John W. Basore, Loeb Classical Library 310 (Cambridge, MA: Harvard University Press, 1935), 4, 9.

16. Seneca, *Epistles*, volume 3: *Epistles 93–124*, 5, 19, 114, 25.

17. Seneca, *Controversiae*, volume 2, trans. Michael Winterbottom, Loeb Classical Library 464 (Cambridge, MA: Harvard University Press, 1974), 1, 12.

18. Pliny, *Natural History*, volume 33, Loeb Classical Library (Cambridge, MA: Harvard University Press, 1952), 95.

19. Seneca, *Epistles*, volume 3: *Epistles 93–124*, 114, 115.

20. Pliny, *Natural History*, volume 37, Loeb Classical Library (Cambridge, MA: Harvard University Press, 1962), 29.

21. Seneca, *Controversiae*, volume 2, 1, 13.

22. Seneca, *Epistles*, volume 1: *Epistles 1–65*, trans. Richard M. Gummere, Loeb Classical Library 175 (Cambridge, MA: Harvard University Press, 1917), 5, 17; *Epistles*, volume 2: *Epistles 66–92*, trans. Richard M. Gummere, Loeb Classical Library 76 (Cambridge, MA: Harvard University Press, 1920), 71, 23.

23. Tacitus, *Annals: Book 2*, trans. Clifford H. Moore and John Jackson, Loeb Classical Library 249 (Cambridge, MA: Harvard University Press, 1931), 1, 33, 432–433.

SELECTED BIBLIOGRAPHY

Braudel, Fernand. *La Méditerranée et le monde méditerranéen à l'époque de Philippe II.* 2 vols. Paris: Armand Colin, 1990.

De Romanis, Federico, and André Tchernia, eds. *Crossings: Early Mediterranean Contacts with India.* New Delhi: Manohar, 1997.

Di Giacomo, Giovanna. *Oro, Pietre preziose e perle: Produzione e commercio a Roma.* Rome: Edizioni Quasar, 2016.

Dubois-Pelerin, Eva. *Le luxe privé à Rome et en Italie au Ier siècle après J.-C.* Naples: Collection du Centre Jean-Bérard, 2008.

Fontanella, Elena, ed. *Luxus: Il piacere della vita nella Roma imperiale.* Turin: Museo di Antichità, 2009–2010; Rome: Istituto Poligrafico e Zecca dello Stato, 2009.

Lapatin, Kenneth. *Luxus: The Sumptuous Arts of Greece and Rome.* Los Angeles: John Paul Getty Museum, 2015.

Schneider, Pierre. "Erythraean Pearls in the Roman World. Features and Aspects of Luxury Consumption (Late Second-Century BCE–Second-Century CE)." In *The Indian Ocean Trade in Antiquity: Political, Cultural, and Economic Impacts*, edited by Matthew Adam Cobb, 135–156. London: Routledge, 2018.

MANUSCRIPTS
Exempla and the Freedom of Copyists at the End of the Middle Ages

Marie Anne Polo de Beaulieu

The notion of contagion, as it occurs in the manuscript tradition, is a crucial issue for philologists required to explain their methodology in editing ancient texts. The term that philologists prefer is "contamination," and it has the same negative medicalized connotations as "contagion" when applied to the process whereby texts were copied and transmitted. When a work was recopied from two distinct models, that is, when the copyist had two different manuscript versions of the same work before him and his copy was based on a reconciling of the variants across the two versions, what was produced was a new version of that work with alterations that might be for good or ill. Our present inquiry goes beyond such a narrow notion to examine all forms of textual contagion in the manuscript tradition of collections of sermon *exempla*. These collections were groupings of stories—*exempla*—intended for insertion in sermons. They were generally told in the vernacular when preached to listeners but were conserved in Latin.

The *Scala coeli* (the ladder of heaven) is an example of this sort of compendium.[1] Its title speaks of the spiritual course that begins with confession of sins and leads the believer to salvation. It was put together by John Gobi the Younger in the years 1327 to 1330 at the Dominican friary of Saint-Maximin, where he held the post of *lector* (reader).[2] The collection is easily recognizable through its consistent title and precisely structured contents: a thousand or so *exempla* are divided into 122 chapters ranging alphabetically from *Abstinence* to *Usury*. Moreover, the author puts his name to the work in the prologue, which is unusual. Another identifying feature is an alphabetical subject index. Some forty manuscripts of the *Scala coeli* have survived and are currently known. The manuscripts' fluid tradition gave rise to various sorts of textual contagion. This study of its contaminations is based on fourteen manuscripts, shown in table 1.

Examination of the manuscript tradition of the *Scala coeli* reveals manuscript families that often correspond to regional areas—Germanic and Polish areas in particular—but also Provence or northern France. Geographical proximity thus favors textual contagion.

The structure of the *Scala coeli* is in the main adhered to by the majority of manuscripts, with a few variations in the placing of the table of contents and prologue. There are, however, two notable exceptions. In a manuscript dating from the end of the fifteenth century and conserved in Avignon's Bibliothèque Municipale, mention is made of the two stiles (side rails) of the "Ladder of Heaven." One is the collection of *exempla*; the other is a universal chronicle. The *exempla* comprise 188 folios, while the short universal chronicle comprises only six. The final table of contents lists the titles of *Scala coeli*'s chapters, followed by the titles of the universal chronicle. A second manuscript, kept at Marseille, also includes an allusion to the

Table 1

Manuscript Location	Date	Shelf Mark
Avignon	15th c.	BM 335
Bamberg	15th c.	Staatsbibl. Theol. 113
Brunswick	15th c.	Stadtsbibl. 10
Brussels	15th c.	BR 3651–3653
Dublin	15th c.	Trinity coll. 128
Göttingen	15th c.	Stadtsbibl. Theol. 140
Liège	15th c.	BU 348
Lons-le-Saunier	15th c.	BM 2
Marseille	15th c.	BM 98
Münster	15th c.	Bibl. Sem. B1 146
Paris	15th c.	BNF lat. 16517
Soest	15th c.	Stadtsbibl. 13, II
Strasbourg	15th c.	BNU 32
Troyes	15th c.	BM 1345

first stile of the ladder but does not mention a second. It has to be wondered whether the phenomenon is the trace of an overlooked initial project or the isolated initiative of a single copyist. Whatever the truth of that matter, the work's structure allowed for the addition of words or expressions in Franco-Provençal, fresh *exempla*, and new chapters. Thus two manuscripts (conserved at Troyes and Strasbourg) included a supplementary chapter, *Dies dominica* (the Lord's day), which represented a limited contamination. Similarly, a chapter entitled *Silentium* (Silence) was transmitted in only three manuscripts (those kept at Avignon, Liège, and Bamberg).

The *Scala coeli* is a substantial work but was adjustable to different formats. Most often it appears as a discrete work in a single manuscript and in "complete" form, that is, comprising between 944 and 1063 *exempla*. In its "medium" (893–923 exempla) and "abridged" (490–881 exempla) forms, it is bound with other texts in a given codex. The *Scala coeli*'s cohabitation with other works in a single codex could give rise to contamination when the work was received. The types of works copied or bound together with the *Scala coeli* give an initial idea of the sort of contaminations that could happen. The space accorded to sermons, *exempla* collections, hagiographic literature, and theological treatises suggests that John Gobi's collection served as a didactic instrument oriented to the education of friars and as a preaching aid complementing the other works in the same codex. It was also possible, when a manuscript was copied, for one collection of *exempla* to contaminate another. Thus the Liège manuscript, which lacks a prologue, was contaminated by Arnold of Liège's *Alphabetum narrationum* (Alphabet of tales), in as much as the latter contributed additional chapters entitled *Abbas* and *Abbatissa*. Even so, this particular contamination did not become established; it is not found in other manuscripts.

Contamination could also occur in the form of extraneous stories entering the *Scala coeli*'s essential structure. Such is the case with two long historical accounts devoid of the characteristics of *exempla*. They do not mention their source, are not introduced by a numbered moral or doctrinal lesson, and do not end with a moral. The first of these stories tells of a Polish knight possessed by seven devils. It appears in five manuscripts of the *Scala coeli* belonging to the Germanic geographical area. In the

Brunswick, Göttingen, and Strasbourg manuscripts, the knight's story is separated from the *Scala coeli* and is placed between the explicit and the table of contents. In the Brussels manuscript, it appears just after the final chapter, followed by displaced chapters and a new chapter. In the Münster manuscript, the story of the Polish knight cuts short the *Sortilegia* chapter, whose theme it shares; it is followed by the table of contents.

It is worth noting that none of the manuscripts of the *Scala coeli* copied or conserved in Poland contain this story of the Polish knight, even though its historic context is Polish, namely, the conflict in 1284–1287 between Henryk IV Probus and the bishop of Wroclaw (Breslau), Thomas II, who was supported by the Dominicans. In the Brunswick and Göttingen manuscripts, the story of the Polish knight is followed by a second tale, a eucharistic miracle dated 1231, set in the town of Waterlere (today's Wasserleben, Germany) in the Halberstadt diocese. It is a classic (albeit still unedited) eucharistic miracle, according to which a host stolen at mass begins to bleed when it is discovered. Unlike the previous story, this one is full of proper names that should permit the discovery of other sources. But in this instance, as in the previous one, the contamination remained limited.

Finally, there are cases where contamination occurred but did not spread. These are instances where limits are attributable to the irreducible specificity of individual manuscripts. Each manuscript in such cases is seen to have been shaped by its copyist or copyists following their own interests. Some copyists on occasion modified the titles of the chapters (thus Paris); sometimes, it is simply the alphabetical order of the chapters that is disturbed (thus Brussels, Dublin, and Soest). Other copyists are seen to have intervened in the text itself by abbreviating certain *exempla* (thus Brussels, Lons-le-Saunier, and Strasbourg). In the Bamberg manuscript, the copyist has much glossed the chapter devoted to the word of God, which is brought to enclose with a long excursus of alternating *exempla* and glosses. The *Scala coeli* here then ends abruptly, being immediately followed by a *Formula of Confession*, as an invitation to pass from meditation to confession, which is actually a recurrent theme of *exempla* collections. Yet this manuscript, the fruit of intense contamination, did not establish a tradition. The same was true of another of the Soest manuscript's innovations: one copyist detached the chapter devoted to female sins from the remainder of the text, while two others interpolated nine exemplifying stories. This configuration similarly is not evident elsewhere in the manuscript tradition.

These various phenomena are linked to the formal characteristics of the *exemplum* and *exempla* collections. Their form was prone to contamination in as much as their composition was a pragmatic exercise that responded to the needs of preaching to the people. Each copyist might modify the collection's structure and the content of the exemplifying tales. If another copyist found such modifications suitable, he was free to copy them. Moreover, when a codex was put together, the *exempla* collection's cohabitation with other texts, most often consisting in material for the work of a preacher, influenced the manuscript's reception. In describing the successive transformations of these texts, the negative medicalized term "contamination" is not, in the last analysis, ideal. It would be better to speak of socially anchored negotiations consigned to writing, arranged in a particular way on the page, and preserved as a manuscript text. This is what Stephen Kelly and John J. Thompson encourage us to do in describing the medieval book: "As a site upon which the contemporaneous activities of readers and writers [*or copyists?*] take place; as, in other words, a site upon which a series of genuinely social negotiations are enacted."[3]

These words are particularly relevant to an *exempla* collection, where such negotiations would have been intense and would have engaged strong community identities harnessed to a momentous endeavor, namely, the salvation of humankind.

translated by Graham Robert Edwards

NOTES

1. Jean Gobi, *La Scala Coeli de Jean Gobi*, edited by Marie Anne Polo de Beaulieu (Paris: Centre national de la recherche scientifique, 1991).

2. Jacques Quétif and Jacques Echard, *Scriptores Ordinis Praedicatorum*, vol. 1 (Paris: Christoph Ballard and Nicolas Simart, 1719–1721); here reprint (Paris: Picard, 1910–1914), 633.

3.   Stephen Kelly and John J. Thompson, "Imagined Histories of the Book: Current Paradigms and Future Directions," in *Imagining the Book: Medieval Texts and Cultures of Northern Europe*, vol. 7 (Turnhout: Brepols, 2005), 1–14, here 2; my insertion.

SELECTED BIBLIOGRAPHY

Bourgain, Pascale, and Françoise Vielliard. *Conseils pour l'édition des textes médiévaux*. Vol. 3 of *Textes littéraires*. Paris: CTHS/École Nationale des Chartes, 2002.

Foehr-Janssens, Yasmina, and Olivier Collet, eds. *Le recueil au Moyen Âge: Le Moyen Âge central*. Texte, Codex & Contexte 8. Turnhout: Brepols, 2010.

Guerreau, Alain, and Marie Anne Polo de Beaulieu. "Classement des manuscrits et analyses factorielles: Le cas de la *Scala coeli*." Bibliothèque de l'École des Chartes 154, no. 2 (1996): 359–400.

Grévin, Benoît, and Aude Mairey, eds. *Le Moyen Âge dans le texte: Cinq ans d'histoire textuelle au LAMOP*. Paris: Publications de la Sorbonne, 2016.

Kelly, Stephen, and John J. Thompson. "Imagined Histories of the Book: Current Paradigms and Future Directions." In *Imagining the Book: Medieval Texts and Cultures of Northern Europe*, vol. 7, edited by Stephen Kelly and John J. Thomspon, 1–14. Turnhout: Brepols, 2005.

Polo de Beaulieu, Marie A. "Incursion d'un chevalier polonais dans la tradition manuscrite de la *Scala coeli* de Jean Gobi le Jeune († v. 1350)." In *Fleur de clergie: Mélanges Jean-Yves Tilliette*, edited by Yasmina Foehr-Janssens, Jean-Claude Mühlethaler, and Prunelle Deleville, 981–1002. Geneva: Droz, 2019.

Tilliette, Jean-Yves. "L'*exemplum* rhétorique: Question de définition." In *Les* exempla *médiévaux: Nouvelles perspectives*, edited by Jacques Berlioz and Marie Anne Polo de Beaulieu, 43–65. Paris: Honoré Champion, 1998.

MICROBES

Understandings of Disease Transmission in the Western World (Fifteenth to Twenty-First Century)

Frédéric Vagneron and Patrice Bourdelais

The notion of contagion implies a relationship of direct or indirect contact, mediated by a living vector or object. In either case, it leaves open the nature of what exactly is transmitted and, initially, the means by which propagation occurs. Knowledge of contagion makes visible the links between entities such as humans, animals, objects, or micro-organisms. It is man, depending on the times, who knows or ignores, stimulates, alters, or breaks these links voluntarily or not. Contagion raises a tricky question: how does one contract a disease? Even today, many queries remain as to the modes of contagion of diseases that have either been around for centuries or are emerging.

First appearing in sixteenth-century medical literature, use of the term contagion reached a peak in the nineteenth century, when it structured debates between supporters and defenders of infection and miasma theory——or the so-called anticontagionists. It was not until the end of the century that notions of contagion and infection became almost synonyms with the rise of microbiology. Today, the concept of infectious and communicable disease has taken over. In the Western world, the idea of contagion is linked to contexts of state-building, the development of medical practices and knowledge, the professional interests of physicians, and later to the emergence of biological knowledge in medicine.

In Western medical thought long dominated by Hippocratic-Galenic theory, the notion of contagion has been secondary. The idea of contracting a specific disease is at odds with a holistic view of health fluctuations.

The latter is the result of a complex equilibrium, of multiple more or less distant causes, depending on humors, environmental, telluric, and even divine influences. Poor state of health is treated by restoring favorable conditions, for each individual, via a medical approach concerned with singular constitution, personal history, and the specific air quality of the place.

The figure of Girolamo Fracastoro, a sixteenth-century Italian physician, is often associated with an early conceptualization of contagion through "fomites" carrying the "seeds" of contagion, at the height of the European syphilis epidemic. If a misreading made his work the precursor of germ theory, while he remained faithful to the Galenic tradition, syphilis did indeed provide a favorable context to observe the transmission of a disease with particularly visible and long-lasting symptoms. Syphilitic propagation in Europe during the Renaissance could be associated with the movement of foreign troops, the frequenting of prostitutes, and a corrupt physical and moral atmosphere.

Smallpox, in the eighteenth century, also exemplified contagion by reproducing characteristic symptoms in the bodies it infected, covered with pustules. Initially fought through isolation, smallpox gave rise to preventive practices, first popular and then medical, which helped support the idea of direct contagion. First came variolation and then inoculation after Edward Jenner's discovery, which established the role of direct contact with a transmissible poison. Nevertheless, the nosological picture of the early nineteenth century remained dominated by the refinement of fever categories, linked to the constitution and topography of places according to neo-Hippocratic theory. Syphilis and smallpox were just two exceptions.

In the nineteenth century, discussions focused on knowledge and public action against contagious, epidemic, and endemic diseases. In its repeated passage through Europe, cholera caused a constant readjustment of medical theories. Such theories were ultimately put to rest by both the triumphant discovery of the role that water contaminated by fecal matter played in the disease's transmission (John Snow in 1848 in London) and later of Koch's bacillus. The succession of epidemics, and the fears and coercive measures they provoked (quarantines and *cordon sanitaires*), fueled controversy between proponents of contagion and anticontagionists. The first insisted on the chains of contagion between patients from the epidemic outbreaks in the East. The latter observed that the simultaneity of the cases and the number of individuals who escaped contagion could only mean other local, atmospheric, or social factors. These theoretical debates were based on new knowledge emerging from clinical medicine: the anti-contagionists saw "internal inflammation" as the root of the disease, each patient becoming host to a radiating infectious ailment. The "seeds" of the disease, familiar since antiquity, had become visible in the eyes of observers, who called them viruses, animalcules, germs, miasmas, or microzyme. Nevertheless, these theoretical positions often hinged on one another and were contingent on the observation that contagion could be preceded by infection and vice versa.

The work of Robert Koch in Germany and that of Louis Pasteur in France inherited these theories of germs and infection. The new microbiological discipline showed that the seeds of contagion were living things, which could be isolated and cultivated in the controlled conditions of the laboratory and produce similar diseases in the body. By experimentally disqualifying the theory of spontaneous generation, Pasteur transformed the role of air from a driving force to a vector of contagion, transporting microbes like water for Vibrio cholera. With medical microbiology, the specific disease "that one catches" became an independent and reproducible entity. Disease was understood to be the result of the infection of bodies by distinct microbes, invisible to the naked eye and sometimes even under the microscope, which could multiply in susceptible hosts before colonizing other organisms and producing the same symptoms.

Epidemiological investigation, which had long been a meticulous collection of the factors singularizing each local medical constitution, became an adjunct to laboratory science at the end of the nineteenth century. Observation of the circulation of bacteria shed light on multiple forms of contact: directly through expectoration and indirectly from objects soiled with microbes or by insect vector. Thus "modern" rail transport was identified as a transmitter of influenza via travelers, water supply networks disseminators of typhoid, and pilgrimages to Mecca vehicles of possible cholera attacks in Europe. The detection, surveillance, and isolation of patients bearing germs became top public health policy priorities. Two decades before the First World War, the "battle" against the microbial enemy, both metaphorically and practically, gained new momentum; meanwhile the Spanish flu (1918–1919) and its tens of millions of deaths were left out of discourse of unprecedented victory against (other) epidemics in military campaigns.

While the effectiveness of preventive measures is indisputable, they are difficult to evaluate. The effectiveness of antibacterial therapies only became apparent when new drugs were produced in the late 1930s. The association led to the drastic reduction of infectious diseases after the war and established the market for modern medicine. Public declarations were made about the future disappearance of infectious pestilence. The eradication of smallpox, a symbolic historical disease, embodied the success of a global intervention led by the World Health Organization in 1978. Yet, shortly thereafter, the appearance of HIV-AIDS marked a break in public opinion. It reflected in the return of fear, discriminatory discourse, and measures against certain social groups and populations. The pandemic brought an end to dreams of complete control over contagion through scientific progress.

The power to treat infectious diseases faced new challenges in the last third of the twentieth century. Biomedical knowledge shifted understanding to the level of molecular exchanges between human, animal, and plant species to the environment. The chain of contagion became infinitely complex: viruses constantly mutate, contact with wild animal species spreads unknown diseases, and genes and bacteria acquire resistance to therapeutic agents massively produced by an industrial complex supported by public funding and consumed as intensively in medicine as in agriculture. Thus, the use of antibiotics became a "historical environmental event,"[1] giving rise, at the biological level, to a new articulation between infection and heredity—a direct consequence of the massive therapeutic fight against infectious diseases.

In this contemporary configuration, the international mobilization against "emerging and reemerging diseases" launched in the 1990s evoked both a comeback of microbial threats to the policy agendas of rich countries and the no less political recognition of emergences inextricably linked to the unprecedented exploitation of nature and transformations induced by the latter. After having long been considered sources of infection, hospitals, paradigmatic places of victory against infectious diseases, once again became the possible weak links in chains of contagion. In the fight against the COVID-19 pandemic, they are the very last resort of a care system whose curative orientation is structurally threatened by the new contagions.

translated by Maya Judd

NOTE

1. Hannah Landecker, "Antibiotic Resistance and the Biology of History," *Body and Society* 22, no. 4 (2016): 19–52.

SELECTED BIBLIOGRAPHY

Ackerknecht, Erwin H. "Anticontagionism between 1821–1867." *Bulletin of the History of Medicine* 22 (1948): 562–593.

Anderson, Warwick. "Natural Histories of Infectious Disease: Ecological Vision in Twentieth-Century Biomedical Science." *Osiris* 19, no. 1 (2004): 39–64.

Bourdelais, Patrice. "La construction de la notion de contagion: Entre médecine et société." *Communications* 66 (1998): 21–37.

Landecker, Hannah. "Antibiotic Resistance and the Biology of History." *Body & Society* 22, no. 4 (2016): 19–52.

Mendelsohn, J. Andrew. "Typhoid Mary Strikes Again: The Social and the Scientific in the Making of Modern Public Health." *Isis* 86, no. 2 (1995): 268–277.

Pelling, Margaret. "Contagion/Germ Theory/Specificity." In *Companion Encyclopedia of the History of Medicine*, vol. 1, edited by William F. Bynum and Roy Porter, 309–334. London: Routledge, 1993.

MIGRATION

Migration Networks: Mapping and Theorizing Mobility

Paul-André Rosental

"Migration is patently more complex than that merely reshuffling of heads which is assumed by crude economic 'push-pull' models."[1] With these words, in an article published in 1964, John and Leatrice MacDonald attacked the most simplistic economistic explanation of migration processes. Financed by the Population Council, an organization founded twelve years earlier by John Davison Rockefeller III out of an obsessive fear of world overpopulation, the MacDonalds made use of the rich sociological material available on Italian immigration into the United States. They concluded that it was interpersonal networks that had enabled such long-distance mobility. Their key idea, featured in their title, was by its nature contagionist. Thus "chain migration can be defined as that movement in which prospective migrants learn of opportunities, are provided with transportation, and have initial accommodation and employment arranged *by means of primary social relationships with previous migrants.*"[2]

The MacDonalds' assessment would be repeated over and over again in succeeding decades by demographers, sociologists, and other geographers. They were to "rediscover," with the kind of pride that is born of ignorance, that the mere existence of an economic differential between two places was not sufficient to produce a migratory flow from one to the other. Their target was the so-called push-pull model (PPM), established in the 1920s, which observed a statistical correlation between the economic cycle and flows of migration to the United States.[3] The model was a typical piece of social scientific "objectivity," giving an impression of total empirical solidity that was nevertheless only partial when subjected to analytical scrutiny. It appealed to an undeniable reality that, when they considered migrating, people would think it worth moving toward locations where opportunities, economic and other, were more abundant than in the area they left.[4] It became the model of reference used by economists, international organizations, and those who feared a mechanical overflow of population from the south toward the countries of the north. It thus resisted the recurrent demonstration of an equally durable phenomenon that it was incapable of explaining: the fact that, since human beings were not atoms, the spatial distribution of their movements was not reducible to differentials in electric power. Its "irregular" cartography, as the MacDonalds pointed out, revealed the limits of the PPM: "Why did immigrants from certain towns in Southern Italy settle together in certain localities in the United States? These immigrants were not distributed among the 'Little Italies' by chance."[5]

These two sociologists were not content to replace a macroeconomic reading of the situation by a micro social one. As if anticipating the sort of criticism that would meet an approach ideologically suspected of individualism, they did not restrict themselves to opposing economic or political factors by an appeal to interpersonal relationships. They also took into account both labor market organization models and the institutional and legal frameworks governing migratory flows, thereby proposing a sociohistorical model, valid in situations and periods where international migration was relatively free. Away from naive optimism of interpersonal solidarity, the "link" could result from a strict hierarchy in the form of, for example, ethnic patronage likely to be obtained between a "patron"—or employer—and their employees.[6]

Clearly, then, the MacDonalds' article was an important milestone in understanding the interactions among migrants as a factor affecting long-distance mobility in very many instances. To treat migration as a potentially contagionistic mechanism therefore ought to count among initial hypotheses of any empirical study of the phenomenon, though it needed to be acknowledged, as did the MacDonalds, that it was not of universal application. Such being the case, the model's modalities and effects called for debate. If contagion was at work, how did it start and operate? And what did it lead to?

One layer of bibliographical ignorance can mask another. Funnily enough, these questions had been raised and settled in the ten years running up to the MacDonalds' 1964 article, but it was in a country and in a discipline that did not have the centrality of American sociology. The most powerful formulation of the contagionistic interpretation of migration had already emerged from Sweden's "Lund Geography School" through one of the volumes[7] and one of the periodicals (*Geografiska Annaler*) that provided the fullest treatment ever given of the theory and observation of migrations.

Sweden shared with the MacDonalds' Italy the characteristic of being a nation whose massive emigration toward the United States in the early twentieth century had given rise to a substantial literature. Two authors delved into it and derived from it a conceptual construction that was exceptional in its blend of the empirical with social theory, cartography with statistics, and *Landschaftskunde* (landscape studies) with phenomenology and land use planning. One of these was the Estonian geographer Edgar Kant (1902–1978), an ardent nationalist who was exiled in Sweden after holding office during the Second World War as rector of the prestigious University of Tartu. At the University of Lund, Kant was to train Torsten Hägerstrand (1916–2004). Apart from a major book on the spread of innovation, Hägerstrand created the notion of "migration area" to promote the analytical centrality of preferred destinations in the formalizing of migration flows.

How, then, can it be explained that, other things being equal, that is, for a given distance and volume of economic opportunities, one rural commune should send out masses of emigrants to a particular city rather than to another? Hägerstrand initiated his study at exactly the point where the MacDonalds would end theirs a few years after speaking of "Little Italies." He could already see that a challenge of this kind severely undermined the PPM, but he then proceeded to explain why. In so doing, he proposed a more powerful model in which unevenness of spatial distribution was to be seen not as exceptional but rather as a given that called for explanation.

Hägerstrand proposed a statistical simulation of migratory move-ments, basing these on a simple hypothesis: given a certain distance and level of opportunities, there would be a greater probability for a person to leave their village to join (as a "passive migrant") a fellow former resident who had already emigrated than to go (as an "active migrant" or "pioneer") to a wholly new destination. By implementing a theoretical "pioneers" (attractive) versus "passives" model, he was able to observe the step-by-step emergence of uneven spatial configurations. With the passage of time, the initial choices of the earliest migrants became solidified. Granted the spatial distribution of resources, the destinations chosen by the earliest migrants attracted future migrants at the expense of other places. Thus the spatial unevenness that could be observed was not fortuitous but the result of a long process that was not reducible to a strictly interpersonal reading. Migratory contagion set up enduring flows that could solidify in the form of institutional links such as transport networks.[8]

Finally, Hägerstrand's model shows in two very different ways how important history is. On the one hand, as with an epidemic, to appreciate the orientation of a flow of mobility one needs to track back as far as pos-sible and identify its "pioneer" or "first migrant," a quest facilitated in the Swedish case by the richness of the nominative data, which were inherited from a tight system of population registration by the Lutheran Church.[9] On the other, space cannot be reduced to the distribution of resources among different locations. As their respective "migrant areas" reveal, each one over a period of time evolved a profile peculiar to itself.

Here lie the scope and twofold value of the model created by Kant and Hägerstrand. It not only pioneered a way of defining, quantifying, and thereby universalizing spatial and migratory processes but also belonged within a long Central European tradition that blended *Heimatskunde* (so to speak, the "science of small homelands") and nationalism in the face of especially Russian menace. Indeed, Hägerstrand's mentor, Edgar Kant, was himself trained in Tartu by the Finn Johannes Gabriel Granö (1882–1956), whose "pure geography" was fundamental to his country's claim to independence.[10] Lund's school of geography, which has always been of service both to history and to the social sciences, is today finding enhanced political relevance in a world torn between universalist and localist political claims.

The career of Kant, its inspiration, also embodied this duality. An Estonian nationalist in orientation, he had nonetheless experienced a scientific tour through Budapest, Szeged, Vienna, Saint-Gall, Hamburg, Amsterdam, Paris, and Grenoble, thereby gaining personal access to the European academic community and its claim to universalist culture. Knowing as he did the work of Gabriel Tarde, Kant was even able to point out to Hägerstrand in 1953, when Hägerstrand defended his thesis, that his model amounted in fact to a formalization of the French sociologist's model, being at one and the same time a symbol of the close links between "contagion" and "imitation" and the dialectic between universality and frontiers.[11]

translated by Graham Robert Edwards

NOTES

1. John S. MacDonald and Leatrice D. MacDonald, "Chain Migration, Ethnic Neighborhood Formation and Social Networks," *Milbank Memorial Fund Quarterly* 42, no. 1 (January 1964): 82–97, here 82.

2. MacDonald and MacDonald, "Chain Migration, Ethnic Neighborhood Formation and Social Networks," 82.

3. Harry Jerome, *Migration and Business Cycles* (New York: NBER Books, 1926).

4. Samuel A. Stouffer, "Intervening Opportunities: A Theory Relating Mobility and Distance," *American Sociological Review*, vol. 5, no. 6 (December 1940): 845–867.

5. MacDonald and MacDonald, "Chain Migration," 84.

6. On these issues, see: Gérard Noiriel, "Les espaces de l'immigration ouvrière, 1880–1930," in *Villes ouvrières, 1900–1950*, edited by Susanna Magri and Christian Topalov (Paris: L'Harmattan, 1989), 171–186; Manuela Martini, *Bâtiment en famille: Migrations et petite entreprise en banlieue parisienne au XXe siècle* (Paris: CNRS Éditions, 2016).

7. David Hannerberg, Torsten Hägerstrand, and Bruno Odeving, eds., *Migration in Sweden: A Symposium* (Lund: Gleerup for the Royal University of Lund, 1957).

8. Sven Dahl, "The Contacts of Västerås with the Rest of Sweden," in *Migration in Sweden*, 206–243.

9. John G. Rice and Robert C. Ostergren, "The Decision to Emigrate: A Study in Diffusion," *Geografiska Annaler, Series B, Human Geography* 60, no. 1 (1978): 1–15.

10. Olavi Granö, "J. G. Granö and Edgar Kant: Teacher and Pupil, Colleagues and Friends," *Geografiska Annaler, Series B, Human Geography* 87, no. 3 (2005): 167–173.

11. From an interview of Torsten Hägerstrand by the author, May 24, 1992.

SELECTED BIBLIOGRAPHY

Burmeister, Stefan. "Archaeology and Migration: Approaches to an Archaeological Proof of Migration." *Current Anthropology* 41, no. 4 (2000): 539–567.

Ellegård, Kajsa, and Bertil Vilhelmson. "Home as a Pocket of Local Order: Everyday Activities and the Friction of Distance." *Geografiska Annaler, Series B, Human Geography* 86, no. 4 (2004): 281–296.

Latour, Bruno. *Où Atterrir?* Paris: La Découverte, 2017.

MacDonald, John S., and Leatrice D. MacDonald. "Chain Migration, Ethnic Neighborhood Formation and Social Networks." *Milbank Memorial Fund Quarterly* 42, no. 1 (January 1964): 82–97.

Rosental, Paul-André. "Les formalisations spatiales de la mobilité: Fragments pour l'histoire longue d'une non-réception." *Genèses* 29 (1997): 75–98.

Rosental, Paul-André. *Les sentiers invisibles.* Paris: Éditions de l'EHESS, 1999.

Rosental, Paul-André. "Où s'arrête la contagion? Faits et utopie chez Gabriel Tarde." *Tracés: Revue de sciences humaines* 21 (December 2011): 109–124.

MYTH

The Neanderthal Jew: A Structure That Gives Meaning to the Subjugation of the Other

Ron Naiweld

A few years ago, I was studying the history of the monotheistic myth, from the genesis of the myth as it is attested in the Hebrew Bible until its dissemination into the world at the end of antiquity. My initial intuition, based on personal experience, was that the biblical god had the power to inhabit the individual's inner language and to occupy a sovereign space. In this view, the monotheistic god would be akin to a virus; that is, a structure composed of the same raw material as rational thought but with its own internal logic and its own desire to multiply. By inserting itself into the individual's inner language, this god would transform the individual into its contaminating agent in the world of humans.

If we take into account the singular context in which the biblical stories were written, by Hebrew scribes in Jerusalem during the period of Persian domination, it was by no means preordained that they should be disseminated throughout the Greco-Roman world. The myth's viral power could thus explain how they successfully reached the diverse range of people who inhabited the ancient world.

My inquiry focused on the ancient world, with the Epistles of Paul as the endpoint, because it was Paul who successfully gave the myth of the biblical god its multiethnic and international renown. It was he who best exploited the myth's potential virality. But I kept an eye on the contemporary world, looking for places where the power of the myth could still be found today.

Around the same time, I heard about a book by Yuval Noah Harari called *Sapiens: A Brief History of Humankind*. Based on the author's lectures at the Hebrew University of Jerusalem for a course entitled "General Introduction to History," the book was published in Hebrew in 2011 and has since been translated into dozens of languages. It has been a worldwide success. In France, the book was on the list of the twenty bestselling nonfiction works for more than three years. I thought to myself, "Here is another book, written in Hebrew, in Jerusalem, that tells the story of humanity, as seen from this corner of the world. And humanity can't get enough of it." The coincidence prompted me to read the book.

The story put forth by Harari, whose initial works show a fascination with the experience of war, begins with human speech, at a turning point that he calls the linguistic revolution. Sapiens were not the only Hominidae with language, but they were the only ones to use language to create myths that federated a very large number of individuals. This was what enabled them to triumph over other "Homo" species, most notably the Neanderthals. Neanderthals communicated in small groups, like other primates, whereas Sapiens created symbolic structures flexible enough to enlist a multitude of individuals in a common project. The linguistic revolution was not the invention of language but of new, very powerful uses for language through which our ancestors, who were physically weaker than the Neanderthals, populated faraway lands and made us the most powerful species on the planet.

It is instructive to view this story as a myth in the sense that the author gives to the word, and the book's popularity is an invitation to do so. The myth of Harari would represent a dynamic structure that produces violence by dividing humans who share the same space into two groups. The dynamic structure creates cohesion through the division of humans into two species, only one of which earns a place in history.

The same dynamic structure appears at the end of the book, where the author focuses on the present. Sapiens have successfully dominated the planet and eliminated the possibility of their extinction. According to Harari, we are now living between two eras. We are at the close of the long period during which our species fought for survival and at the dawn of another in which we are realizing our age-old dream of becoming God. A new battle is brewing, between the new humans who have realized the dream and the old humans who are stuck in the preparatory stage with ideas and values to which the godlike humans no longer subscribe.

The dynamic structure expressed by Sapiens, which gives history a beginning and an end, has itself a long history. One of its first written descriptions can be found in a Latin text written at the beginning of the third century. Titled *Against the Jews*, it is one of the first Christian treatises of its kind, the first one in Latin in any case. It is attributed to Tertullian, a Carthaginian jurist and Christian apologist. This text was to inspire many other Christian writers over the course of the following centuries.

The point of departure in *Against the Jews* is a Judeo-Christian dispute witnessed by Tertullian. At the time, Christians were persecuted by the Roman Empire mostly on a local level and in many places could debate publicly and openly with Jews. Tertullian does not say who won the debate or even what the content was. For him, the outcome was a foregone conclusion. He mentions a detail of the debate, however, that the person defending the Jewish cause was a convert to Judaism. "In fact, this is enough—that the Gentiles are able to be admitted to the law of God—for Israel not to pride itself still that the Gentiles are counted as a drop in the bucket or as dust from the threshing floor.'"[1]

For Tertullian, the fact that a man who was not Jewish by blood could become Jewish marked a new era in the history of mankind. Before the advent of Christ, only the Jews could disseminate the word of their god into the world. Their patronizing sayings with regard to the Gentiles, such as those of the prophet Isaiah, whom Tertullian quotes in this text, were not completely wrong. But now it was no longer only Jews by blood who could carry the word of their god. Gentiles could also carry it, and according to Tertullian and the other Christian apologists, they generally did so in a more authentic manner than did the Jews, in a way that better corresponded to their god's divine nature, giving them historical consistency. They could no longer be considered a drop of water or a historical detail. They were full participants in history and not only as the divinity's passive instruments.

Tertullian wrote this text because in his time, everyone knew of the Jewish origin of this god, and many people believed that to be included in his promises, they had to become Jews and obey Jewish law. In Tertullian's time, there were thus two groups vying for the love and support of the same god, for the privilege of being his "people." The stakes were high. The winner would carry the word of the god into history. Tertullian's fear was that the ancient people would win out and the new people would become a footnote to history; that human history would not advance or would advance without them.

To calm his fears, Tertullian looked to the Old Testament, the collection of stories where this god's promises were recorded. He went back to the origin of the story to demonstrate that the new people must triumph over the old. He found a multitude of examples of the biblical people's problematic behavior. And to the extent that the Jews of his time identified with this people, it was very easy for him to show their disloyalty to their god, that they were an obstinate, stiff-necked people who did not deserve their status of elders. The new people were loyal to the divine father and were therefore more deserving of his love.

The pivotal moment in history for Tertullian was not the advent of Christ but the birth of Christianity as a social movement, that is, the presence of a large number of Christians in the world, a new people that better complied with the creator's plan than did the ancient people. This is why Tertullian believed it was natural for the new people, loved by the master of the universe, to dominate the ancient people.

Tertullian's conclusion is frightening, especially in light of the way it was subsequently implemented in Christian countries. The story he told became the ideology that served to justify persecution of the Jews in many ways and in many contexts. The Christian view of the Jews became a skewed one, with Christians ready to condemn the Jews for adhering to an archaic and decadent concept of humanity's divine mission.

A question remains. How did the Judeo-Christian structure evolve between the time of Tertullian's text and Philip the Fair's expulsion of the Jews from France in 1306, to give but one example? This is where we can think of a history of contagion. Tertullian, who formulated an idea in Latin that had already circulated in Greek, would be an important contaminating agent in that history. His words contaminated other Christian authors who succeeded him, then decision-makers, kings, emperors, and judges, all the while reinforced by other sources embracing the same ideology.

This mythical structure limited the representation of social reality and led to the conclusion that one people could dominate and possibly eradicate another. So it can be beneficial to study how the structure came to contaminate humanity. The objective of such a study would not be to describe the trajectory of the structure from one agent to another overtime but to reconstruct the historical instances of contagion so as to demonstrate the free will of the individuals involved.

translated by Steven Sklar

NOTES

1.   Tertullian, "Against the Jews (Adversus Judaeos)," in Geoffrey Dunn, *Tertullian* (London: Routledge, 2004).

SELECTED BIBLIOGRAPHY

Harari, Yuval N. *Homo Deus: Brief History of Tomorrow*. New York: HarperCollins, 2016.

Harari, Yuval N. *Sapiens: A Brief History of Humankind*. New York: HarperCollins, 2015.

NAMING

Lineages of Choice among the Artists of the Renaissance

Christiane Klapisch-Zuber

What does the idea of contagion bring to the study of renaming, that is, the borrowing and adoption of a part or the whole of a name of one individual by another? I investigated this question within the framework of a fairly well-defined social category: the milieu of Italian artists whose careers were described by Giorgio Vasari in his *Lives of the Most Excellent Eminent Painters, Sculptors, and Architects* (1550 and 1568 editions). The period covered is generally called the Renaissance, although its dates vary considerably according to the country under discussion. For Italy, according to Vasari, this period is usually placed between the fourteenth and sixteenth centuries. The author relates facts concerning anthroponymy for only a fraction of the hundreds of artists whose lives and works he records. This is enough, however, to understand the mechanisms of name-changing. This practice was not unknown in other contexts. For example, the successor to the leadership of a commercial or industrial company was sometimes known by the name of his predecessor. As perpetual migrants, artists accepted changes in how they were called. Can we compare this passing of names from one person to another outside of biological ties to a phenomenon of contagion? Or should we consider anthroponymic shifts rather as coming from another kind of transfer, the contamination of one model of kinship for another?

This is not a study of the mode that can affect the field of onomastics. In this approach "contagion" is mentioned when we study this "taste experienced as individual, but [which is] in fact socially determined."[1] Various sociological and historical studies of different societies, among them the medieval world, have shown the characteristics of the spread of a particular given name, or groups of names, sharing certain aspects. We can take as examples names of Christian saints, names of a political nature, or names of powerful figures.

What I have observed with Italian artists of the Renaissance eludes this notion of mode. Nor, at first glance, does it seem to have much to do with a phenomenon of contagion. One example is that of the painter "Michele di Ridolfo Ghirlandaio" (1503–1577). At birth, his *cognome* (the collective and hereditary family name) was "Tosini," which came from his biological father. He was at first the student and then later the associate of Ridolfo di Domenico del Ghirlandaio (1463–1561), another painter who came from the dynasty of artists named "(del) Ghirlandaio." Vasari, who knew Michele well, writes that these two men, Michele and Ridolfo "lov[ed] each other like father and son" and that Michele "was so beloved by him, that, as one belonging to Ridolfo, he has ever been and still is known by no other name than Michele di Ridolfo."[2] Beyond this patronymic nickname ("di Ridolfo") showing lineage, he also inherited the *cognome* "del Ghirlandaio" from Ridolfo's father (Domenico, 1449–1494). This *cognome* was the professional nickname[3] of the master of this father's brother, a nickname oddly given the status of *cognome* in the descent of the Bigordi sibling group (Domenico, Davide, and Benedetto Bigordi alias del Ghirlandaio) and taken up again by an associate such as Michele Tosini himself. Except for his baptismal name, Michele underwent a complete change of identity.

Within this selection of anthroponymic transfers, we also find cases of family names originating in place transmitted from master to student, even when the latter came from somewhere else entirely. This is how the sculptor Andrea Sansovino (1465/70–1527), son of a poor peasant named Domenico Contucci from Monte Sansavino, was known across the whole of Italy by the name of his native land, il Sansovino. One of his apprentices was a certain Jacopo d'Antonio Tatti (or del Tatta) (1486–1570); According to the life of Jacopo Sansovino, "the reciprocal friendliness and love between these two, as it were between father and son, [was such] that Jacopo in those early years, began to be called, no longer Tatti but Sansovino and," Vasari adds, "so he has always been, and always will be."[4]

So names were transferred, in part or in whole, from a master to his student, disregarding the normal rules of anthroponymy prevalent in this region of Italy. Indeed, such transfers question connections between men, as expressed in kinship terms borrowed from biological family (father/son, grandfather/grandson) or from chosen family (godfather/godson, adoptive father/adoptive son). According to Vasari, these relationships were sealed by specific habitual affects expected in these artist couples and that he groups together under the word "love."

For this author, the relations that upset the rules of kinship were founded on an affective relationship that in turn upset various social codes. As long as we do not conceive of the word "contamination" in an essentially negative way, the term can capture fairly well this relationship of individual to individual as expressed by the passing of a name from one to the other.

The transfer of a name from the master to a particular student implied something shared between them: the sharing of techniques of the one, of his style (of his "grace" writes Vasari, taking up the Christian notion). Beyond that, it also reflected the transfer of notoriety toward the student. In this contamination, the *vox publica* intervened. Be it the given name, the nickname (of origin, of profession, sobriquet) or of the master's family name, this *vox publica* diffused it, anchoring it into an artistic lineage. In a society of interknowledge where personal relations were based on neighborhood, profession, and gossip, these processes were subject to almost collective choices. Thus the beneficiary of the master's name then internalized and displayed the name, prior to sometimes transmitting it in turn to the following generation of his own students.

Such was the case of Giovanni Antonio Bazzi (1472–1549), a painter burdened with the nickname "Sodoma" by the people of Sienna. "Far from being sad and furious, he made it a source of pride" and carried it off with an air. In a show of bravado, he had his nickname proclaimed in the town streets when his horse won the *palio*.[5] One of his students, Giomo Magnani, was commonly called "Giomo del Sodoma," taking up, perhaps against his will, a moniker "so vile" (according to Vasari) as a patronymic nickname. Another example shows how the acceptance of a name suggested by the entourage could promote the man who received and adopted it. The architect Giuliano Giamberti complained to his patron Lorenzo the Magnificent that he and his courtiers constantly called him "da Sangallo." He accepted this nickname and transmitted it to kin and disciples when Lorenzo assured him that a reference to one of his works was worth more than the name of his ancestors who had nothing to do with it.[6]

In its effects, this contamination from person to person, as relayed and amplified by the *vox publica*, corresponds to ways of considering the individual and the collective from which it borrows much of its meaning, as if by contagion. When Vasari speaks of a master's "grace" transferred to a disciple by means of his name, he places the phenomenon he is describing on a spiritual plane, drawing a parallel between the master/disciple relationship and that of godfather and godson. Or again when, to his eyes, the "love" between two men justifies such an anthroponymic transfer, we cannot but recall the centuries-long debate opposing paternal and maternal love. We are also reminded of the debates concerning the love of an adoptive father for an adopted child and that of the biological father of the latter. These are all themes explored in the period's literature, by way of so many scenes that turn on reunions and recognition of children by their parents.

Interferences between situations engendered by spiritual kinship, adoptive kinship, or the apprentice relationship are thus reflected, as if by contagion, in the anthroponymic shifts observed among artists that affect and animate their tenor. Their anthroponymy reclaims several models of kinship current at the time, but it deliberately breaks the usual rules, the better to express a career and the human relationships upon which success was founded. It corresponds to a need for individualization in a larger society rather than to a desire for social distinction. If there is indeed contagion, it happens through the proximity of these practices with those that prevail in other social spheres and that imply models such as spiritual lineage acquired by baptism, by aesthetic, by intellectual and economic interests tied to apprenticeship, or by adoption procedures.

translated by Vicki-Marie Petrick

NOTES

1. Dominique Schnapper, "Essai de lecture sociologique," in *Le prénom, mode et histoire: Entretiens de Malher 1980*, ed. Jacques Dupâquier, Alain Bideau, and Marie Élizabeth Ducreux (Paris: Éditions de l'EHESS, 1984), 14.

2. Giorgio Vassari, *Le vite de' più eccellenti pittori, scultori e architettori nelle redazionni del 1550 e 1568*, ed. Rosanna Bettarini with commentary by Paola Barocchi (Florence: Sansoni, 1966–1994). English translation: GiorgioVasari, *Lives of the Most Excellent Painters, Sculptors, and Architects*, vol. 8., trans. Gaston Duc de Vere (London: MacMillan and Company and Medici Society, 1912–1914), 66.

3. A *Ghirlandaio* is the craftsman who makes the ornaments for women's he ads called *ghirlande*, hence the name of the dynasty of the Ghirlandaio.

4. Vasari, *Lives of the Most Excellent*, 31 (vol. 5) and 187 (vol. 9).

5. Vasari, *Le vite de' più eccellenti*, vol. 5, 231 and 235.

6. Vasari, *Le vite de' più eccellenti*, vol. 5, 170.

SELECTED BIBLIOGRAPHY

Dupâquier, Jacques, Alain Bideau, and Marie-Élizabeth Ducreux, eds. *Le prénom, mode et histoire: Entretiens de Malher, 1980*. Paris: Éditions de l'EHESS, 1984.

Klapisch-Zuber, Christiane. *Se faire un nom*. Paris: Arkhé, 2019.

NUCLEAR
Visualizing the Nuclear Contamination of the Planet during the Cold War

Sebastian V. Grevsmühl

Today, pollutants of anthropogenic origin, starting with microplastics, are everywhere on our planet, deposited in the ice of the polar regions, dispersed in the upper atmosphere, and transported to the ocean depths. Scientific awareness of the global distribution of these pollutants is not new; our knowledge of the contamination of the world developed considerably throughout the nineteenth century and has continued to expand. The focus here on the monitoring, surveillance, and study of the numerous nuclear tests during the Cold War is but a very recent manifestation. Nevertheless, this was a crucial historical step, as it led to the publication of the first global maps of the nuclear contamination of the world, making visible and palpable some of the effects of a possible nuclear war. Even more importantly, these new global views have reinforced our understanding of the entire biosphere as a radically interconnected ecological space. They thus strengthened the global environmental knowledge that forms the pillars of our current environmental concerns.

Two maps, published in 1956 in the midst of the Cold War by three US Weather Bureau researchers in *Science*, reflect this important historic process. Later becoming iconic (figures 1 and 2), they made it possible to trace the trajectories of radioactive particles around the globe. Thus, figure 1 shows the global and relatively rapid atmospheric diffusion of radioactive particles, originating from a small atoll in the Pacific and that, once injected into the stratosphere, continued on their way around the planet. Figure 2 complements these global diffusion pathways with a more quantitative

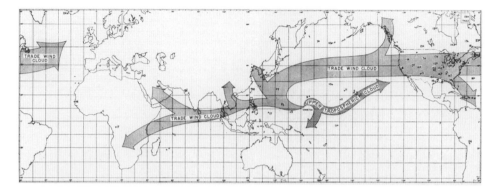

Figure 1
Map illustrating the global atmospheric movement of radioactive particles following the "Mike" test of November 1, 1952. *Source*: Author's own collection.

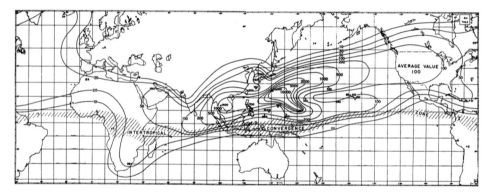

Figure 2
Map of Isolines showing the overall dispersion of radioactive particles and their concentration. *Source*: Author's own collection.

map, consisting of isolines that indicate the average rates of concentration of radioactivity in the air as well as an "intertropical convergence zone" thought not to be crossed by these radioactive particles.

These two maps represent key scientific results of the first atmospheric nuclear tests conducted under the auspices of the Atomic Energy Commission (AEC) in the Pacific. They demonstrated the power of the new global atomic fallout monitoring network established by the United States and its allies in the late 1940s. For its authors, the discovery of the world's radioactive contamination was not foremost a source of concern but rather the realization of a long-held aspiration, namely the possibility of tracking volatile but easily identifiable tracers in the atmosphere. Previously, only exceptional and very large-scale events, such as the explosion of the volcano Krakatau in 1883, had made this possible. Of course, these are not the first maps of this kind; the visual tradition of illustrating atmospheric flows on a large scale dates back at least to the seventeenth century. Other earlier reports had, in fact, presented similar maps, but they remained long inaccessible, being classified as "top secret" defense matters. The publication of these two maps in the open literature thus testifies to the establishment of a new policy of the diffusion (certainly still very partial) of geophysical knowledge previously under security restrictions.

Their publication was accompanied by a strong underlying tension that, since the beginning of the nuclear age, characterized all publications in this sector that were considered highly sensitive. Different observation techniques emerged out of a desire on the part of nuclear powers to closely monitor foreign atomic activities. The first observation networks set up to detect nuclear activities were obviously military. They came into being at the end of the Second World War when the United States sought to determine the German nuclear program's progress by measuring xenon-133 in air samples collected over suspect sites using military aircraft. Institutionalized as the AFOAT-1, this research unit, under the direct supervision of the Central Intelligence Agency and the AEC, saw its mission rapidly expand to include the monitoring of all nuclear activities, including not only nuclear tests but also nuclear reactor use and plutonium production. Thus, as early as 1949, it ran two scientific laboratories and had four squadrons of B-29 bombers dedicated to collecting air samples and twenty-four ground stations spread around the globe. Moreover, close collaboration with the British military made it possible to expand the network, allowing the unit to localize the Soviet Union's first nuclear test in 1949. The accuracy of the network was subsequently considerably improved by the integration of all detection methods (i.e., seismic, radiological, and sonic), techniques that were continually evaluated as part of the US nuclear tests in the Pacific.

The two maps thus evoke both the past and the future. They point to the past in that they are based on the long legacy of military surveillance of foreign nuclear programs, activities that have remained largely secret. But they also point to the future because they make visible two complementary structural aspects of the Cold War. First, the publishing of the maps in an "open" journal indicates the growing public pressure exerted on US agencies following the radioactive contamination of the population of the Marshall Islands and of nearby Japanese fishermen in the Castle Bravo nuclear accident in March 1954. This event resulted in strong indignation on the part of Japanese as well as the international press, prompting several countries to implement nuclear counterexpertise around which various nascent environmental movements were organized.

The second aspect concerns the emergence of new global environmental knowledge. Indeed, nuclear tests led to the creation of key tools for better understanding atmospheric and oceanic planetary flows as well as to the exchanges of energy and matter that take place therein. This new geophysical knowledge forms the foundation of our current global atmospheric and oceanic circulation models. Importantly, in tracking the diffusion of radionuclides both through the atmosphere and through plants, animals, and human populations, scientists could demonstrate the integration and interconnectedness of the entire biosphere. Unsurprisingly, in her influential book *Silent Spring* published in 1962, Rachel Carson drew directly on such studies to denounce the circulation and accumulation of chemical pollutants, particularly the pesticide DDT, throughout the biosphere.

We can thus see how the publication of these two maps of nuclear tests marks a historic moment in the construction of the idea of the world's contamination on a global scale. Beyond their documentary value, the maps offer new perspectives on what the process of contamination means since the Cold War. Through them, we see the birth of a new world lastingly transformed by the massive injection of radioactive particles into the atmosphere during the numerous nuclear tests carried out in the Pacific and elsewhere. It is precisely this long-term modification of the environment that significantly contributed, throughout the Cold War, to the shift from the earth sciences to earth system sciences.

A historical analysis of our scientific knowledge of the mechanisms of global contamination thus warns us not to view nuclear tests solely from the perspective of atomic annihilation but to account for the historical antecedents that have led to the current diagnosis of environmental crisis, thus favoring a richer and more complex narrative. As is often the case in the sciences, visualizations also played a key role here. Giving visibility to the global processes of contamination enabled an emerging environmental movement to establish close links between very distant events on our planet. In this sense, global visualizations of radioactive contamination have not only contributed to the creation of new geophysical realities, but they have also drawn our attention to the fact that we inhabit extremely uneven geographies and the originators of environmental fears and the places affected by these changes rarely coincide.

translated by Maya Judd

BIBLIOGRAPHY

Doel, Ronald. "What Is the Place of the Physical Environment Sciences in Environmental History?" *Revue d'histoire moderne et contemporaine* 56, no. 4 (2009): 137–164.

Herran, Néstor. "'Unscare' and Conceal: The United Nations Scientific Committee on the Effects of Atomic Radiation and the Origin of International Radiation Monitoring." In *The Surveillance Imperative: Geoscience during the Cold War and Beyond*, edited by Simone Turchetti and Peder Roberts, 69–84. New York: Palgrave Macmillan, 2014.

Higuchi, Toshihiro. "An Environmental Origin of Antinuclear Activism in Japan, 1954–1963." *Peace & Change* 33, no. 3 (2008): 333–366.

Jarrige, François, and Thomas Le Roux. *The Contamination of the Earth: A History of Pollutions in the Industrial Age*. Cambridge, MA: MIT Press, 2020.

Machta, Lester. "Finding the Site of the First Soviet Nuclear Test in 1949." *Bulletin of the American Meteorological Society* 73, no. 11 (1992): 1797–1806.

Masco, Joseph. "Bad Weather: On Planetary Crisis." *Social Studies of Science* 40, no. 1 (2010): 7–40.

Lutts, Ralph. "Chemical Fallout: Rachel Carson's Silent Spring, Radioactive Fallout and the Environmental Movement." *Environmental Review* 9, no. 3 (1985): 210–225.

PLAGUE

Processions at Beaune amid the Wars of Religion: A Word against Which Evil?

Diane Carron

When, on July 25 and 26, 1584, the inhabitants of Beaune sought God's assistance by walking in procession behind the canons of Notre-Dame, their intention was threefold, namely "for the goods of the earth, for the unity of the Church, and against contagion."[1] The word "contagion" has an ambivalent look in a context where Beaune's canons could conceivably reckon contamination of the body and that of the mind as equal dangers. Indeed, the severe plague outbreak that struck Burgundy like most of the rest of the kingdom between 1580 and 1586 provided as much a reason to be fearful as did the ecclesiastical divisions occasioned by the reformation at Beaune, where a Protestant congregation had been established prior to 1569. The Edict of Poitiers (1577), which imposed restrictions on the Protestant religion, had already aggravated tensions between Beaune's Catholics and Reformed.[2] On July 7, 1585, a month before the signing of the Edict of Nemours revoked all the edicts in favor of toleration, Beaune's inhabitants were walking in procession again "to extirpate heresy."[3] The confessional dissent attacked by the Catholic clergy was not an isolated phenomenon. It was paralleled in the political sphere by a conflict that saw a newly formed (1584) anti-Protestant league supported by Burgundy's governor, Charles of Mayenne, brother to Henry of Guise, opposing the king's legitimist partisans.

Can we be sure what sort of "contagion"—medical or religious—the canons of Beaune were seeking to defend themselves against? The standard Christian, and especially heresiological, vocabulary that employed the term "contagion" to connote the fear of the spread of subversive or heterodox notions went back to the twelfth century. While the term was not frequently used concerning religion over the centuries that followed, we do find it in politico-religious contexts, as in, for example, La Boétie's *Mémoire inédit concernant l'édit de tolérance de janvier 1562* (Original memoir concerning the Edict of Toleration of January 1562). In that same year, Catherine de' Medici ordered the lieutenant governor of Burgundy to "cleanse the entire land of Burgundy of this vermine of preachers and ministers who have put the plague there."[4] She thus resorted to prophylactic imagery to reference Reformation ideas, even if she did not use the term "contagion" as such. Recourse to the polysemic "contagion" also figured in written correspondence, including among Protestant writers, like the Burgundian Theodore Beza. The word *contagio* appears some thirty times in Beza's correspondence between 1556 and 1591, eighteen of these in a medical sense (having regard to fatal illness) and twelve times regarding the propagation of ideas that he repugned. In 1587, for example, he feared the spread of Claude Aubéry's false doctrines in the church at Geneva "lest this contagion emanate even unto us."[5] Equally, he observed that a sickness spread only "lightly and without any progress of contagion" in the city, enabling prophylactic measures to be lifted.[6]

To gauge the type of physical or ideological contagion envisaged by the chapter of Notre-Dame at Beaune, as also to trace more broadly the spread of the word itself within a comparable documentary corpus (i.e., beyond the narrow topo-chronological confines of the town of Beaune alone), we here offer an analysis of thirteen hundred stated intentions of collective processions that occurred in a number of towns in Burgundy and Champagne. They appear in the chapter registers of the cathedral chapters of Langres and Chalon-sur-Saône, in the collegiate chapters of Beaune and Saulieu, and among the deliberations of the municipalities of Dijon and Nevers. Such practices are detectable in the source material from the 1390s onward, with one or two extraordinary processions per annum in each locality. The number rises markedly in the sixteenth century with ten to a dozen such processions taking place each year, equivalent to two-thirds of the total; however, the phenomenon sharply diminishes in the seventeenth century, becoming a marginal practice from the 1740s.

Taking the long view makes it possible to assess how frequently the word "contagion" occurred and any variations of nuance between medical and religious frames of reference. The terms "contagion" and "contagious" (*contagieux*) occur only eight times between 1584 and 1714; thus their use is very rare in this body of material (i.e., less than 0.01 percent). They do not figure at all between 1396 and 1583, and their actual use is essentially concentrated into the forty-five-year period between 1584 and 1629. Geographically, they are confined to the area bounded by Dijon, Beaune, and Saulieu (all in the present-day Archives départementales de la Côte-d'Or, the Departmental archives of Côte-d'Or). These eight occurrences are expressed as shown in table 1.

Apart from the last mentioned, late occurring case, which refers explicitly to the epizootic of the rinderpest virus that struck cattle in Europe between 1709 and 1717, the seven other cases are more ambiguous. They suggest the usefulness of extending the analysis by opening it up to the use of other words related to sickness on the one hand and heresy on the other. These eight occurrences are reported in table 2 in relation to medical and religious vocabulary.

Words relating to sickness were used before, during, and after the period in which the word "contagion" occurs. On the other hand, this last period slightly overlaps the period in which the words "heretic(al)" (*hérétique*) or "heresy" (*hérésie*) were used and goes substantially beyond 1592, which marks abandonment of the word *hérétique* (simultaneous with the conversion of Henry IV). Although the word "plague" (*peste*) might be used metaphorically to connote the spread of Reformed ideas, such cannot be clearly determined on the basis of this body of material. Besides which, the word was in use both well before the Reformation took root and after the revocation of the Edict of Nantes. Moreover, the word "vermine," which is used four times between 1540 and 1605 in the procession records, always concerns harm done to crops (*gâtant la vigne*, "spoiling the vine"; *dévastant les biens de la terre*, "laying waste to the goods of the earth") and never refers to persons suspected of heresy.

Within the present body of material, it therefore remains difficult to gauge the exact meaning of the word "contagion." The elliptical character

Table 1

Use of the terms "contagion"/"contagious" (*contagieux*) in the sources for collective processions in Burgundy and Champagne

Date	Place	Intention	Reference
January 20, 1584	Beaune	for the goods of the earth and against contagion (*pour les biens de la terre et contre la contagion*)	Arch. Dép. Côte-d'Or G 2507, fol. 135
July 25 and 26, 1584	Beaune	for the goods of the earth and the unity of the Church and against contagion (*pour les biens de la terre et l'union de l'Église et contre la contagion*)	Arch. Dép. Côte-d'Or G 2507, fol. 176v
August 20, 1585	Beaune	against contagion and sudden death (*contre contagion et la mort subite*)	Arch. Dép. Côte-d'Or G 2508, fol. 18
July 16, 1628	Beaune	against contagion (*contre la contagion*)	Arch. Dép. Côte-d'Or G 2524, fol. 19
June 24, 1629	Beaune	against the contagion affecting the town's surroundings (*contre la contagion qui règne aux environs de la ville*)	Arch. Dép. Côte-d'Or G 44, fol. 52
1635 after Easter	Dijon	thanksgiving for the ending of the contagious sickness (*action de grâce pour la cessation de la maladie contagieuse*)	Arch. mun. Dijon B 272
1636 undated	Dijon	for the ending of the contagion and of all the ills afflicting the people (*pour la cessation de la contagion et de tous les maux qui affligent le peuple*)	Arch. mun. Dijon B 274
July 4, 1714	Saulieu	to seek the cessation of the contagious illness affecting horned beasts (*pour demander faire cesser le mal contagieux sur les bêtes à cornes*)	Arch. Dép. Côte-d'Or G 3145, fol. 31

Source: primary sources for collective processions in Burgundy and Champagne compiled by the author.

of the formulations militate against determining whether physical illness or the spread of ideas was intended. Yet, if we have regard to the historical context, such mentions are nonetheless enlightening. The dates when the word appears coincide precisely with the peaks of deadly epidemics experienced between Auxerre and Mâcon, that is, the plagues of 1584–1585 and 1628–1629 and the typhoid fever and plague of 1635–1636. The correlation of the use of the word with fatal epidemics and the absence of correlation with the episodes of politico-religious strife known to have affected the area suggest a medical rather than religious use in these sources.

Table 2

Distribution of words relating to physical sickness and/or heresy in the intentions of collective processions in Burgundy and Champagne

Vocabulary	Frequency	1400–1449	1450–1499	1500–1549	1550–1599	1600–1649	1650–1699	1700–1749	1750–1799
Sickness	11	X	X	X	X	X	X	X	X
Pestilence/Plague	52		X	X	X	X	X	X	X
Death/Mortality	9	X	X	X	X	X	X	X	
Epidemic	8	X	X	X	X	X	X	X	X
Air	1			X					
Flow	1					X			
Blood	1					X			
Fever	1					X			
Contagion/Contagious	**8**				X	X	X	X	
Heresy/Heretic(al)	39			X	X	X	X		
Huguenots	4				X				
Enemies of the faith	3				X	X			
So-called RPR	1					X			
Lutheran sect	1			X					
False doctrine	1				X				

*"RPR" represents so-called reformed religion, "r[eligion] prétenduement] r[éformée]."

Complementary to this research, analysis of the online inventories of the Departemental Archives of the Côte-d'Or, notably of those of the Chambre des Comptes at Dijon, reveals that the word "contagion" is always explicitly used there to refer to contagious physical disease (the recourse to medical practitioners, burial of people dying of contagion, judicial adjournment due to contagion) and never to the spread of ideas.

The religious sense of the term "contagion" does not therefore seem to have been current in this series of processions, whether they were organized and/or recorded by civil or church authorities; probably the same could be said of remaining acts of administrative practice in Burgundy. These often laconic mentions nevertheless say nothing as to the kind of discourse occurring along the processional routes or in sermons preached at the time, in which the dual sense of the word might circulate.

translated by Graham Robert Edwards

NOTES

1. Dijon, Archives départementales de la Côte-d'Or, G 2507, fol. 176 v: "pour les biens de la terre, l'union de l'Église et contre la contagion."

2. Jacques Fromental, *La réforme en Bourgogne* (Paris: Les Belles Lettres, 1968), 57–58.

3. ADCO, G 2508, fol. 3: "pour l'extirpation de l'hérésie."

4. Quoted in Hector de la Ferrière, ed., *Lettres de Catherine de Médicis*, vol. 1 (Paris: Imprimerie Nationale, 1880), 327: "nettoyez tout le pays de Bourgogne de cette vermine de prédicans et ministres qui y ont mis la peste."

5. Theodore Beza, *Correspondance* (Geneva: Droz, 2006), letter 1901: "ne vel ad nos usque haec contagio emanet."

6. Beza, *Correspondance*, letter 1891: "sed levissime et absque ullo contagionis progressu."

SELECTED BIBLIOGRAPHY

Carron, Diane. "Peuple de saints et pèlerinages dans les diocèses d'Autun et de Nevers, du temps des martyrs au temps des réformes." PhD thesis, Université de Bourgogne, 2006.

Crouzet, Denis. "Recherches sur les processions blanches, 1583–1584." *Histoire, Économie, Société* 1, 4 (1982): 511–563.

Fossier, Arnaud. "La contagion des péchés (XIe–XIIIe siècle): Aux origines canoniques du biopouvoir." *Tracés* 21 (2011): 23–39. https://doi.org/10.4000/traces.5128.

Massoni, Anne. "La participation des chanoines à l'encadrement religieux." In *Structures et dynamiques religieuses dans les sociétés de l'Occident Latin (1179–1449)*, edited by Madeleine de Cévins and Jean-Michel Matz, 85–94. Rennes: PUR, 2010.

POLLUTION

The Chemical Industry: A Barricade against Infection (1770–1830)

Thomas Le Roux

When industrialization began to shape the transformation of European society at the end of the eighteenth century, some of its effects on public health quickly gave cause for concern. The pollution it produced, described at the time in such terms as "corruption," "insalubrity," and "filth," was construed within a cloud of meanings associating morals with medicine. Were the new industrial emanations breeding unknown diseases and threatening the "preservation of citizens" sought by every enlightened public administration? If so, how would these diseases spread, and what measures of prevention or disinfection would be effective? The diagnoses made by the medical profession—and increasingly by chemists, the most conversant with industrial processes—not only shed light on the causation and spread of diseases but also proved to be an essential factor in our society's acculturation to the industrial world in the early 1800s.

Medical perceptions of the sources of disease seem to have been very unfavorable to industrial development for most of the eighteenth century. Neo-Hippocratism, which held that sickness or health was determined by the surrounding environment, dominated at the time and clashed with contagionism, the belief that disease spread through person-to-person contact, although the dividing line between the two theories was highly permeable. Anticontagionist, "miasmatic" medicine insisted on the role of the air, water, and soil in transmitting disease, even for illnesses long known to be contagious through contact (plague, ophthalmia, syphilis, and smallpox). This medical view was widely shared in Europe, especially in Italy,

Great Britain, and German-speaking countries where there was little doubt of the connection between diseases and various climates, atmospheres, and emanations.

The environmental factor was endorsed by the English physician John Arbuthnot, a fellow of the Royal Society, who linked air quality to people's health in his *Essay Concerning the Effects of Air on Human Bodies* (1751) and by the French physician Menuret de Chambaud, who won a prize from the *Société royale de médecine* (Royal Society of Medicine) for his work implicating craft workshop emissions in the propagation of contagious diseases (*Essai sur l'action de l'air dans les maladies contagieuses*, 1781). Since a foul odor ("miasma") was considered to be an indicator of deleterious emanations, it followed that craft or industrial activities processing putrescible matter or chemical substances were regarded with especial dread.

Consequently, in keeping with established jurisprudence, urban police forces used preventive and repressive measures to closely monitor these workshops and factories while relegating them to areas far from homes. The *Traité de la police* (Treatise on the police) authored by Paris police commissioner Nicolas de la Mare in the early eighteenth century was widely applied in continental Europe; it contained an entire chapter on environmental and health regulations for workshops and factories. To protect public health, severe repressive measures were taken, extending even to the demolition of facilities or imprisonment. During epidemics and "in times of contagion," leather and dye works were prohibited, just as blacksmiths were banned from burning coal, in order to not spread infection.

However, between 1770 and 1830, a dramatic change in attitude occurred. Acid vapor was no longer perceived to be aggressive but healthy; coal smoke, due to the sulfur it contained, was welcomed by some as a disinfectant, and putrefaction was no longer held to be the source of mortal miasmas. Decisive strides toward a new definition of harmlessness, though it remained a subject of dispute and much controversy, were spurred by eminent chemists with medical training, such as Antoine Fourcroy, Jean-Antoine Chaptal, and Claude-Louis Berthollet. In this circle revolving around Antoine Lavoisier, Louis-Bernard Guyton de Morveau initiated the paradigm shift. In 1773, at the request of the bishop of Dijon, he fumigated the city's cathedral, using hydrochloric acid to eliminate the foul odors produced by the decaying corpses in the burial vaults. The experiment yielded spectacular results: the stench completely disappeared. Seen as a victory over putrid infection, the method had a tremendous impact.

The following year, acid fumigations were prescribed to treat epizootic diseases; to purify the air in hospitals, ships, and prisons in both France and England, and to fight yellow fever in Spain. In 1801, having become a member of the French Academy of Science and a prominent figure under the consulate, Guyton de Morveau published his *Traité des moyens de désinfecter l'air, de prévenir la contagion et d'en arrêter le progress* (Treatise on the ways to disinfect air, prevent contagion and stop its progress), in which he strove to demonstrate the superiority of his methods of disinfection. Chaptal, the then interior minister, lost no time in having the publication distributed to all prefectures.

The crusade for the purification of air did not lead to a radical change in the frontier between contagionists and anticontagionists in the medical world, but it influenced how the causes and spread of disease were diagnosed: industry, which had been suspected of proliferating insalubrious air, was in fact a means of salvation. As a result, urban police forces found themselves confronted with chemists' new and unprecedented expertise, which contradicted jurisprudence and clashed with local regulations. During the peak of the conflicts that pitted chemical factories against their neighbors and the local police, the Council of State regularly intervened by granting exceptions enabling these facilities, especially those manufacturing sulfuric acid, to operate.

The trend deepened in 1804 and 1809, when, in reports to the Academy of Science on factories that discharged foul odors, the chemists Chaptal, Guyton de Morveau, Fourcroy, Nicolas Deyeux, and Nicolas-Louis Vauquelin exonerated the chemical industry from harmfulness. Their reports paved the way for the 1810 law on pollution, which gave free rein to industrial development. The Paris Health Council (Conseil de salubrité), created by Chaptal in 1802 and mainly active after 1806, took charge of spreading the new theories. Accordingly, when the synthetic soda industry flourished after 1809, releasing quantities of noncondensed hydrochloric acid fumes, the Health Council recommended locating these factories near areas of putrefaction (such as excrement heaps and workshops using organic matter) to purify the air. These ideas opportunely coincided with the industry-friendly political economy of the time as well as with the growth of international trade; disinfection with acid could potentially destroy the germs of contagion on people and goods alike, thereby enabling quarantine restrictions to be reduced.

Around the same time, the Health Council affirmed that coal smoke was not as harmful as believed. Although it indeed contained sulfur, the latter was the active ingredient in treating respiratory diseases. On this basis, some even recommended spending time near chemical plants during cholera outbreaks to avoid contagion. Going further still, the Health Council's commissioners eventually demonstrated that putrescent material and factories handling animal matter, then perceived to be "hotbeds of contagion,"[1] were less dangerous than had been imagined. In observing cases of intermittent fever that occurred between 1807 and 1812, they attributed its causes to marshes and stagnant water rather than to the particularly rank leather, strong glue, and tallow factories. Regarding the latter, the veterinarian Jean-Baptiste Huzard wrote in 1812 that the vapors emanating from melting vats were "not only . . . not unwholesome, but on the contrary . . . enrich those who live among them, and they were even regarded as effective in the healing of pulmonary phthisis."[2] In 1818, Charles Marc, the future president of the French Academy of Medicine, made a compelling demonstration in Asnières, where residents blamed a local gut factory for triggering an epidemic of ophthalmia. Marc refuted the claim, pointing his finger instead at the level of humidity in homes. His theory was confirmed when the illness disappeared the following year, even though the factory continued to release its unpleasant odors into the city's air.

Consequently, even malodourous workshops such as tanneries and curriers, which processed animal hides, were allowed in urban centers. In the 1820s, the Health Council expanded its arsenal of disinfectants to include chlorinated products, which could at least eliminate troublesome odors (although the smells were no longer deemed unhealthy). In a gut factory in Clichy, the pharmacist Antoine Germain Labarraque, who was also a member of the Health Council, found that immersing the animal matter in a solution of chloride of lime would immediately clear the putrid smell. The chemical became popular, and after 1823 the police prefecture encouraged its use. This product of modern hygiene was also closely linked to the chemical industry, since it resulted from the industry's byproducts.

Therefore, although medical etiologies saw little change in the first decades of industrialization, a radical shift in thinking occurred among anticontagionists: not only was industry not harmful, but in some cases it could even be an excellent safeguard from contagion, as could the many chemical substances it produced. These new theories facilitated the acculturation to the industrial world. By proclaiming the innocuity of industry, advocates of public hygiene ultimately allowed industrial development that, in the guise of modernity, would lead to new forms of contamination over the next two hundred years.

translated by Elaine Holt

NOTES

1. Archives Nationales (French national archives), F1cIII Seine 20, table of the situation of rural municipalities in the Seine Department, based on responses from mayors and deputies to the circular of 16 Brumaire Year IX.

2. Archives of the Police Prefecture, Health Council report, January 28, 1812.

SELECTED BIBLIOGRAPHY

Baldwin, Peter. *Contagion and the State in Europe, 1830–1930*. Cambridge: Cambridge University Press, 1999.

Coleman, William. *Death Is a Social Disease: Public Health and Political Economy in Early Industrial France*. Wisconsin: University of Wisconsin Press, 1982.

Hamlin, Christopher. *Public Health and Social Justice in the Age of Chadwick, 1800–1854*. Cambridge: Cambridge University Press, 1998.

Janković, Vladimir. *Confronting the Climate: British Airs and the Making of Environmental Medicine*. New York: Palgrave Macmillan, 2010.

La Berge, Ann Fowler. *Mission and Method: The Early-Nineteenth-Century French Public Health Movement.* Cambridge: Cambridge University Press, 1992.

Le Roux, Thomas. "Du bienfait des acides: Guyton de Morveau et le grand basculement de l'expertise sanitaire et environnementale (1773–1809)." *Annales historiques de la Révolution française* 383 (March 2016).

Le Roux, Thomas. *Le laboratoire des pollutions industrielles: Paris, 1770–1830.* Paris: Albin Michel, 2011.

Riley, James C. *The Eighteenth-Century Campaign to Avoid Disease.* London: Macmillan, 1987.

PRISON

"Prison Is a School of Crime": Proselytism in the Jails of the Ancien Régime

Natalia Muchnik

"Give me a Christian prisoner and I will give him back to you Jewish."[1] This claim, attributed to a Portuguese inquisitor, reported in 1625, appears to be corroborated by Abraham Idaña, a Spaniard who converted to Judaism in Amsterdam and who, in a text of 1683, commented wryly on the role of inquisitorial jails: "a number of those whom they [the inquisitors] detained, going into prison without having ever having known [any life other] than that of Christians, came out as Jews."[2] While no doubt excessive, these declarations express one aspect of the reality of the carceral world of the ancien régime, namely that jails come forth as places of proselytism for prisoners charged with crimes of faith, such as those accused of crypto-Judaism (the Marranos) or crypto-Muslim practices (the Moriscos) in Spain, of (crypto-)Protestantism in France following the revocation of the Edict of Nantes, or of (crypto-)Catholicism in reformed England. That which constituted then, in the eyes of repressive authorities, a form of cultural contagion, in fact concerned just as much those "potentially" belonging to the minority group in virtue of the charges against them as it did the jailers and their families living *in situ*, as well as prisoners charged with other offenses. Such was the case with a mercenary and two "poisoners" imprisoned at Newgate in London who converted to Catholicism in the 1610s as a result of the proselytism of their fellow prisoners.

The sense of "contamination" or "corruption" in prisons, not only spiritual (moral and religious) but also physical (due to sickness and deprivation), was not exclusive to those charged with crimes of faith. It was perceived by the wider body of actors in the carceral world in that period; the terms that evoke it, readily drawing on bodily (and epidemic) vocabulary to describe the evolution of souls, appear in numerous sources. Stains and infections are commonplace when describing the jails in which many saw the reign of barbarity. On the prisoners' side, they were the result of overcrowding where men were heaped in with women and with delinquents of every social origin. Honor suffered in consequence, as it did with the upheaval in the social order where the observation of precedence, at that time the mark of civility, ceased to hold. The savagery of the carceral world ran throughout their correspondence, their petitions, and their literary writings. On the side of visitors alarmed by conditions, they provoked disgust, indeed, avoidance, or, conversely, protest at the "good" (socioeconomic élites and those accused of crimes of faith) being mixed with the "bad" (paupers and delinquents).

The authorities, for their part, oscillated between differing postures according to the resources available to them. While overcrowding, the principal source of "contagion," was often used as a means of repression, they occasionally attempted to remedy it, notably in the matter of gender distinction. By the same token, they periodically attacked, more broadly, the corruption of jailers prosecuted, among other things, for allowing banned religious practices to proliferate in their establishments. Moreover, the risk of contagion accounts for partitioning progressively coming to prominence in the nineteenth century with the emergence of the cellular model and hygiene as an instrument of order. Indeed, for a number of eighteenth-century reformers, such as John Howard and Louis-Michel Lepeletier de Saint-Fargeau, isolation was conducive to repentance and amendment, thus avoiding moral "corruption" by other prisoners.

Inside jails, especially for prisoners of crimes of faith, "contagion" was at the same time internal ([re-]activation and recidivism) and external (corruption and spreading), active (through persuasion) and passive (through example). It was fostered by the modalities of incarceration given that the accused and the condemned were often confined in collective rooms from the sixteenth to the nineteenth century and could, by and large, circulate within the jail, either officially or clandestinely. This spreading appeared, in short, to be an inevitable consequence of the forms of overcrowding, even though contact could also be made in furtive encounters or by a voice carried from room to room. More broadly speaking, prisoner state of mind likewise offered propitious terrain for conversion, in forms resembling phenomena of the intensification of the religious in contemporary prisons. Deprivation, the anguish of waiting without knowing when it would end, the fear of physical suffering (notably torture), and death promoted a greater closeness with the divine.

Moreover, the authorities, aware of the risk of proselytism stemming from the presence of the heterodox among the rest of the prisoners, made attempts to isolate them. Certain places of confinement were singled out for them, such as, in the case of those accused of Protestantism in France, the Tower of Crest in the Dauphiné region and the Tower of Constance at Aigues-Mortes. In London, Catholics and priests in particular seem to have been often incarcerated at Newgate, the (Westminster) Gatehouse, the Clink, the Fleet, Marshalsea, and the Tower of London. For those who, usually dispersed on the outside, had few opportunities to meet their coreligionists and, even less, their spiritual guides, prisons provided hitherto unknown possibilities for reinforcing their faith.

The modalities and intensity of carceral proselytism depended on the numbers present, on individuals' knowledge, on their past functions in the group, and on their origins. In Spain, Muslims (notably slaves) and Jews born of the diaspora and converted to Christianity, as well as renegades educated under the Ottoman Empire, could have a significant cultural impact on their fellow prisoners. Other prisoners could avail themselves of external contributions or items of worship, especially books. The latter circulated widely in jail, for internal usage, or, when required, they were sent out to coreligionists of the diaspora. Prisoners, above all English Catholics and French Protestants, often penned religious writings or devoted themselves to copying works to be disseminated on the outside.

"Contagion" was not limited to prison walls and their prisoners; it also affected free people to be found alongside prisoners in their jails: visiting families, suppliers, servants, and slaves. In 1586, a "gentleman" familiar with Newgate alerted the authorities to the "pernicious" role of jails in the spreading of Catholicism. "If you mean to stop the stream," he argued, "choke the spring, for . . . The prisons of England are very nurseries of papists Banish them [the Catholics] or let them remain close prisoners, that they may not daily poison others."[3] That was especially the work of priests living in reclusion and who celebrated masses and marriages indoors, sometimes in the presence of visitors, or even instructed the children who were sent to them. In France, where arrested pastors were normally held in isolation, it was the family members who then took over that education, as is illustrated by the case of Poitevin Hudel. Thrown into the Bastille in 1690 and subsequently into the castle of Loches, he was next transferred to the castle of Saumur where, it is said, "he was at liberty to see his wife and children and . . . he kept two of his children at Saumur so as to be able to instruct them in his religion." As late as 1698, it was still insisted upon that "he should not be allowed the instruction of his children, lest he give them the wrong one; therefore, he must not see them."[4]

It should be pointed out that the places of detention at that time, in the greater part of Europe, were particularly porous. They allowed for comings and goings, usually after money had changed hands, with or without warders accompanying prisoners outside. They could often be structurally open for part of the time, as was the case with the penitential prisons of the Inquisition in Spain that the condemned could leave during the day to earn their living. Those prisons were often housed in preexisting buildings (including urban gateways, watchtowers of ramparts, monasteries, palaces, private dwellings) and were frequently located in the heart of town, close to local inhabitants. Moreover, the latitude given was often even greater; certain Morisco prisoners condemned by the Inquisition of Granada in the second half of the sixteenth century were allowed outside to work their land, on condition that they brought back a certificate of proof and returned on certain occasions, notably on Sundays and Catholic feast days.

This serves to underline that the fear of physical and spiritual "contamination," which would gradually lead to reforming the places of detention and their standardization, was seen as founded, as regards the accused and condemned, "on the grounds of faith." The prospect of "contagion" was held to be all the sharper when it escaped over the prison walls, for jails were hotbeds of proselytism and instruction in faiths forbidden to their coreligionists on the outside, not only face-to-face but at a distance, through prisoners' writings and the examples they set.

translated by David M. Thomas

NOTES

1. January 10, 1625; Madrid, Archivo Histórico Nacional, Inquisition, Legajo 134 (18).

2. Benjamin N. Teensma, "Fragmenten uit het amsterdamse convoluut van Abraham Idaña, alias Gaspar Méndez del Arroyo (1623–1690)," *Studia Rosenthaliana* 11 (1977): 127–156, especially 152–153.

3. London, British Library, Harley MS 286, fol. 97 (no. 60), quoted by Peter Lake and Michael Questier, *The Antichrist's Lewd Hat: Protestants, Papists and Players in Post-Reformation England* (New Haven: Yale University Press, 2002), 203.

4. François Ravaisson-Mollien, ed., *Archives de la Bastille*, vol. 10: *Documents inédits; Règne de Louis XIV 1693 à 1702* (Paris: A. Durand and Pedone-Lauriel, 1879), 245–247.

SELECTED BIBLIOGRAPHY

Lake, Peter, and Michael Questier. *The Antichrist's Lewd Hat: Protestants, Papists and Players in Post-Reformation England*. New Haven: Yale University Press, 2002.

McClain, Lisa. *Lest We Be Damned: Practical Innovation and Lived Experience among Catholics in Protestant England, 1559–1642*. London: Routledge, 2004.

Muchnik, Natalia. *Les prisons de la foi: L'enfermement des minorités (XVIe–XVIIIe siècle)*. Paris: Presses universitaires de France, 2019.

Perelis, Ronnie. "Prison Revelations and Jailhouse Encounters: Inquisitorial Prisons as Places of Judaizing Activism and Cross-Cultural Exchange." In *Religious Changes and Cultural Transformations in the Early Modern Western Sephardic Communities*, edited by Yosef Kaplan, 137–153. Leiden: Brill, 2019.

Salle, Grégory. "La maladie, le vice, la rébellion: Trois figures de la contagion carcérale." *Tracés: Revue de sciences humaines* 21 (2011): 61–76. https://doi.org/10.4000/traces.5148.

PROGRESS

The Battle of Wheat: An Ideological Tool for Fascist Italy

Niccolò Mignemi

The *Battaglia del grano* (Battle of Wheat) was the first mass mobilization campaign launched by the Fascist regime in Italy in 1925. To break Italy's dependence on imports and in the name of achieving food self-sufficiency, it promoted agricultural intensification and the rationalization of cereal production and led the government to collaborate with scientists and professional organizations—of farmers and of food industries. The extent to which their combined efforts permeated the local level will be examined here. In all evidence, the widespread dissemination of the campaign's productivist message to farmers cannot be entirely attributed to the Fascist regime's repressive tactics. An exploration of the financial incentives employed, such as subsidies and loans, and the measures of propaganda used, which included prizes, conferences, and demonstration fields, provides some insights into how the diffusion of agricultural innovations supported a reactionary modernism in which scientific and technological progress were pillars of the regime's nationalist plan.

The province of Parma, in Emilia-Romagna, offers historians an especially rich field for observing these dynamics at the local level. First, the province featured a diversity of farming environments, ranging from the fertile Po plain to the Apennine mountains. Second, an agricultural extension office (*cattedra ambulante di agricoltura*), headed by Antonio Bizzozero and funded by both the public and private sectors, had regularly been providing advice and assistance to farmers in the region since 1892. Local experts and modernizing elites had established its legitimacy among the rural population by promoting a democratic program of agricultural reform. However, attracted by Fascist promises, they shifted their support to a productivist agrarianism, in which the peasant-entrepreneur was seen as a factor of economic growth and social stability.

The Parma extension office therefore put its weight behind the *Battaglia del grano*, promoting the campaign and monitoring its implementation. It helped to turn biological innovation into a tool that could leverage past experience and also into a fundamental driver of the green revolution announced by the Fascist regime. Since the end of the nineteenth century, Italian scientists had been working intensively on the hybridization and genetic selection of cereals, which led to the development of new early ripening and high-yielding varieties in the 1920s and 1930s. The seeds were then presented to farmers as their most valuable asset, requiring a limited investment but quickly leading to a profit. The new varieties were not just a product of agricultural research but also an instrument of state intervention, since the regime sought to ensure their massive dissemination and widespread use.

With the assistance of local farmers, the extension office set up demonstration fields, ranging in size from a few hundred square meters to up to a hectare, in a variety of locations in the Parma province. The plots were planted to display the benefits of using the new varieties and fertilizer in different environments and with different crop rotations. The efforts of the local cooperative and expanded access to credit facilitated farmers' investment in the purchase of the selected seeds. Meanwhile, public funding made it possible to install sieving machines, in hilly and mountainous areas in particular, and to establish a system in which selected seeds were distributed to small farmers in exchange for an equivalent amount of wheat landraces. Substituting new varieties for traditional ones was not the only goal, however. More importantly, the selected seeds became a means to influence the technical choices made by farmers and to shift the focus of the extension office's expertise to maximizing yields.

Technical experts and government authorities disseminated propaganda in enthusiastic waves, successively promoting the elite varieties called Ardito, Villa Glori, and Damiano Chiesa. Nevertheless, diffusion of these seeds remained limited because their potential yield depended largely on soil fertility, the quality of plowing, and the use of inputs. Instead, farmers seemed to prefer the Mentana: although it did not promise the exceptionally high yields of the three other elite varieties, it was more resistant and demanded less investment. The extension office's experts deduced that the Mentana was chosen because it was better adapted to the poorer-quality soils typically found in the hills and mountains of Parma; however, statistics showed that smallholders preferred the Mentana even in the plains. In fact, the only area where the high-yielding varieties flourished were the prosperous farms in the lowlands, which had both the soil conditions and the investment capital required. This local pattern of dissemination of the selected seeds confirms the idea that the various social groups were unequal in their ability to benefit from the grain intensification campaign, a fact that the region's heterogeneous environments had tended to conceal. Despite these differences, the *Battaglia del grano* succeeded in standardizing the quality of the seeds provided to farmers and constructing a new metrology to compare yields in a consistent manner. Thanks to the contributing role played by the extension office, the cultivated land became a vast source of practical experience that could provide additional data to complement the scientists' laboratory and field trial findings.

In the same way as for peanuts in Senegal, plant breeding proved to be a powerful conveyor of cultivation standards that intended to rationalize agricultural practices and intensify farming systems. The monthly bulletin published by the Parma extension office regularly reminded farmers that the selected seeds were not effective without deep plowing; the use of root crops and vegetables such as tomatoes, beets, and tobacco to prepare and improve soils; abundant fertilization using chemicals; various operations to facilitate the nitrification process in winter; mechanization; the use of a precise calendar for late, high-density line sowing; and last, early harvesting to accelerate the frequency of crop rotations.

As they worked to disseminate innovation, the proponents of the *Battaglia del grano* had to constantly balance their desire to impose standard models with their awareness of the need to develop solutions that were adapted to the diverse environments and the social groups being targeted.

This pull of opposing forces can be perceived in the national competition held each year to reward best practices and to celebrate the wheat intensification campaign's biggest producers. The agricultural extension offices took part in defining each province's selection criteria for the three prize categories: small, medium, and large farms. Although it was expected that each of these subgroups would have its own specific characteristics, comparisons—despite the use of yield per hectare as a common denominator—could prove to be difficult. The competition nonetheless aimed to spread the idea that the regime's policies enabled farmers of every size to take part in the modernization, to their own extent.

In connection with the national competition, local prizes funded by local authorities, landowners, credit unions, and local industries were also awarded. In Parma, for example, the province's farmers' union launched a special contest for sharecroppers in 1931, which received considerable national attention. In addition to being the only one of its kind in Italy, the initiative was of interest for two reasons. On the one hand, it reached out to a social class overlooked by traditional competitions targeting landowners and tenant farmers. On the other hand, it drew a clear distinction between sharecroppers and farmworkers, against the backdrop of the 1930s trend toward proletarianization. This recognition of sharecroppers was meant to rally their support for the cereal intensification policies and to indirectly pressure landowners to invest. The regime did not rely solely on the modernizing elite—who benefited the most from the wheat subsidies and protectionist measures—to drive agricultural progress. Instead, the implementation of this initiative demonstrates the regime's desire to win over the widest possible support—even if unenthusiastic—from the mass of small farmers who saw the promise of social ascension in the dissemination of innovation and the tools of productivist propaganda.

Although Mussolini proclaimed it a victory in 1933, the *Battaglia del grano* proved to be only the first stage of an overall intensification program that would spread to all agricultural production in the country. This larger plan aimed to expand the combination of technical solutions, economic incentives, and advisory services that formed the core of the strategies developed since 1925. Propelled by the regime's policies, the productivist agricultural rhetoric successfully permeated throughout the Parma province. However, this could never have been achieved without the participation of organizations that had for many years operated as spaces for mediation between the efforts of scientists, the food industry's needs, and the solutions developed by local farmers. This network of influence was gradually incorporated by the state and ensured the Fascist regime's control over practices and innovation models, by targeting both conservative landowners and hesitant peasants in the march toward agricultural progress.

translated by Elaine Holt

BIBLIOGRAPHY

Bonneuil, Christophe. "'Pénétrer l'indigène': Arachides, paysans, agronomes et administrateurs coloniaux au Sénégal (1897–1950)." *Études rurales* 151–152 (July-December 1999): 199–223.

Bonneuil, Christophe, and Frédéric Thomas. "Purifying Landscapes: The Vichy Regime and the Genetic Modernization of France." *Historical Studies in the Natural Sciences* 40, no. 4 (2010): 532–568.

D'Onofrio, Federico. "The Microfoundations of Italian Agrarianism: Italian Agricultural Economists and Fascism." *Agricultural History* 91, no. 3 (2017): 369–396.

Harwood, Jonathan. *Europe's Green Revolution and Others Since: The Rise and Fall of Peasant-Friendly Plant Breeding.* London: Routledge, 2012.

Henke, Christopher R. *Cultivating Science, Harvesting Power: Science and Industrial Agriculture in California.* Cambridge, MA: MIT Press, 2008.

Herf, Jeffrey. *Reactionary Modernism. Technology, Culture, and Politics in Weimar and the Third Reich.* Cambridge: Cambridge University Press, 1984.

Moser, Peter, and Tony Varley, eds. *Integration through Subordination: The Politics of Agricultural Modernisation in Industrial Europe.* Turnhout: Brepols, 2013.

Saraiva, Tiago. *Fascist Pigs: Technoscientific Organisms and the History of Fascism.* Cambridge, MA: MIT Press, 2016.

PROPHYLAXIS
Singing to the Virgin for Protection from the Plague

Sergi Sancho Fibla

Since antiquity, many sources bear witness to prophylactic or curative practices implemented by song and instrumental music. This phenomenon is particularly seen in preventing the propagation of disease. The case of the antiphon *Stella Coeli* illustrates this practice against the spread of the plague, one of the most fatal diseases of the medieval and modern West. It is a Latin text extant in the fifteenth century in handwritten form, addressing a petition to God, asking him to put an end to an epidemic. The antiphon never had an official melody in liturgical books, but its wide circulation over the centuries has given rise to various local usage in the forms of songs, music, prayers, and processions.

At the end of the Middle Ages, the therapeutic power of music and song was rooted in concepts transmitted by Greco-Arab medicine, which mixed cosmology, natural philosophy of the elements, and study of the human body. For example, in *De artibus liberalibus*, Robert Grosseteste (circa 1175–1253) claims that healing illnesses is based upon restoring order and regularity, an exploit that may be achieved with sound. According to Grosseteste, the world order is made of audible measures and proportions, which when calculated precisely, may correct bodily and spiritual ailments.[1] The same notion of bodily harmonization through music is found in several writings of the time or later, such as the celebrated *Declaratio musicae disciplinae* by Ugolino of Orvieto (circa 1380–circa 1457).[2]

The proliferation of liturgical and devotional songs in the fourteenth and fifteenth centuries may be interpreted as so many ritualized responses to the consequences of the Black Death. Compositions of Italian *laude* and German *Geissler lieder*, originally sung by groups of flagellants, are noted examples. These practices are linked to the will to purify humans from sin and epidemics. At the same time, within church and monastery walls, a series of offices and prayers is developed with the same purpose. Characters to whom songs of popular piety and liturgical services are addressed are identical to devotional images: Saint Bartholomew, Saint Roch, Saint Sebastian, and especially Mary, who intercedes between human and divine realms. The antiphon *Stella Coeli* appears in this context. It is inscribed in votive images dedicated to the Virgin and these saints. For example, frescoes in the Church of San Martino in Fiume in Cesena, Emilia-Romagna, dating from the early sixteenth century, contain a series of paintings produced at the request of worshipers. Among these is the figure of the *Madonna del Latte*, the Nursing Madonna, over which a banner bears the first few words of the antiphon. Below, an inscription states that the image was commissioned in 1508 by Andrea de Bexache to thank the Virgin for having been spared during the plague epidemic.

This precise image of Mary breastfeeding Jesus is at the textual heart of the antiphon *Stella Coeli*. The song's subtitle mentions the challenge of the composition "against the contagious plague." A fifteenth-century book of hours explicitly defined the song as a prayer "contra pestem."[3] Thus, the antiphon was born and propagated against this principal scourge, although it has also been used against other contagious diseases. The text begins with an allusion to Mary, star of the sky, thereby establishing a correlation between cosmological harmony and the account of humanity's salvation. From its beginning, the song presents a dichotomous vision of the universe, articulated between order and chaos. Mary is praised for eradicating sin by breastfeeding Jesus Christ. This redemptive act reorders the chaos of contagion; it is the remedy against the "plague and ulcers of death" and against the "battle of the constellations," or cosmological disorder. The different strata of chaos are directly linked, with the stellar imbalance, moral debauchery of Christians, and disruption of physical health, causing contagion. In a symmetrical way, as more than just a model of virtue, the Virgin is a pure breastfeeding body and a star superior to all others. She is the effectual agent attaining equilibrium in all strata, that is to say, ending the epidemic.

The antiphon text was circulated orally and in handwritten and printed form. It was gradually included in liturgical and spiritual collections. Franciscans played a decisive role in its dissemination by early commitment to managing plague crises. Furthermore, the female branch of the order, especially the Order of the Poor Clares of Coimbra, is associated with a legend about the antiphon's origin. This story spread in the sixteenth and seventeenth centuries, found in many Franciscan chronicles as well as in loose sheets next to the printed text of the antiphon. Legend associates the creation of the antiphon with a miracle that would have occurred in Santa Clara-a-Velha in 1480, at the height of the plague epidemic in Coimbra. When the nuns were about to abandon the convent out of fear of contagion, a beggar whom they identified as Saint Bartholomew presented himself at the portal and gave the abbess the text of the *Stella Coeli*, stating that it must be sung each day. The abbess followed the instructions and the building was protected. Some versions even indicate that the entire city was healed. The effect of the antiphon thus oscillates between prevention and cure; by its range of action, it affects participants and their surroundings. The legend about the convent of Coimbra was then inserted in a chronicle of the Franciscan order by Fr. Gonzaga, published in Rome in 1587. This deed was undoubtedly the catalyst for a new impetus in circulating the antiphon among ecclesiastics, monks of all orders, and even laypeople. Some loose leaves and prints made in different European countries cite the chronicle, thereby bringing official recognition to this remedy against contagion.[4]

Like other devotional practices, including prayers, processions, and offerings of oblations, the antiphon has often been set to music for local usage and incorporated in the practice of abstinence. Several musical manuscripts from before the fifteenth century include a version. One of these has become a relic in the Santa Clara Convent where it is believed to have been written. In 1677, the nuns established a new house, Santa Clara-a-Nova. The altarpiece of the new building presents an image of the abbess and beggar, as well as two altars dedicated to the same saint, in the choir and church. According to a chronicle by Fr. M. de Esperança from 1666, the nuns sang the antiphon every day and organized an annual procession in homage to the saint. The monastery thus actively maintained the memory of its own legend. These practices may have been inherited from the old convent; perhaps they are also the result of reestablishing the rite in 1598 after a new plague epidemic. Either way, the antiphon then became the primary remedy against contagion and gradually spread across Europe.

In the seventeenth century, the antiphon was used again in the city of Barcelona during another plague epidemic. A ruling in 1651 bears witness to the decision by priests of the church of Santa Maria del Pi to sing the antiphon in thanks for their salvation. The song is then defined as a "custom of yesteryear of this church," suggesting a repeated use spread across time, according to necessity and epoch.[5] Here again, the practice is fixed in a ritual and enduring manner, to protect from future contagion but also to celebrate the Virgin to whom the institution is dedicated.

The use of the song against the epidemic is thus halfway between prophylactic practice, healing action, and memory process. The thin border separating sacred from profane spaces in which it could be exercised, as well as the vagueness of its radius of action, allowed it to be widely diffused in space and time, adapting to local situations and serving in protean form as an amulet, remedy, and commemoration against contagion.

translated by Benjamin Ivry

NOTES

1. Ludwig Baur, ed., *Die Philosophischen Werke Des Robert Grosseteste, Bischofs Von Lincoln* (Münster: Aschendorff, 1912), 4–5.

2. Albertus Seay, ed., *Ugolini Urbeuetanis, Declaratio Musicae Disciplinae*, vol. 1 (Rome: American Institute of Musicology, 1959), 15–16.

3. Paris, Bibliothèque nationale de France, lat. 18029, fol. 119v.

4. Among others, Père Léonard de Paris, "Office," in *La règle du Troisième Ordre* . . . (Paris: C. Huart, 1721), 115; *Breviarium Romanum ex decreto Sacro sancti Concilii Tridentini* . . . (Antwerp: N.p., 1752); separate sheet of the ASMP (Barcelona): C 699, uncatalogued.

5. Barcelona, Arxiu Parroquial de Santa Maria del Pi, B-362, Delib. 1651–1659, 8v–9r.

SELECTED BIBLIOGRAPHY

Esperança, Fr. Manuel de. *Historia Serafica da Ordem dos Frades Menores* . . . Vol. 2. Lisbon: Antonio Craesbeeck de Mello, 1666.

Gonzaga, Francesco. *De origine seraphicae religionis Franciscanae eiusque progressibus* . . . Roma: N.p., 1587.

Horden, Peregrine. *Music as Medicine: The History of Music Therapy since Antiquity.* Aldershot: Ashgate, 2000.

Macklin, Christopher. "Plague, Performance, and the Elusive History of the Stella Celi Extirpavit." *Early Music History*, 29 (2010): 1–31. https://doi.org/10.1017/SO26112790000057.

Sandon, Nick. "Mary, Meditations, Monks and Music: Poetry, Prose, Processions and Plagues in a Durham Cathedral Manuscript." *Early Music* 10 (January 1982): 43–55. https://doi.org/10.1093/earlyj/10.1.43.

RACE

The Discourse on "Blood Contamination" in Colonial Britain

Silvia Sebastiani

The notion of "contamination" is discernible in the vast array of eighteenth-century writings that attempt to address the issue of the differences among peoples. The line of thought exposed by Edward Long (1734–1813), an English-born planter in Jamaica, in his *History of Jamaica* (1774) is paradigmatic in this respect. His use of the terms "contamination" and "contagion" in reference to both diseases and mixed unions between Black and white people help show how theories on the risk of contamination of the blood of white people were prevalent in mixed societies at a time when the first abolitionist legislation was being developed.

Samuel Johnson's *Dictionary of the English Language* (first edition, 1755) defines the verb *to contaminate* as "to defile; to pollute; to corrupt by base mixture," while the word *contamination* was explained as "pollution; defilement."[1] In the eighteenth century, a contamination was therefore a corruption, a perversion, a deformation, a disturbance, a stain, and an infection, directly evoking the notion of contagion and the spread of disease. Both the verb and noun forms were ubiquitous in language describing the construction of racial categories at that time. Johnson's dictionary also defines *race* as "family descending," "a generation," "a collective family," and "a particular breed": in so doing, it makes traditional associations with lineage and procreation.

To talk about *race* in the eighteenth century was to tread on shifting and unstable semantic terrain, because the term was used with multiple, ambiguous meanings in a wide variety of sources. An interest in race was not the exclusive territory of any one group—even less so of scholars—and could be observed in very diverse social settings. These entangled layers of discourse led to many language associations, as attested by the word *contamination*.

The notion of race was rooted in the belief that the foundations of the differences among human groups were not (only) social but (also) natural. Within this framework, the moral or social characteristics of both individuals and peoples were passed down from generation to generation through various body tissues or fluids (blood, sperm, milk). As a result, individuals remained locked into behaviors embedded in their physical bodies. Racial thinking imprisoned individuals in the "race" to which they were supposed to belong; this assignment, in turn, outweighed any differences in their social experiences. The idea of physiological transmission was therefore central to racial discourse: this could be taken literally (i.e., inherited qualities were actually carried in the blood) or more metaphorically (referring to a vague notion of inheritance incorporating both the physical attributes and the social effects of belonging to a lineage).

The ancient idea of fluids being able to corrupt and contaminate progeny took on a new meaning in the Enlightenment, when, for the first time, humans were integrated into the animal kingdom and classified as such. Carl Linnaeus's *Systema Naturae* (first edition in 1735) and Buffon's *Histoire Naturelle* (1749–1788) show this process well: although they used conflicting methods, both considered humanity outside the biblical framework. With this radical new approach, they shifted the focus to the human body, placing it within the same system of knowledge as the rest of the natural world. Consequently, physical dissimilarities became markers of essential differences. The naturalization of humans and even the possibility of studying them as a natural entity contributed to the division of humanity into distinct "races."

The race-related vocabulary of the Enlightenment became part of the colonial empire's everyday language. This was best illustrated by Long, who also served as a judge in Jamaica's Vice Admiralty Court, the court having local jurisdiction in British colonies. As one of the most fervent defenders of the slave trade and the institution of slavery, Long has been called the father of English racism. After living in Jamaica from 1757 to 1769 to manage his family's plantations, he returned to England to find a different political atmosphere, one that was more favorable to antislavery views and challenged the "right" to own enslaved people. Long's *Candid Reflections* were his immediate protest against the Somerset ruling (1772), which extended *habeas corpus*—a right previously afforded only to the British—to the enslaved. In the pamphlet, he accused the judge Lord Mansfield of inventing "the art of washing the Black-a-moor white."[2] In his *History of Jamaica*, published two years later, Long borrowed from the legal language of the colonists' rights and freedoms to defend Jamaica's significant contribution to England's prosperity and the necessity of slavery to maintain it. To justify the "servitude" of Africans, however, Long used the medical vocabulary of a contamination of "white blood."

For the polygenist Long, "Negroes" formed a distinctly different species of humanity and were by nature inferior to the "White man." Pointing to the close similarity between Africans and orangutans, insisting on their mating and consanguinity, and alerting to the dangers of sexual intercourse between Black and white people, he warned against the social disintegration of Jamaica, England, and all of "white civilisation." Although he saw "races" as fundamentally unchanging, timeless, and static, he believed they could be altered through degeneration and interbreeding. Africans were placed outside of history, yet they could enter it indirectly by causing a decline of the "white race." "Contamination" was therefore a key concept in Long's worldview, marked by an obsession with the sexual relations of "white men of every rank cohabiting with Negresses and Mulattas, free or slaves," which produced "a vast addition of spurious offspring of different complexions" and a "yellow offspring not their own." The mixing of "black and white" went against nature, since they were "two tinctures which nature has dissociated, like oil and vinegar."[3]

This wake-up call to the dangers of degeneration through contamination was sounded against the backdrop of Jamaican laws, which recognized the children of third-generation Africans as having the same privileges and immunities as whites. As Long deplored, these descendants "are called English, and consider themselves as free from all taint of the Negroe race."

The example of Spanish America provided a historical reference: due to their failed colonization, the Spanish had produced "a vicious, brutal, and degenerate breed of mongrels." To avoid a similar fate, Long encouraged the "white men of that colony" to free themselves from the "goatish embraces" of "black women" and "perform the duty incumbent on every good citizen, by raising in honourable wedlock a race of unadulterated beings."[4]

In *Candid Reflections*, Long addressed the issue of the tainting of blood, not just in the colonial world but also inside his home country. England itself was already contaminated, or at least so were its lower classes. In addition to differences between races, he pointed out differences between social classes, mixed with a dose of sexism: the staining of the "race" was the doing of white women of lower classes who engaged in intercourse with Black men, the latter being assimilated with horses or donkeys. Thus, between Africans and apes, a continuum between humans and animals took shape, with positions determined by race, social class, and gender. According to Long, mixing could transform "the whole nation" into "the Portuguese and the Moriscos in complexion of skin and baseness of mind. This is a venomous and dangerous ulcer, that threatens to disperse its malignancy far and wide, until every family catches infection from it."[5] For Long, the integration of Black people in England, the country of freedom, would unleash a sickness on the entire society.

Proslavery planters were not alone in their alarm over the contamination of "white blood." Infection was also a central concern for the founding fathers of the United States. Although he supported the emancipation of the enslaved, Thomas Jefferson presented the corruption of blood of white people as a new dilemma for the history of humanity, in his *Notes on the State of Virginia*. Unlike the (white) enslaved of the Roman world, the Black enslaved, once freed, must be forbidden to intermingle: "When freed, he [the Negro] is to be removed beyond the reach of mixture." The corollary of this reasoning was that the difference between whites and Blacks was fixed in "nature."[6] However, an assertion that Black people were naturally inferior did not automatically translate into an approval of slavery—not in Jefferson's case nor for the majority of polygenists, ranging from Voltaire to David Hume.

Monogenism did not settle the issue of color either. Benjamin Rush, a physician in Philadelphia, active abolitionist, and professed monogenist, considered Black skin to be the sign of a treatable disease. In his "Observations," which he shared with the American Philosophical Society as of 1792 before their publication in 1799, Blackness was caused by a hereditary illness, leprosy, of which Africans could be cured if put in a favorable environmental and social setting.[7] "Race" had become a medical problem: it was the role of the physician to find a treatment to rid Black people of the "infection" and to end contamination. Seen as a physical question coupled with a risk of contagion, the "race" issue prompted not only a division between human groups but also a hierarchy among them, by separating those who were "pure" from those who threatened the purity of others.

translated by Elaine Holt

NOTES

1. Samuel Johnson, *A Dictionary of the English Language* (1st ed., 1755), 6th ed. (London: J. F. And C. Rivington, et al., 1785).

2. Edward Long, *Candid Reflections upon the Judgment Lately Awarded by the Court of King's Bench in Westminster Hall on What Is Commonly Called The Negroe Cause, by a Planter* (London: T. Lowndes, 1772), iii.

3. Long, *The History of Jamaica*, vol. 2 (London: T. Lowndes, 1774), 327–328, 332.

4. Long, *The History of Jamaica*, 328.

5. Long, *Candid Reflections upon the Judgment*, 48.

6. Thomas Jefferson, *Notes on the State of Virginia*, ed. William Peden (Chapel Hill: University of North Carolina Press, 1955), queries VI and XIV.

7. Benjamin Rush, "Observations Intended to Favor a Supposition That the Black Color (as It Is Called) of the Negroes Is Derived from Leprosy," *Transactions of the American Philosophical Society* 4 (1799): 289–297.

SELECTED BIBLIOGRAPHY

Curran, Andrew. *The Anatomy of Blackness: Science and Slavery in an Age of Enlightenment.* Baltimore: Johns Hopkins University Press, 2011.

Hall, Catherine. "Whose Memories? Edward Long and the Work of Re-Remembering." In *Britain's History and Memory of Transatlantic Slavery*, edited by Katie Donington, Ryan Hanley, and Jessica Moody, 129–149. Oxford: Oxford University Press, 2016.

Lafont, Anne. *L'Art et la race: L'Africain (tout) contre l'œil des Lumières*. Dijon: Les Presses du réel, 2019.

Müller-Wille, Staffan, and Hans-Jörg Rheinberger, eds. *Heredity Produced: At the Crossroads of Biology, Politics, and Culture (1500–1870)*. Cambridge, MA: MIT Press, 2007.

Newman, Brooke N. *Dark Inheritance: Blood, Race, and Sex in Colonial Jamaica*. New Haven: Yale University Press, 2018.

Schaub, Jean-Frédéric. *Pour une histoire politique de la race*. Paris: Éditions du Seuil, 2015.

Sebastiani, Silvia. "Challenging Boundaries: Apes and Savages in Enlightenment." In *Simianization: Apes, Gender, Class, and Race*, edited by Wulf D. Hund, Charles W. Mills, and Silvia Sebastiani, 105–137. Berlin: Lit Verlag, 2015.

Seth, Suman. *Difference and Disease: Medicine, Race, and the Eighteenth-Century British Empire*. Cambridge: Cambridge University Press, 2018.

RED GUARDS
August 1966: Social and Ideological Violence in Mao's China

Sebastian Veg

Throughout the Red August of 1966, violence carried out by groups of students against holders of authority (teachers, party cadres, intellectuals) or politically proscribed individuals spread across Peking. It took the form of public "struggle" sessions, home searches, and physical acts of violence, claiming over one thousand lives in one month against a backdrop of mass demonstrations by Red Guards on Tiananmen Square. Both witnesses and historians often describe this revolutionary violence as "contagious." What, then, were the social and intellectual mechanisms for mass mobilization and the spreading of violence? The historiography of the Cultural Revolution has undergone a significant renewal over recent years, which we shall attempt to examine here.

Students began to mobilize on campuses during May 1966, echoing attacks against three intellectuals accused of having criticized Mao. It was among the students that the term "Red Guard" first appeared, on a *dazibao* (big character poster) at the secondary school attached to Tsinghua University. On May 25, professors in the department of philosophy at Peking University, encouraged behind the scenes by an emissary of Mao, pasted up the "first Marxist-Leninist *dazibao*," accusing the university's president of counterrevolutionary sympathies. The text was immediately reprinted by the *People's Daily* and broadcast on radio on Mao's initiative.

Throughout June, work teams were sent to universities by the central government. The work teams generally joined the students in attacking heads of administration and academic authorities. Acts of violence then occurred on campuses, notably in struggle sessions where the accused were made to wear a dunce's cap. Yet the teams also attempted to control the student movement, even locking up some radical students. Mao seized on this pretext to come out of his southern retreat, return to Peking on July 18, and give orders to all work teams to withdraw from campuses and release the arrested rebels. At the eleventh Plenum of the eighth Central Committee that opened on August 1, Mao violently took to task president Liu Shaoqi and praised the *dazibaos* pasted up on campuses, in comments published on August 5 under the title "Bombard the Headquarters." The "Decision of the Central Committee on the Great Proletarian Cultural Revolution" (also known as the "Sixteen Points") was adopted on August 8 and was immediately broadcast on radio and published in the press; its fourth point called for "the liberation of the masses by themselves" without fear of provoking "chaos." A directive adopted by the Central Committee on May 16 had already emphasized that the fight against the bourgeoisie was a "life and death" struggle and designated five categories of targets: professors, teachers, artists, journalists, and publishers. When the Plenum drew to a close on August 12, mass violence was spreading in Peking, an outbreak that historians directly attribute to Mao's injunctions to the Red Guards.

Red August began with a sadly famous incident. On August 5, at the secondary school for girls attached to Peking Normal University (attended by the daughters of high-placed party leaders, notably Deng Xiaoping), the deputy headmistress Bian Zhongyun was tortured for several hours by fifth-form pupils before being subjected to a hail of blows and left for dead in a refuse trolley. By the time someone had finally plucked up the courage to transport her to the neighboring hospital, she was pronounced dead on arrival. One of the pupils involved in the violence, according to several witnesses, was Song Binbin, the daughter of General Song Renqiong, member of the Politburo.

The first mass demonstration of Red Guards occurred on August 18, hailing Mao in front of the Gate of Heavenly Peace (Tiananmen). At the rostrum, Song Binbin presented Mao with a Red Guard armband, receiving his congratulations. In the course of the month following August 18, it is estimated that 114,000 homes were searched and 44.8 million yuan in cash and objects of value confiscated as well as 2.3 million books and 3.3 million paintings. Some books were publicly burned. Violence reached a climax in the last week of August with roughly 200 deaths per day. The official count was established at 1,772 deaths in August and September in Peking.[1]

How have historians gone about documenting and explaining the violence? Two classic interpretations have been put forward. A group of sociologists (around Anita Chan and Jonathan Unger), working at the end of the 1970s from interviews with former Red Guards who had taken refuge in Hong Kong, places the emphasis on conflicts between social strata within communist society. In the secondary schools of Canton, growing tension set the children of the "intelligentsia" against those of the red political elite who had ended up monopolizing the opportunities for entering the Communist Youth League and universities. The emergence of two factions of Red Guards mirrored the fracture between the children of high cadres (joining "loyalist" Red Guards, often tied to the league) and the children of the intelligentsia whose achievements at school were good but whose political pedigree was only average (joining the "rebels" taking issue with the privileges of the authorities in place, and notably with the parents of their loyalist fellow pupils). If the summer of 1966 was dominated by the loyalists, the excessive drift toward caste discrimination (the "theory of blood lineage") was disavowed by Mao, to such an extent that the rebels regained the upper hand in the autumn. Viewed through this prism, factional violence is understood as the expression of a "class war."

The converse thesis, defended by another sociologist, Andrew Walder, insists on the importance of networks and political clientelism. Examining the Red Guard newspapers published on the university campuses of Peking, Walder holds that there was no direct correlation between "class" membership (in the sense of the categories applied by the regime) and the constitution of Red Guard factions. It was, rather, the reaction to political events on the campuses (the arrival of work teams) and beyond (factional struggles at the party summit) that determined students' choices in seeking to maximize their own interest by interpreting as best they could the coded signals emanating from the seat of power. As proof of this, Walder points to the fact that, as soon as one group landed a decisive victory over another, the victorious group in turn split into factions. Viewed through this prism, it was, above all, the endless factional conflicts that generated the ever-increasing violence.

Drawing on recent interviews with former Red Guards, the historian Xiaowei Zheng has attempted to go beyond this dichotomy and reintroduce the dimension of individual choice, through the study of Tsinghua University in Peking. Zheng stresses the importance of ideological convictions and the sincerity of political commitment of certain students. It was, for example, their passion for the contradictory aspects of Mao's thought, she argues, that led them to clash in the name of different ideals. She also underlines that students were responsible for acts that were increasingly remote from their convictions.

The historian Youqin Wang has conducted several hundred interviews with former secondary school and university students. For her, it was the verbal violence of the *dazibaos* that unleashed the physical violence on the campuses. The decision by Mao to withdraw the work teams at the end of July opened the way to an escalation, encouraged by the authorities (Jiang Qing), which spread from the campuses to the entire town and then to the whole country, targeting administrators, teachers, people with "political problems," and anyone who might have offended a Red Guard. Participation in acts of violence was seen as a privilege reserved to the "reddest" students, others having to settle for tasks such as surveilling prisoners. The collective dimension of violence consequently fostered rivalry among group members as well as a sense of impunity for individuals taking part in the collective.

These conclusions are confirmed by research based on oral history (Sang Ye) and memoirs published in informal journals such as *Jiyi* (*Memory*) or semi-official ones such as *Yanhuang Chunqiu* (*Annals of the Yellow Emperor*), which, until muzzled in 2016, contained a special section entitled "Confessions." It published the accounts of numerous perpetrators of violence, ranging from a sixth-form pupil who killed a classmate by throwing a brick at his head to another who denounced a fellow boarding school student by stealing his diary and handing it in to the authorities to a man who denounced his mother, thus leading to her execution. Violence penetrated to the very heart of families.

If "contagion" is perhaps not the best metaphor for describing the spread of political violence, it is because such violence follows social and intellectual mechanisms. The ideological and linguistic violence propagated in official documents throughout the Mao era, the underlying class conflicts in communist society, and a group logic that made violence into an object of rivalry and exculpated individuals from all responsibility are the three aspects most clearly established by historians.

translated by David M. Thomas

NOTE

1.   *Beijing Daily*, December 20, 1980.

SELECTED BIBLIOGRAPHY

Chan, Anita, Stanley Rosen, and Jonathan Unger. "Students and Class Warfare: The Social Roots of the Red Guard Conflict in Canton." *China Quarterly* 83 (September 1980): 397–446.

MacFarquhar, Roderick, and Michael Schoenhals. *Mao's Last Revolution*. Cambridge, MA: Belknap Press of Harvard University, 2006.

Sang, Ye. *1949, 1989, 1999*. Hong Kong: Oxford University Press, 1999.

Su, Yang. *Collective Killings in Rural China during the Cultural Revolution*. Cambridge: Cambridge University Press, 2011.

Veg, Sebastian. "Confessing and Repenting: The Chanhuilu Column of Yanhuang Chunqiu." In *Transitional Justice without Transition*, edited by Daniel Leese, forthcoming, 2021.

Walder, Andrew. *Fractured Rebellion: The Beijing Red Guard Movement*. Cambridge, MA: Harvard University Press, 2009.

Wang, Youqin. "Student Attacks against Teachers: The Revolution of 1966." *Issues and Studies* 37, no. 2 (March/April 2001): 29–79.

Zheng, Xiaowei. "Passion, Reflection, Survival: Political Choices of Red Guards at Qinghua University, June 1966–July 1968." In *The Chinese Cultural Revolution as History*, edited by Joseph Esherick, Paul Pickowicz, and Andrew Walder, 29–63. Stanford: Stanford University Press, 2006.

RELICS
Contagious Virtue of Sacred Bodies
Nicolas Sarzeaud

In June 1619, while exorcizing several demons in the Champagne region, Father Prinet was afflicted by sudden illness. His acolyte Blaise Mahon recalled that the priest had carried with him a "small image of the Holy Shroud [of Besançon], sanctified by having touched the sacred model." The image soothed Father Prinet and liberated the possessed people. In 1624, Jean-Jacques Chifflet, a man of letters from the Franche-Comté region, reported this miracle, asking "Why, if a magnet has the power to communicate its attractive property to iron that is applied to it, wouldn't Holy Relics possess the same honour?"[1]

In Christianity, the bodies of holy persons, dead or alive, are charged with a miraculous energy or *virtus*, transmitted to things surrounding them. This principle is found in the Gospels, with the episode of Jesus healing the bleeding woman whose hemorrhage ceases when she touches his cloak (Matthew 9:20–22, Mark 5:25–34, Luke 8:46–48). Like a magnet, a thaumaturgical energy is drawn from the body of Christ that is transmitted through the textile interface, since Christ says, "Someone touched me; I know that power [*virtutem* in the Vulgate] has gone out from me" (Luke 8:46).[2] The Acts of the Apostles report that "God did extraordinary miracles through Paul" (Acts 19:11) and "handkerchiefs and aprons that had touched him were taken to the sick, and their illnesses were cured and the evil spirits left them" (Acts 19:12). A chain of virtue is thereby organized, from God who is the source, through Christ, Saint Paul, and the objects they touch.

Ethnologists have created models of these energy flows. Alfred Gell, discussing the sympathetic magic of James Frazer (*The Golden Bough*, 1890–1935) proposes the concept of a *distributed person* pertinent to our purpose: the saint's *virtus* is distributed through the objects he touched. We can also use the concept of contagion, advanced by Deleuze and Guattari as an alternative to the concept of a world through filiation: "The vampire does not filiate, it infects. The difference is that contagion, epidemic, involves terms that are entirely heterogeneous: for example, a human being, an animal, and a bacterium, a virus, a molecule, a microorganism."[3] This is one of the distinctive features of the thaumaturgical economy of relics: it does not merely diffuse between objects of the same nature, from body to body or image to image. From the beginnings of Christianity, pilgrims bring back soil from sacred places and holy water from the Jordan River or sanctuaries as well as shards infected with the *virtus*' factors in sacred history. Throughout the Middle Ages, shrines produced pilgrim flasks, or ampullae, that could contain holy matter or pilgrim badges made of lead alloy, cast with images evoking the holy person and applied against reliquaries. They are efficacious souvenirs, used as devotional supports and amulets protecting their wearers.

In the year 594 CE, Gregory the Great (Pope Gregory I) apologizes to Constantina, empress consort of Maurice of the Byzantine Empire, for being unable to send the skull of Saint Paul that was venerated in Rome.[4] Gregory affirms that Roman custom is to not divide relics but rather to touch them with strips of cloth (*brandea*) before depositing them into their intended shrine as contact relics. The argument is primarily intended to reject the impossible request by the empress of the Byzantine Empire. Contrary to what Gregory claims, Latin Christianity does divide relics; nevertheless, the distribution of textile fragments that had touched relics of a saint is well attested during the Middle Ages. For example, in several sanctuaries, fragments are found of the twill damask that enveloped the prestigious remains of the Three Kings of Cologne.

Since the era of the Gospels, linens have been privileged objects for transporting *virtus*, by their bodily intimacy and permeability, but many other substances may become *supramaterial* in the sense that Caroline

Walker Bynum used that word. For example, there are distillations, holy water in which bones have been left to infuse. We can cite the exceptional case of the water of Saint Thomas, in which the blood of the martyr of Canterbury who has just died is diluted. Texts describe the protective role of these ampullae suspended in churches and houses and the wonders of Canterbury medicine (*medicina Cantuariensis*). When a devotee is in grave danger, like Everard, Chaplain of St. Mary's in Winchester, water of St. Thomas is sought in the vicinity and is consumed as a remedy.[5] Just as shrines produce and market wine ampullae and pilgrim badges, the faithful also create relics by touching sacred bodies with their wands, rosaries, and other objects. Evidence of this may be seen in sixteenth-century prohibitions against throwing objects at relics during their ostension.

How do these objects work? In Chifflet's narrative, the image of the shroud is the conductor of the *virtus* of the model that it imitates and has touched. The shroud is a distributed relic, operating remotely through its replica. In some cases, we observe a change in status and in the nature of the object experienced; *virtus* does not just circulate, it also transmits. Gregory states that when any doubt existed about the quality of *brandea* as relics, his predecessor Leo the Great (St. Leo I) would make an incision in them until they started to bleed. This signals a profound change in the very materiality of linen, which not only captures energy, sanctifying it, but in turn becomes a miraculous body. The Besançon shroud is itself a copy of the Shroud of Turin but emerged after its first appearance in 1523 as a relic independent of its model; here, the transmitted body is equivalent to the body that transmitted it, not simply a conductive stone but rather a new magnet.

Due to this infectious *virtus*, the sacred bodies multiply, parallel to the Eucharistic economy to which they are linked; on the one hand, there is a ubiquity of relics, capable of acting through third-party objects, and on the other hand an overall inflation of sacred material. The Christian world conversion project includes materials turning into sacred bodies, bit by bit.

In a naturalistic society, relics and images do not function, because only humans are gifted with intentionality. In animism, the environment is populated with spirits, images, and bones that therefore contain an effective personality. According to Philippe Descola, until the seventeenth century, the Christian West was marked by a tendency to analogy, an intermediate ontology: in Creation, there is not a direct continuity between the human and his environment but "a chain of beings" hierarchized by games of analogies and resemblances, for example, between the functioning of the human organism and that of the elements or planets.

What about our contaminated items? In *Le corps des images*, Jean-Claude Schmitt recalls the way in which theologians anxious to avoid idolatry, that is, the veneration of the image of the saint and not of the saint himself, justify the bodily life of these weeping images, speak, bleed, care: for them, images and relics are simple auxiliaries allowing intercession. What occurs in the melee between the faithful and the image or the remains of the saint is only the terrestrial reflection of a miraculous operation strictly celestial. Both the correspondence between distinct spheres and the constitution of chains of objects correspond to an analogical ontology. However, during these virtuous contagions by which relics transform multiple objects into holy bodies, given to touch, to make touch, to ingest, it is in matter that clerics and the faithful draw energy from the saint. These practices therefore result from a tension between analogism, as defined by Descola, and an animism of images and objects.

If the Council of Trent (1545–1563) strictly confines images and relics to a role of auxiliary of intercession, there are always many cases, in the post-Tridentine period and in modernity, of objects brought into contact with relics and working miracles. However, we can spot a mutation using the introductory example of the Shroud of Besançon, a copy that has become a relic. In the miracle reported by Chifflet, his image is only the conducting channel of his virtues, but the image does not become a new relic. Thus, the shrouds are always copied and their images loaded by contact with the relic, but from the seventeenth century, none of these copies became a new Holy Shroud.

The entry into the modern era does not therefore mark the end of the virtuous contagion, which continues to operate. But this contagion no longer has the appearance of the vampire contagion, dear to Deleuze and Guattari, which induces a metamorphosis of the contaminated object. It seems to be limited to a magnetic contagion, to use Chifflet's formula. The relic acts through conductive objects. We can read there a rigidification of the analogical hierarchy between the saint with the celestial stay, his terrestrial remains and the objects having touched his remains, parallel to the rigidification of the dualism of the soul and the body that leads to contemporary naturalism.

translated by Benjamin Ivry

NOTES

1. Jean-Jacques Chifflet, *Hierothonie de Jésus-Christ, ou Discours des saincts suaires de Nostre Seigneur* (Paris: Cramoisy, 1631), 74 and 76, translation of *De linteis sepulchralis*, 1624. See Paola von Wyss-Giacosa, "Between Erudition and Faith: Jean-Jacques Chifflet's Tract on the Shroud of Besançon (1624)," *Journal for Religion, Film and Media* 5, no. 1 (2019): 47–68. The magnetic metaphor is also present in writings by Wilhelm Gumppenberg. See Ralph Dekoninck, "Une science expérimentale des images mariales: La *Peritia* de l'*Atlas Marianus* de Eilhelm Gumppenberg," *Revue de l'histoire des religions* 2 (2015): 135–154.

2. [All citations from Scripture are from the New International Version.—Trans.]

3. Gilles Deleuze and Felix Guattari, *A Thousand Plateaus: Capitalism and Schizophrenia*, vol. 2, trans. Brian Massumi (Minneapolis: University of Minnesota Press, 1987), 266–267.

4. Gregory the Great, "Epistolae," IV. 30, Patrologia Latina, 77, col. 702 A–B.

5. Several of these miracles are recounted in "Passio et miracula S. Thomae Cantuariensis" by Benedict, Abbot of Peterborough as discussed by Pierre-André Sigal in "Naissance et premier développement d'un vinage exceptionnel: L'eau de saint Thomas," *Cahiers de civilization médiévale* 44, no. 173 (2001): 35–44.

SELECTED BIBLIOGRAPHY

Bruna, Denis, ed. *Enseignes de pèlerinage et enseignes profanes*. Paris: Réunion des Musées Nationaux, 1996.

Bynum, Caroline. *Christian Materiality: An Essay on Religion in Late Medieval Europe*. New York: Zone Books, 2015.

Deleuze, Gilles, and Félix Guattari. *A Thousand Plateaus: Capitalism and Schizophrenia*, vol. 2. Trans. Brian Massumi. Minneapolis: University of Minnesota Press, 1987.

Descola, Philippe. *Par-delà nature et culture*. Paris: Gallimard, 2005.

Frank, Georgia. *The Memory of the Eyes: Pilgrims to Living Saints in Christian Late Antiquity.* Berkeley: University of California Press, 2000.

Gell, Alfred. *Art and Agency: An Anthropological Theory.* Oxford: Clarendon Press, 1998.

Martiniani-Reber, Marielle. "Le rôle des étoffes dans le culte des reliques au Moyen Âge." *Bulletin du CIéTA* 70 (1992): 53–58.

Sarzeaud, Nicolas. "Les tombeaux ouverts: Montrer les corps saints à la fin du Moyen Âge." *Images Re-vues* 16 (2019). http://journals.openedition.org/imagesrevues/6911.

Schmitt, Jean-Claude. *Le corps des images: Essai sur la culture visuelle au Moyen Âge.* Paris: Gallimard, 2002.

REVOLUTION

The "French Contagion" and "Jewish Jacobinery" in the Writings of Italian Antirevolutionaries

Davide Mano

The medieval stereotype of the "Jewish dog," the Jew at the margins of society who was filthy and contagious, the origins of which go back to the twelfth century, was a tenacious stereotype that endured well beyond the Middle Ages. It was at the root of anti-Jewish accusations in the mid-fourteenth century following the pandemic of the Black Death. It still played a role at the beginning of the Early Modern period when the first ghettos were created—places of enforced confinement for Jews alone, designed to achieve a physical separation from their Christian neighbors. It reappeared in various forms at the very end of the Early Modern period with the upsurge in anti-Jewish violence during the revolutionary transition, most notably in the context of counter-revolutionary riots. The image of "Jewish contagion" was at that time used to demonize "the Jew," not only by reference to his religious conviction (held to be "obstinacy" in falsehood) or to his marginal par excellence nature but also by reference to his political vision, namely his presumed desire to destroy Christianity, to overthrow its power system and its model of social order.

The fear of political overthrow lay at the root of Italian antirevolution-aries' anxieties and obsessions. Coming into being from 1789–1792, the idea of an anti-Christian revolutionary conspiracy reached its apogee in 1796–1797 with the first Napoleonic Italian campaign and again in 1799–1800 with the second campaign, which was particularly marked by violent internal riots designated as "counterrevolutionary." These manifestations of violence had a very important anti-Jewish aspect. In the eyes of the "Holy

Faith" rioters, the stereotype of Jewish contagion was, in effect, the cumulation of various vectors of contamination: those coming from external enemies, that is, "French (moral and political) depravity," combined with those coming from internal enemies, that is, Italian "Jacobins" or "patriots" holding sympathy with transalpine ideas.

In characterizing the "French contagion," antirevolutionary language frequently drew on medical vocabulary. Among the best-known publications it is worth mentioning *L'épidémie française*, a satire published in 1790 and translated into Italian three years later.[1] As for the *Annali di Roma*, a periodical likewise camped on antirevolutionary ground, in 1792 they portrayed the situation of the Austrian Empire following the premature death of Leopold II as being that of a power attacked by "an epidemic illness" that had "contaminated the air" and whose progress "had to be halted" so that "the French contagion does not spread over all of Europe and cause thrones to topple."[2] According to one Venetian literary journal, among the consequences of the French contagion, account had to be taken of the "perversion of the organisation of the body" and of "the influence of moral and religious perversion" spilling over to "the physical." It went on to say that "once the sentiments of religion are lost, man becomes atheistic or deistic or materialistic," he "abandons himself to the empire of passions" and to "the predominance of voluptuous pleasure."[3]

In the eyes of antirevolutionaries, this disorder was equally the result of a "perverted" dress code and "immoral" economics. French fashion, as well as the "dissolute mores and customs of the French" provoked profound disquiet among the conservative writers of Europe. This "abominable French fashion" transformed "women into prostitutes and men into sodomites while destroying the rusticity of national dress." To the same extent, partisans of free trade were identified as "wreckers of homes," labeled "fucking barons rigged out as enemies of humanity" and "cannibals" at the head of a "plague-striking Hydra."[4]

The condemnation of revolutionary mores included description of the debauched activities of Italian Jacobins. In the clubs frequented by "Jews, dissolute youths and libertines of every class," one felt free to attack "with impunity the sacred dogmas of the Religion of our ancestors." "Depravity of the soul" and "corruption of the heart" were rife there, and "exercises in seduction, scandal, impiety, irreligion, subversion and infamy" were common practice.[5]

The French contagion was ultimately synonymous with an irreligious "fanaticism" manifested in the form of a "persecution" of the Christian religion.[6] Jacobinism was bound up with Jansenism to form a "superb machination" whose objective was to bring down Christian tradition. For antirevolutionaries they were dealing with a veritable conspiracy where "the Jews" counted among its foremost partisans "not people merely different in their beliefs with respect to Catholic Religion, but conspirators and occult co-operators seeking to bring it down," obstinate followers of the "contempt for Religion, that is to say, of the Tree of mad political liberty" that they "tended in order to nail to it and hang from it the faithful disciples of Our Saviour Jesus Christ."[7]

The infidelity of Jews, considered particularly "ignominious," constituted the synthesis of all the evils peddled by revolutionaries to the greater detriment of Catholic tradition. For some Italian antirevolutionary authors, "Jewish Jacobinery" condensed in a single "body" the most extreme social expressions of irreligiousness and anti-Christian conspiracy, combining the Frenchman, the Jacobin, and the Jew. One of those authors, Giovan Battista Chrisolino reproved the Jews twice over in calling them "bi-Jacobins, that is to say, by birth and by choice of side." Their irrevocable fault was compared to that of certain "sick people having only themselves to blame for their misfortune," for "he who has come out of Egypt and has been delivered from the barbarian people yet who desires to return there, in the image of Jewish madmen, is not a man of probity but a true Egyptian."[8]

"Opinion," or the fact of taking the side of Revolution, was portrayed as a kind of substantial physical and moral infirmity from which it was far from easy to recover. Such an infirmity had spread by contagion, or, in the singular case of the Jews, it had been inherited from birth. In a satirical play published in Milan in 1799, two "citizens" called Gradasso and Sbrega meet up to take the thermal waters and treat their decidedly modern malady:

Sbrega   What, then, is your illness?

Gradasso   It is, I imagine, of the same nature as the illness of all those who, like we two, still support the chimerical system of equality, and that in spite of universal hatred and execration.

Sbrega   And would you call it a physical illness?

Gradasso   Well, what synonym would you give for it, then?

Sbrega   An opinion which makes us more inclined to one system rather than another, you judge that to be an illness, do you?

Gradasso   Every time systems are not linked to reason, justice and the universal good, it is to be feared that this very same reason can suffer from dizziness and that the frequency of these dizzy spells can progressively take on the character of a chronic illness known by the name of infirmity of opinion. . . . When the mass of blood is already corrupted by an inveterate habit it is most difficult for a cure lasting only a few days to restore to good health a patient who has been infected by this baneful epidemic.[9]

The use of the notion of "contagion" in the writings of Italian anti-revolutionaries thus rests on an implicit comparison with illness. As an event that went "against the nature of things," Revolution brought about a disorganization of man's vital functions, irreparably altering his physical and moral health. The sole remedy envisaged by the counter-revolutionary rioters of 1799 was violence and murder, seen as a treatment for the traditional community that would purify it through the putting to death of the spreaders of contagion, the external and internal enemies. First and foremost, that meant the *bi-Jacobins*, which is to say the Jews.

translated by David M. Thomas

NOTES

1.   *La epidemia francese, ovvero La monarchia e la religione quasi distrutte dall'Assemblea nazionale* (Da una Città Anti-Anarchica l'anno 1793 nella Tipografia della Verità).

2.   *Annali di Roma: Da gennaro a tutto aprile dell'anno 1792*, vol. 6 (Rome, 1792).

3.   *Memorie per servire alla storia letteraria e civile*, May 1796, Venice.

4. Municipal Archives of Pitigliano, *Vicariato, 1799–1800*, booklet 3/F, Proclamation "Digitus Dei Est Hic" by Pietro Ceccarelli (Orvieto, July 10, 1799).

5. Giovanni Chrisolino, *Insurrezione dell'Inclita e Valorosa Città di Arezzo mirabilmente seguita il di 6 maggio 1799 contro la forza delle armi e delle frodi dell'Anarchia Francese* . . . (Città di Castello: Francesco Donati e Bartolomeo Carlucci, 1799), 34.

6. *Il fanatismo della Lingua rivoluzionaria* . . . *Opera interessante di Gian Francesco Laharpe, volgarizzata a disinganno degl'Italiani* (Cristianopoli, 1798).

7. Giovanni Chrisolino, *Insurrezione dell'Inclita*, 283.

8. Chrisolino, *Insurrezione dell'Inclita*, 323 and 346.

9. *La commedia del giorno, ossiano I giacobini ai bagni di Lucca*, Milan, 1799.

SELECTED BIBLIOGRAPHY

Gainot, Bernard, ed. "L'Italie et la Révolution française." *Annales historiques de la Révolution française* 339, 2005.

Guerci, Luciano. *Uno spettacolo non mai più veduto nel mondo: La Rivoluzione francese come unicità e rovesciamento negli scrittori controrivoluzionari italiani (1789–1799)*. Torino: UTET, 2008.

Mangio, Carlo. *I patrioti toscani fra "Repubblica etrusca" e Restaurazione*. Florence: Olschki, 1991.

Martin, Jean-Clément, ed. *La Contre-Révolution en Europe: XVIIIe–XIXe siècles. Réalités politiques et sociales, résonances culturelles et idéologiques*. Rennes: Presses universitaires de Rennes, 2001.

Salvadori, Roberto G. *1799: Gli ebrei italiani nella bufera antigiacobina*. Florence: Giuntina, 1999.

Stow, Kenneth. *Jewish Dogs: An Image and Its Interpreters*. Stanford: Stanford Studies in Jewish History and Culture, 2006.

Todeschini, Giacomo. "Fra stereotipi del tradimento e cristianizzazione incompiuta: Appunti sull'identità degli ebrei d'Italia." *Zakhor* 6 (2003): 9–20.

Turi, Gabriele. *Guerre civili in Italia, 1796–1799*. Rome: Viella, 2019.

RITUAL
Emergence of Meaning in Medieval Liturgy
Vincent Debiais

Determining the mechanisms at work in the creation of medieval images ineluctably leads us to ponder notions of source, illustration, and translation. Ultimately, it leads us to establish a more or less strict dependence of the image on textual material. The image would then seem to be illustrating or commenting upon the text, particularly when such translation deals with the visual components of liturgy and theology.

Liturgical practice in the Middle Ages, meaning the ensemble of Christian worship practices regulated by norm and tradition in the medieval West, shared a theoretical stability with contemporaneous practices of the image. Paradoxically, however, these were both in fact highly fluid. The apparent rigidity transmitted by texts ordering the ritual could be tempered by the permanent phenomena of change, augmentation, retreat, sampling, and synthesis. New celebrations were created and others disappeared. At one and the same time as the seemingly absolute eschatological framework of the immutable staging of the *imitation Christi*, there was also insertion, transformation, and superposition. This occurred without any sense of contradiction.

As for the practice of the image, it was subjected to a constant tension between three elements. For one, there was theology's regulation of the meaning and practice of representation. Second came the necessarily contextual form and content of what was being shown. Third was the creative dynamic of those who "made" the image, between translation, innovation, and rupture. Liturgy and image, two supreme forms of ordering the world, were constantly intersecting in the Middle Ages: first through "environment," as images were mobilized in the time and the place of the liturgy, and then through "motif," as liturgy and image inflected the same themes according to their respective modalities of meaning. From this meeting of environment and motif come similarities of form and content. The method of iconographical analysis interprets these similarities as source effects in the methodological pervasiveness of placing text over image. In this view, the image was an aftereffect of the liturgy. The text supposedly furnished material for the visual, its practice, its sequencing, and so forth. The relationship between the two thus seems to be one of replication or of transfer. In short it seems to be based on a kind of faithfulness to the model, altered only by a change of medium.

We can free our understanding from this deterministic paradigm of a straight line leading from source to illustration by turning to the notion of contagion. This concept first describes, then qualifies, the phenomenon at work between liturgy and image, and with this model we can instead take note of the relationship created between carriers by the contagious agent. The relationship is first and foremost based on a circulation from one carrier to another, of a transfer without loss of either content or meaning—the liturgy still exists after the contagion of the image by motif. In this sense, let us take the example of the full-page painting showing the Mass of Saint Erhard of Regensburg in the famous Uta Codex (figure 1). Although it is entirely liturgical by both environment and motif, in all its complexity, it demonstrates that one is not traced from the other. The borrowing of specific elements of the ritual—such as furniture, vestments, or inscriptions—comes into play, in fact, in the creation of a complex discourse on the real presence of Christ in the Eucharist.

It seems risky to apply the notion of contagion to the circulation of theological elements through images. Indeed, this notion is by and large negatively connoted in medieval writing. It recalls, among other things, taint and illness, sin and sacrilege. And yet we can see that these theological elements are propagated by contact between objects or by a rebound in ideas from ceremony to book, from ritual to object, or from treatise to image. The inability of the art historian to place a specific text to each

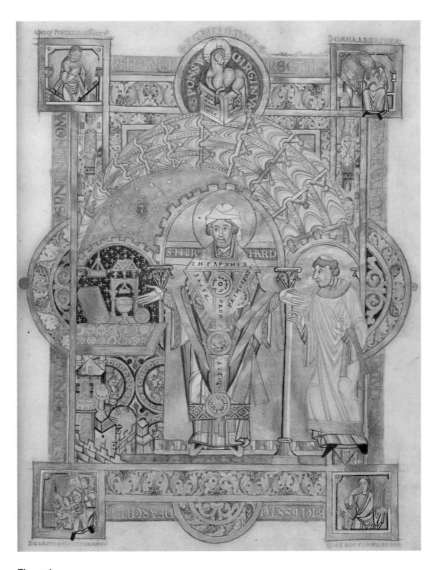

Figure 1

Mass of Saint Erhard. *Source*: Uta Codex. Munich, Bayerische Staatsbibliothek, Clm. 13 601, fol. 4.

image is tied to this diffuse and free from the propagation of ideas in a social context. Thus the Eucharistic context of the Uta Codex is also a context possible for a vast number of images that are, apparently, directly dependent on the liturgy.

Crucifixion scenes associated with the T initial in the *Te igitur* prayer in the sacramentaries, particularly for the High Middle Ages, can serve as an example. For instance, the text pronounced by the priest does not constitute the source of the painted image in the Gellone sacramentary circa 800 (figure 2). This picture of a suffering man bleeding on the starred wood of the cross does not correspond to the words of the liturgy. Instead, it translates, in a liturgical environment, contemporary reflections on the presence of Christ at the altar at the moment of the canon of the Mass, or again on his body's power of mediation (as can be found specifically in the writings of Alcuin and Theodulf of Orléans). In the Uta Codex, putting the very large Crucifixion (figure 3) face to face with the Mass of Saint Ehrard suggests an original and large-scale expression of the modalities of contagion of this theological principle to liturgical images. Opening the double page, the image produces a mirror effect between liturgy and its exegesis.

Furthermore, the canopy pictured above the altar in the scene on the right hand folio is inscribed with a quote from John 6:51 ("I am the living bread which came down from heaven"). This passage can be found precisely at the heart of developments by Alcuin and Theodulf affirming the presence of Christ at the altar, this very Christ wearing a sacerdotal stola in the image on the left-hand folio of the Uta Codex. The rhizomatic structure of the references from text to image, from image to gesture, from gesture to context corresponds to the complex schema of a contagion that does not suppose any other dependence than that of an analogous use of form and content.

With this we come to the notion of a "source of infection" inherent to the principle of contagion, a place that in this context is sometimes precise, sometimes hazy, sometimes even mysterious. Its possibility allows us to read the relationships between theological elements and their translation to images with neither genealogy nor hierarchy, their point of origin difficult to identify and pinpoint. Contagion works precisely along the lines of the rhizome; it invites us to abandon the problematic notion of lineage.

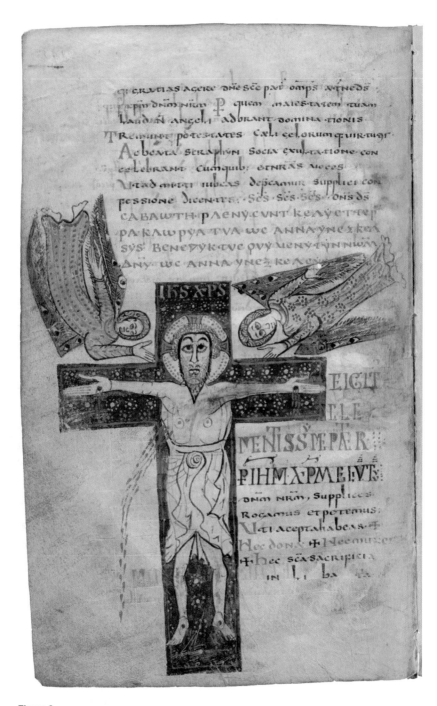

Figure 2

Initial of *Te igitur*, Gellone Sacramentary. *Source*: Paris, Bibliothèque nationale de France, MS lat. 12048, fol. 143v.

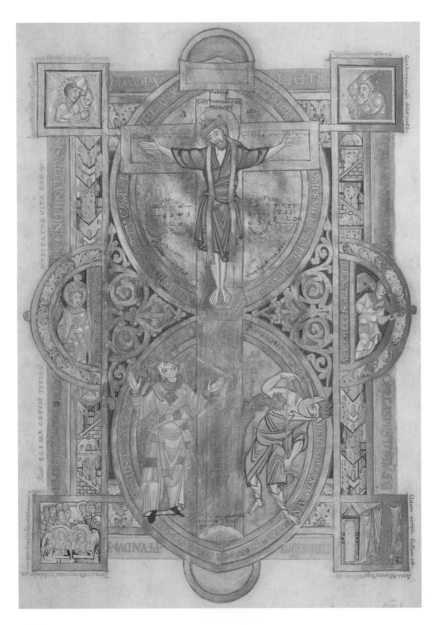

Figure 3

Symbolic crucifixion. *Source*: Uta Codex. Munich, Bayerische Staatsbibliothek, Clm. 13 601, fol. 3V.

There is the question, for instance, of the monumental Chi-Rho sculpted on the tympana of churches in the Pyrenees during the twelfth and thirteenth centuries. The theological content of the motif is incredibly complex, being a synthesis of paraphrases of Christ's words (peace, king, alpha, and omega) and connoting the consecration ceremony of the building (the seal of God marking the body of the church). Its diffusion on these churches eludes all stratification. The specific localization of the phenomenon to either side of the Pyrenees, the restricted chronology of that diffusion, the diversity of buildings concerned, and the object's formal variation will bring any attempt at a linear reading from one example to another to naught. If the structure of the alphabetic composition and its meaning surely change little within the corpus of some three hundred Chi-Rhos, then still their form, for its part, does become modified (it mutates, so to speak) under the influence of exterior elements. It adapts the message of the Trinity and the Incarnation in the figure of the templet to social, political, and intellectual contexts of medieval communities.

At the Jaca Cathedral (in Spain), a poem surrounds the Chi-Rho. The texts called upon to explicate the epigraphical allusions to the peace of Christ in this poem surrounding the Chi-Rho of the cathedral do not provide the source of the sculpted motif (figure 4). Rather, they make up the literary "source of infection," the conditions allowing for the contagion that is afterward limited only by the framework of medieval creativity. These are the "paths of creation" that André Grabar posited as a counterpoint to supposed "origins" in Christian iconography. In no way are we attempting here to suggest that the creation of images with liturgical or theological content acts by way of spontaneous generation. Rather we consider that the appearance of the motif resists the archaeological establishment of an origin and further yet resists the causes of this origin. This amounts to saying that in its form, the motif does not contain the elements that would allow us to link it to a source, to a causality. The object is anchored in a moment in history, and it is history that must describe it first, set it in its rhizomatic structure, and finally explicate it in its anthropological dimension.

Free in this way from a genetic constraint, which consists of seeing in the medieval image only an "evolved" product of the images preceding it,

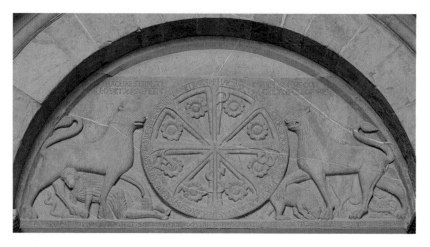

or indeed the illustration of the texts and ceremonies that it accompanies, the existence of the image might be considered as a blossoming or sudden emergence into history. This modality of the appearance of an image draws an analogy with the exegetical principle at work in both liturgy and theology. It resides in taking the hidden content of the text and the ritual and bringing it back to its meaning, and it is lifting the veil on a reality present in its essence but disguised in its form. In any event, the contagion happens through detail, evocation, and sinuous networks. The relationship between image and theology have more to do with symptom than with transfer, with the implicit rather than the explicit. As for research in the humanities and social sciences, it is a question of finding the contextual clues of a participation shared by both the image and the liturgy in the manifestation of the ties between the social and the transcendent, rather than reading the two phenomena in a state of complete dependence on each other. In other words, it is a question of returning to medieval images the poietic modalities of their functioning.

translated by Vicki-Marie Petrick

BIBLIOGRAPHY

Arasse, Daniel. *Le détail: Pour une histoire rapprochée de la peinture.* Paris: Flammarion, 1992.

Baschet, Jérôme. "Inventivité et sérialité des images médiévales: Pour une approche iconographique élargie." *Annales: Histoire, Sciences Sociales* 51, no. 1 (1996): 93–133.

Chazelle, Celia. *The Crucified God in the Carolingian Era: Theology and Art of Christ's Passion.* Cambridge: Cambridge University Press, 2001.

Deleuze, Gilles, and Félix Guattari. *A Thousand Plateaus: Capitalism and Schizophrenia.* Translated by Brian Massumi. Minneapolis: University of Minnesota Press, 1987.

Grabar, André. *Les voies de la création en iconographie chrétienne: Antiquité et Moyen Âge.* Paris: Flammarion, 1979.

Sperber, Dan. *La contagion des idées: Théorie naturaliste de la culture.* Paris: Odile Jacob, 1996.

Wirth, Jean. *L'image médiévale: Naissance et développements (VIe–XVe siècles).* Paris: Klincksiek, 1989.

SANCTITY
Roseline de Villeneuve or the "Invisible Action of the Spirit"

Sergi Sancho Fibla

The word contagion defines not only the spread of disease but also the transmission of moral character. Most often, this "contagion of the soul" expresses a negative view point; that is, it is linked to the notion of developing vices or sins. Roman sources already attest to the use of this formula by the Stoics, although the Fathers of the Church used it more frequently. In explanations of Christian mythology by the latter, original sin is inherited by Adam and Eve. It is therefore the impure germ that contaminates all people. This transmission would explain the spread and persistence of sin and evil, intrinsic to men and, even more, to women.

In the Middle Ages, this concept was developed exponentially in doctrinal and normative documents. We find the term contagion designating the expansion of thoughts contrary to Christian doctrine, described as schismatic or heretical. This association is reproduced ad infinitum in chronicles of religious history up to the twentieth century. Thus, Marcelino Menéndez Pelayo uses this expression on numerous occasions in his well-known *A History of the Spanish Heterodox* (*Historia de los heterodoxos españoles*, 1880–1882), especially when he explains the influences of the mystic and quietist theologian Miguel de Molinos, sentenced to death as a heretic in 1687. According to the author, Molinos is said to have been "contagioned" by Italian *alumbrados*.[1]

In this context, in 1867, a few years before the publication of Menéndez Pelayo's pamphlet, Benoît-Hippolyte de Villeneuve-Flayosc published *The Story of Saint Roseline de Villeneuve*, a hagiography of a medieval saint around whom a significant popular cult developed in the Var region during the modern era. This text uses the term contagion several times. However, contrary to what one might expect from a work of this kind, contagion here takes on a positive connotation, completely reversing traditional usage. The author uses it to designate the transmission of holiness, even rejoicing in the "beautiful contagion of the sacrifice, which won over all who witness edit."[2]

How may we explain such a use of the word contagion? A product of the Provençal nobility, Villeneuve-Flayosc receives a scientific education and works as a researcher and geology teacher. His background permits him to be at the forefront of scientific knowledge of his era in terms of diseases and their transmission. For example, he is interested in the prevention of cholera and closely follows contemporaneous research by Louis Pasteur. Perhaps the inevitability of contagion incites him to expand the lexical field into a completely different subject, when he begins to write his life of the saint.

The notes and hagiographies previously written about Roseline de Villeneuve, which the present author has consulted, do not use the vocabulary of contagion to elucidate the rapid spread of her cult. The use of this process is explained by the ambitions of Villeneuve-Flayosc. Indeed, he presents Roseline de Villeneuve as a member of his own family and seeks to prove that she inevitably became a key figure who enabled the development of Christianity in Provence and around the world. Referring to contagious holiness serves the purposes of his story. It highlights an order that we could define as teleological and redemptive, in which Christianity promotes the civilizing development of the human species. This is why he devotes 210 pages of prologue to a contextualization of the chronological development of Christianity during the Middle Ages, while the hagiographical account occupies only 151 pages. The use of contagion also brings closer to each other the respective efforts to collect medical knowledge and language, as seen in scientific treatises from the same era. Thus, *The Story of Saint Roseline de Villeneuve* is intended to convince the reader of the proven existence of a religious contagion of the world.

According to Villeneuve-Flayosc, Christian civilization is based upon the initial sacrifice of Christ, which has spread throughout time and space. This sacrifice is presented as the germ that allows contagion, while Roseline and her order, the Carthusians, are described as contagious agents: "The movement of expansion of the Carthusian family could only occur in a gradual, progressive manner; salutary contagion of eremitic austerity and clerical continence had to fill monasteries with new initiates [namely, those who made professions of faith]. . . . Each triumph of civilizing ideas represented by the papacy . . . was to make a new Carthusian flower bloom."[3]

For Villeneuve-Flayosc, the sanctity of Roseline prolongs that of Bruno of Cologne, founder of the Carthusian Order. It represents the feminine development of a civilizing project that began with the monk from Cologne. What Bruno established with Pope Urban II, at the time of the implementation of the Crusades and founding of military orders, continues due to the influence of Roseline upon the Eighth Crusade in 1270, the last major crusade, and upon Knights Hospitaller, an influence that Villeneuve-Flayosc deems decisive. In fact, Hélion de Villeneuve, Roseline's brother, was a member of the Order of Malta, and this kinship bond is a starting point, leading him to likewise develop the cult of Roseline in modern times. Bruno and Roseline thus appear as two agents of propagation reach in gall of Christendom, both in body and mind, in the temporal and spiritual orders. They are temporal because Bruno helps Urban II to launch the Crusade and Roseline allegedly contributes to creating the Order of Malta's coast guard. They are also spiritual, insofar as Bruno establishes the Carthusian Order and Roseline helps to spread the message. In this sense, his sanctity was contagious, because it sparked the development of Christian civilization.

In Villeneuve-Flayosc's text, the semantic field of contagion is not cited in connection with Bruno's actions, since he contributed to the civilizing project by tangible means of the Crusades and education. The former emphasizes the Carthusian Order's intellectual leadership, based upon copying books and devotion at monastic schools. On the other hand, Roseline's contribution is made by the miracles of holiness, prayer, and contemplation. The emanation of virginal holiness is transmitted invisibly. Therefore Villeneuve-Flayosc broaches the theme of contagion in this context, by reversing the notion of contagion of vice: "Is not the idea of reversibility of grace a truth felt by all souls who approach a type of holiness? I don't believe that a single person in the world can have escaped the supernatural influence of exceptional merits. If we proclaim the contagion of vice, it is because we recognize the sacred expansion of virtue."[4]

The use of this concept for the expansion of female Carthusian spirituality finds another motivation in its powerfully regional nature. Apart from two establishments, all the female charterhouses were founded between Provence and the Dauphiné. Villeneuve-Flayosc is aware of this distribution, which affects geographic areas in proximity, hence his use of the term contagion to describe the phenomenon. Roseline is said to have contaminated other people who became figures of popular spirituality in the region: Elzéar of Sabran, Jacques Duèze (Pope John XXII), and even Bishop Josselin d'Orange.

In short, Roseline would be an agent of the religious contagion of the world, just as disease-causing bacteria may be. By appealing to the notion of contagion, Villeneuve-Flayosc seeks to show the inevitable nature of the Catholic religion: for him, the world tends toward an increasingly complete harmony due to the "invisible action of the mind."[5] The same discourse is found in his other scientific works, such as *Studies on the Harmony of Terrestrial Forms* (*Études sur l'harmonie des formes terrestres*, 1865), in which he emphasizes that the cosmos tends toward an order of perfection: "What we call the world's revolutions is not one of increasingly standard coordination; each cataclysm was a perfection or improvement."[6]

In this manner, in a universal order, Roseline's contagious sanctity occurs invisibly and inevitably. This idea is consistent with the notion of social progress conceived as a form of positive contagion, according to the way in which virology, an emerging science in the nineteenth century, shows that contagion is an involuntary, intangible, and transmissible phenomenon.

translated by Benjamin Ivry

NOTES

1. The author is referring here to the Italian equivalent of Spanish *alumbrados*. Miguel de Molinos, *A History of the Spanish Heterodox: Book One* (London: Saint Austin Press, 2009), translated by Eladia Gomez-Posthill from *Historia de los heterodoxos españoles* (Madrid, 1880–1882).

2. Benoît-Hippolyte de Villeneuve-Flayosc, *Histoire de Sainte Roseline de Villeneuve, religieuse chartreuse et de l'influence civilisatrice de l'ordre des chartreux avec pièces justificatives* (Paris: Libraire Saint-Germain-des-Prés, 1867), 244.

3. Villeneuve-Flayosc, *Histoire de Sainte Roseline*, 234.

4. Villeneuve-Flayosc, *Histoire de Sainte Roseline*, 207.

5. Villeneuve-Flayosc, *Histoire de Sainte Roseline*, 14.

6. Villeneuve-Flayosc, *Histoire de Sainte Roseline*, 12.

SELECTED BIBLIOGRAPHY

Goldstein, Jan. "'Moral Contagion': A Professional Ideology of Medicine and Psychiatry in Eighteenth- and Nineteenth-Century France." In *Professions and the French State: 1700–1900*, edited by Gerald L. Geison, 181–222. Philadelphia: University of Pennsylvania Press, 1984.

L'Hermite-Leclercq, Paulette, and Daniel Le Blevec. "Une sainte cartusienne: Rosaline de Villeneuve." In *La femme dans la vie religieuse du Languedoc XIIIe–XIVe siècle*, 55–76. Cahiers de Fanjeaux 23. Toulouse: Privat, 1988.

Robert, Aurélien. "Contagion morale et transmission des maladies: Histoire d'un chiasme (XIIIe–XIXe siècle)." *Tracés: Revue de sciences humaines* 21 (2011): 41–60.

SMALLPOX

Inoculation or Quarantine? A Scientific Debate in Europe during the Enlightenment

Jean-Baptiste Fressoz

Smallpox inoculation, or variation, is a minimalist technique, which consists in deliberately causing a healthy person to contract smallpox in order to prevent that person from infection during a dangerous epidemic. In the eighteenth century, at the cost of an incision, some pustules, and a few weeks of convalescence, inoculated smallpox offered a lower probability of death (about one in two hundred) than "naturally" contracted smallpox (one in seven).

In spite of these improved odds, variation was a spectacular failure. In France, by 1800, even after a half-century of propaganda from the Enlightenment thinkers known as the philosophes, barely a few thousand individuals had chosen to inoculate themselves. The idea of contagion and its political consequences played a large role in this defeat.

Advocates of variation asserted that the practice was not immoral, since it amounted to a freely chosen, personal risk. The problem, retorted opponents, was that those who elected to be inoculated were spreading, or feeding, smallpox contagion—with unmeasurable consequences. According to Dr. Louis Pierre Le Hoc, a physician of the Paris Faculty of Medicine, a single person could transmit the disease "to twenty thousand individuals, to the whole of France, to the entire universe." Disagreeing with the champions of variation who advanced the argument of the good of society, he rebutted with another definition of the latter: "What is meant by society? Is it not a multitude of men of all ages, assembled for the most part in cities where *they breathe fresh air*? . . . Allowing a person to be inoculated against the smallpox is akin to saying: *you alone suffice.* Is this not sacrificing the public for the individual?"[1]

The contagion objection was coupled with a social criticism: by inoculating themselves, the elites were spreading smallpox and exposing the populace to an increased risk of infection. Thus, the privileged separated themselves from the common fate at the price of aggravating the risk for others. The criticism was sharpened by the belief that smallpox was a penalty paid for the vices of the ruling class.

Last, variolation raised a relatively new issue: to support it or oppose it could have dramatic consequences for "future generations." Advocates of each side claimed to speak on their behalf. Dr. Antoine Petit of the Paris Faculty of Medicine explained that variolation was a national necessity: "If it came to be that one nation in Europe adopted the widespread practice of inoculating young children, while neighbouring peoples rejected it, then after a very small number of centuries, that nation would inevitably rise above the others and subjugate them without difficulty."[2]

Opponents had dire predictions for future generations as well. Le Hoc reasoned that variolation could render smallpox everlasting, since by spreading contagion it increases the smallpox risk for anyone who is not inoculated and by the same token increases their incentive to get inoculated: "Allow inoculation and render smallpox eternal and universal."[3] Another physician agreed, declaring that "inoculation will perpetuate the disease for centuries to come."[4] The dilemma presented by variolation resembles the prisoner's dilemma, in that an aggregation of decisions made by individuals acting in their own self-interest prompts the group to choose the worst course of action.

Louis XVI's inoculation in 1774 is often heralded as the inoculators' decisive victory. Yet, at the very same time, many police regulations banned variolation in urban areas. In 1778, the Seneschalty of Lyon prohibited it within city limits, making a clear distinction between the royal inoculation, which stood as a symbol of personal bravery, and the public good: "The courageous example, never to be forgotten, shown by our august monarch does not dispense the Crown's preventing the dangers to which the public is thereby exposed."[5]

From the 1770s onward, the tide of popularity ran more in favor of the theories of Dr. Jean-Jacques Paulet, editor of the *Gazette de santé* medical journal and member of the Royal Society of Medicine. Paulet was a fierce objector of variolation. Departing from the neo-Hippocratic theories of his time, which focalized on air, miasma, and circumfusa, or surroundings, he directed his attention to "viruses." The latter had nothing to do with odors, he asserted. Contagion was not spread by the environment but exclusively from person to person.[6] This was proven by the fact that certain isolated villages in the countryside around Montpellier had not seen a case of small-pox for over thirty years, completely changing the light in which the risk of contracting the disease was considered. It was no longer an inevitable "natural disease" caused by mysterious changes in the atmosphere. Conse-quently, the traditional quarantine techniques that had already triumphed against the plague—of which there had been no reappearance in France since the 1720 epidemic in Marseilles—could be equally effective against smallpox. In 1768, Paulet's *Histoire de la petite vérole* (*History of Smallpox*) was a tremendous success. Even Voltaire, the first of the philosophes to campaign in favor of variolation in 1734, conceded that he had had a change of mind after reading the book.[7] Paulet went so far as to found an association, the Ligue contre la petite vérole (League against Smallpox) to win the government over to his point of view.

Referring explicitly to Paulet's publication, several cities did in fact decide to ban variolation, such as Saint-Omer in 1776, followed by Dijon and Lyon in 1778. In Lyon, physicians firmly believed an inoculation had triggered the epidemic that ravaged the small town of Saint-Chamond. In Burgundy, an inoculator was accused of endangering that province's public health. In 1776, the residents of the canton of Bern, in Switzer-land, implemented quarantine measures against their Franche-Comté neighbors, who were overly fond of variolation. The prohibitions did not go unheeded. The Seneschalty of Lyon imposed fines on both givers and receivers of inoculation for violating the 1778 regulation. In 1782, the Parliament of Brittany made it illegal to rent a house for the purpose of inoculation. That same year, despite being in favor of the practice, the lieutenant general of the Paris police, Jean-Charles-Pierre Lenoir, issued a regulation echoing the restrictions placed on variolation by the Parliament of Paris in 1763. The police were also acting to allay fears among the city's inhabitants, alarmed by nearby "inoculation houses." In 1782, the residents of Faubourg Montmartre protested against a surgeon's clinic. In petitions sent to the Parliament of Paris, they described the inoculation houses as unsanitary laboratories contaminating the neighborhood's atmosphere.[8] Variolation was thus perceived as a selfish practice that jeopardized the public good.

Through the lens of the problem of contagion, smallpox inoculation was a concrete illustration of political philosophy's all-important question at the time: how should the hedonistic individual be integrated into the outside world, and how can the individual contribute to the public good? Choosing between inoculation and quarantine seems to be a choice between the advantages and drawbacks of individualism and those of absolutism. Should the public good (the containment of the epidemic) be left to be determined by the aggregation of individual behaviors (inoculations), or should the government take direct action by interrupting the transmission of the virus? For the physicians of the eighteenth century, the effectiveness of quarantine in halting smallpox depended on the nature of the government's power. Quarantine was the appropriate tool in the case of absolute, enlightened power. According to Paulet, "in France, the forces of authority are so closely chained one to another . . . *that a single order from the King can put an end to the contagion. . . .* All governments do not have this degree of ease. England's form of government, for example, seems to constitute an obstruction. The inordinate power of the people, the difficulty of making them see reason and choose a side, are all obstacles that obstruct an enterprise of this nature."[9]

It would seem that inoculation and quarantine corresponded to different political systems. Inoculation was the recourse of loosely governed, individualist countries, in which the self-interest of individuals ruled. In contrast, quarantine was a feasible and desirable solution in well-ordered kingdoms where the monarch's power was absolute, even over a virus.

translated by Elaine Holt

NOTES

1. Louis Pierre Le Hoc, *L'inoculation de la petite vérole renvoyée à Londres*, 1763 (Paris: Gogez, 1801), 47; 35.

2. Antoine Petit, *Premier rapport en faveur de l'inoculation: Lu dans l'assemblée de la Faculté de Médecine de Paris en l'année 1764, et imprimé par son ordre* (Paris: Dessain, 1766), 81.

3. Le Hoc, *L'inoculation*, 39.

4. *Mémoire sur le fait de l'inoculation* (Paris: Butard, 1768), 5.

5. "Jugement de la sénéchaussée de Lyon, 19 Mai 1778," Paris, Bibliothèque nationale de France, Joly de Fleury, fol. 280.

6. Jean-Jacques Paulet, *Histoire de la petite vérole avec les moyens d'en préserver les enfans et d'en arrêter la contagion en France* (Paris: Ganeau, 1768) and *La petite vérole anéantie* (Paris: Ruault, 1776).

7. "Lettre de M. de Voltaire à Paulet au sujet de l'histoire de la petite vérole," *Mercure de France*, July 1768, 97.

8. For these regulations and the case of the Bras dor clinic in Montmartre, see BnF, Joly de Fleury, fols. 195, 277, 289, and 295; and the Lenoir Manuscript Collection, MS 1421 in the municipal library of Orléans.

9. Paulet, *Avis au public*, 87.

SELECTED BIBLIOGRAPHY

Darmon, Pierre. *La longue traque de la variole*. Paris: Perrin, 1985.

Fressoz, Jean-Baptiste. *L'Apocalypse joyeuse: Une histoire du risque technologique*. Paris: Le Seuil, 2012.

Miller, Genevieve. *The Adoption of Smallpox Inoculation in England and France*. Philadelphia: University of Pennsylvania Press, 1957.

Rusnock, Andrea. *Vital Accounts*. Cambridge: Cambridge University Press, 2002.

Seth, Catriona. *Les rois aussi en mouraient, les Lumières en lutte contre la petite vérole*. Paris: Desjonquières, 2008.

SOLITUDE

The Right to Live Alone: A Difficult Path to Acceptance in Contemporary Societies

Marcela Iacub

The word "contagion" can be used in a figurative sense to designate a social phenomenon with negative connotations whose spread is not consciously sought by either individuals or public policies. In fact, "contagion" has two meanings: one is the disease, and the other is an involuntary—or at least partly involuntary—"transmission." In a sociological context, the classic example of a type of behavior that is multiplied through "contagion" is suicide.

Using this definition, the spectacular increase in the number of people living alone in rich, democratic countries in the past fifty years can be linked to the idea of contagion. Although a solo lifestyle does not carry the same degree of negative connotations as the act of suicide, it is not a conscious desire of public policies or mainstream culture. Solo living is not held to be an "ideal" social situation. On the contrary, it is thought to set off the exclusion process known as "isolation"—a sort of social death, which, according to certain researchers, can even accelerate a person's biological death. The many isolated elderly people who died during France's 2003 heatwave are often portrayed as the paradigmatic victims of this social ill, which, according to public statistics, affects all age groups in Western developed societies such as ours, both urban and rural residents alike.

And yet, at the same time, public policies recognize that in certain situations living alone is preferable to living with others as a family, as a couple, or in a specialized institution such as a retirement home. The dangers of isolation are seen to be less serious than those of physical or psychological violence or the lack of autonomy implied by sharing one's residence with other people. As a result, it is not only accepted that solo living can be a genuine choice, but efforts are also being made to facilitate the separation of couples and independent living by young and elderly people. It is as though our society were struggling with conflicting attitudes toward solo living, simultaneously perceived to be both a highly perilous situation and a lesser evil. However, in the past few years, a new school of thought has challenged this approach by advancing the idea that solo living is the most consistent, possibly the most fulfilling, lifestyle choice in a society of individuals. When material conditions allow it, instead of isolating us from others, solo living can open the door to varied and enriching forms of sociability. If we accept this theory, then far from describing these new lifestyles, the word "contagion" emerges as the weapon of an ideology that promotes familial, particularly domestic, socialization as a hegemonic ideal, at the expense of the greater population's happiness.

According to the 2015 census in France, primary residences occupied by just one person represented 35.3 percent of all households. This proportion is higher than that of two-person households (33 percent) or households of three or more (32 percent) and is rising. To gauge the growth of the phenomenon over the past few decades, we must consider that in the 1960s, households with five or more people were as common as one-person households. Today, the former account was for only 4.4 percent of all households. In 1962, households of six people or more still represented 10.8 percent of total households, compared to just 1.7 percent today. Since the 1980s, the rise in the overall number of households has been almost exclusively due to an increase in one- and two-person households. These grew by 2.4 million and 1.4 million people, respectively.

Demographers have identified three main reasons for the sharp rise in single-person households. The first is the longer period of time that young people live alone after leaving the parental home and before moving in with a partner. In France, the number of young people living solo doubled between the 1960s and the end of the 2000s. Additionally, the time interval between a couple moving in together and the birth of their first child is increasing every year. The higher the couple's level of education, the longer the wait.

The second driver of the rise in single-person households is the weaker stability, or decline, of cohabiting couples, although this living arrangement remains the hegemonic model. In 1972, there were 417,000 marriages, compared with just 235,000 in 2018 (including 6,000 same-sex marriages). Between 1964 and 2013, the number of divorces quadrupled. Registered civil partnerships in France (PACS) last, on average, two-and-a-half years. In 2015, 9 percent of families were reconstituted families and 23 percent were single-parent families, whereas the latter represented only 12 percent of families in 1990. Forty percent of people born between 1978 and 1987 had a first cohabiting relationship that lasted less than ten years, compared with 16 percent of people born between 1948 and 1957. Furthermore, the number of desired separations and divorces is potentially higher than the statistics suggest, since some people continue to cohabit simply because they lack the economic means to end the relationship. To get an insight as to how many might be in this situation, we must consider that half of the women in France who live with a partner either do not work or only work part time. Incidentally, among those who separate between the ages of twenty-five and fifty, almost a third do not cohabit again during the next fifteen years. Finally, noncohabiting couples without children currently account for 1.2 million people; among these, 48 percent have a university degree, compared with just 32 percent for cohabiting couples.

The third explanation for the rise in the number of people who live alone is that elderly people are staying in their own homes. In 2013, 21 percent of French men and 48 percent of French women over the age of seventy-five lived alone. In 1968, 40 percent of eighty-five-year-olds lived with a family member, most often a child. By 2015, this proportion had fallen to one in ten. Moving into a retirement institution is still not a common choice. In 2015, barely 6 percent of people aged over sixty-five lived in a retirement home. If pensioners have the "luxury" to do so, it is mainly due to their improved economic situation. In 1960, 45 percent of those over sixty-five years of age claimed the French old-age benefit for low-income individuals, compared with only 4.5 percent today.

As shown by the three reasons described above, the rising proportion of people living solo bears a direct relationship to a radical transformation of family ties. Young people leave the family home without immediately moving in with a partner or having plans to quickly start a family. Marriage among adults is less common and divorce more frequent, while the proportion of people who do not cohabit again as a couple is constantly rising. Elderly people prefer to stay at home and maintain their independence rather than be taken care of by family members, particularly their children. All these factors underscore the extent to which family ties have become less intimate, less self-sacrificial, and less symbiotic, starting in childhood. Even the notion of maternal bonding, often construed through the paradigm of symbiosis and self-sacrifice, continues to erode, a process attributed to women's increased participation in the workforce well as a higher rate of separation among couples. Additionally, smartphones and computers are giving children, very early in life, a space of their own that parents feel apprehensive about yet accept.

All the same, we do not seek to form family-like ties with people outside the family—with friends, for example. Instead, the transformation of family ties has had an impact on all our relationships. Where bonds of friendship were once "profound" and of a limited number, such as those with family members, they are now increasingly superficial and numerous. In France, the fastest-growing form of sociability is the kind we maintain with our neighbors.

Far from being an indication of our isolation, a form of weakness or a social ill, solo living is in fact a sign of our individuality, which should be better preserved to foster a greater openness to others. Even so, public policy makers and members of the mainstream culture have the greatest difficulty in accepting and assuming responsibility for something that they nevertheless continuously promote, namely the protection of our personal autonomy in all respects. That is why they disapprove so strongly of the dramatic increase in people living alone and fail to help the disadvantaged members of society enjoy the "luxury" that the more privileged individuals afford themselves with much satisfaction. Therefore, rather than deplore the isolation "epidemic" that has struck us, public policies should make it a universal right for everyone to be able to not share their residence with another person, that is, the right to live alone.

translated by Elaine Holt

BIBLIOGRAPHY

Flahault, Erika. *Une vie à soi: Nouvelles formes de solitude au féminin*. Rennes: Presses Universitaires de Rennes, 2009.

Iacub, Marcela. *Les Architectures du bonheur: De Charles Fourier aux Grandes Voisins*. Paris: Cent Mille Milliards, Descartes and Cie, 2019.

Kaufmann, Jean-Claude. *Piégée dans son couple*. Paris: Les Liens qui Libèrent, 2016.

Klinemberg, Eric. *Going Solo: The Extraordinary Rise and Surprising Appeal of Living Alone*. New York: Penguin Books, 2012.

Le Bras, Hervé. *Se sentir mal dans une France qui va bien*. Paris: Éditions de l'Aube, 2019.

Storr, Antony. *Solitude, Les vertus du retour à soi-même*. Paris: Robert Laffont, 1991.

SPIRITUALITY

Contaminated and Contagious Passions: From Devout Ecstasy to Demonic Possession

Antoine Roullet

Could the lexicon of contagion be used to describe female mysticism, which was a widespread phenomenon from the fourteenth to the eighteenth century and deemed to be at the margins of "heresy"? Ambivalent expressions such as "waves of possessions," "hotbeds of ecstasy," or "conventicles of devotees" vouch for the idea of women living outside any kinds of control and invading ecclesiastical space. These women sometimes were recognized as saints when they were approved and then consecrated by the institutions. Yet they were more often condemned, either officially or not. In all circumstances they were all taunted for their contagiousness.

As a category of analysis, "contagion" convokes a normative lexicon and a largely disqualified relic of the history of social sciences: Gabriel Tarde's "laws of imitation," a theory less remotivated for its own qualities than for the desire to put aside other theoretical traditions. The notions of imitation and invention on which Tarde established his theory seems to adapt easily to the dynamics of spiritual distinction at the beginning of the modern era, according to which charismatic individuals—religious virtuosos—tended to attract around them a loosely institutionalized community whose members shared a common will to emulate and imitate the charismatic model. Examples of such include small Anabaptist communities; the beguines in Flanders; or the *beatas* (members of a pious association of women) in Spain, Italy, or Portugal, some nuns who were credited with supernatural powers or some groupuscules that the Inquisition judged as "illuminists" in Spain or in America. In the analysis of this type of configuration, the notion of "contagion" would here easily complete today's dominant paradigm, which was inspired by Weberian sociology.

Commenting on Tarde in the introduction of his *Economy and Society*, Max Weber underscores that imitative behaviors are not included in the field of social action as he understood it. Imitation pulls the interpretation toward the other side and sheds light on detoured pathways, as the subjects involved could be unconscious of the power that the *virtuoso* exercised upon them. Since Tarde himself elaborates little on the question of religion, one of his most famous readers and his successor to the chair of modern philosophy at the Collège de France, Henri Bergson, goes back to the notion of imitation when analyzing sainthood as a model. There is a Christian genealogy of imitation, obvious for any historian of Christianism, which, according to Bergson, was very explicit at the time when Tarde's model had its apogee, at the beginning of the twentieth century. The notion of imitation can represent the reformulation of a devout and pastoral tradition whose most accomplished model is the imitation of Jesus Christ. However, in the early modern world, imitation also encompassed a whole series of models of sainthood, proper to each state of life.

What can one say about "contagion" in this context? Revisiting Tarde, Paul-André Rosental reminds us that contagion has narrower and interindividual implications than imitation, which has more ambiguous and larger ones. In that respect, Tarde also uses the term for his analyses of a whole other scale. Although he seems to use the two terms as synonyms—talking about "imitative contagions"—on the plane of values, "contagion" remains as the pejorative twin of "imitation." Each term puts the reverse emphasis on the role attributed to the individual: whereas imitation can stand for a choice, one becomes subjected to contagion, and whereas imitation would call for reason and free will, contagion affects us. Devaluation of the latter term in relation to the former is merely one more formulation of the devaluation, within the Occidental tradition, of the body in relation to the soul or that of reason in relation to emotions.

Just like "imitation," "contagion" has also its proper genealogy within early modern religious rhetoric, which was prompt to denounce heresy as a contagious plague or a venom, these linguistic elements being particularly obvious in the case of Protestantism that was explicitly identified with the notion of contagion, even though the term already had a long history. The prophylactic nature of the measures that were taken to fight against the propagation of "heresy" is quite eloquent from this point of view, if one looks at such examples as censure, public burning, and controls effectuated at the frontiers or ports in an attempt to prevent the propagation of Martin Luther's books. This heretical contagion was based on an anthropology that did not separate the body from the mind: the venom of heresy was thought to be communicated through bodies, and the "breath of heretics" was a *topos* of this literature. Heresy would enter into the body by the door of senses to contaminate the reason and therefore the soul, beginning with the hearing, which justified the attempts to silence heretics at all cost, even by tearing off their tongues on top of stakes. Contagion was based on a more general representation about the relation of man to the world, the demon, and the flesh, a sinful trinity that raped the body in order to dominate the soul. Once heresy broke in the soul of the believer, the worm was in the fruit and it pursued its corruptive work.

These elements, reminded in the historiography with a tersely yet quite circumscribed manner, commanded a whole network of metaphors, the first of which describing the soul as a fortress. They also required a whole series of protection techniques as the counterpart of political measures taken to restrain heresy, by way of locking the body up against all external influences and working on each of the five senses through specific mortifying exercises. This anchorage on the body and the intrusive, irrepressible character of the rhetoric of contagion reveals its difference with the Christian lexicon of imitation, which is more clearly tied up with the will of individuals and with their alleged desire to emulate a model, when that of contagion would break open their will. Evidently, the distinction is rather weak; to refer to just one example among others, a devout education cultivated from a very young age onward an almost nonreflexive imitation of

Christian canons. Where was the reflexivity of imitation in such common cases? One shall not take the opposition between contagion and imitation as a positivist distinction between two categories of phenomena but as a prescriptive categorization destined to decide dualistically between a good and a bad manner of imitating.

Hence, the stake of demonic possession was considered to open up the body, not merely to seize a soul but to make it contagious, notably within female communities. The famous case of the possessed from the city of Loudun, which gained a great historiographic and cinematographic fortune, illustrates this to the point of caricature: at the beginning of 1630s, a whole convent of Ursulines were possessed by hordes of demons through the intermediary of a priest accused of sorcery, Urbain Grandier. Both the contemporaries and the medical tradition that seized upon the case at the end of the nineteenth century considered Loudun as a case of demonic and hysterical contagion. In the monastic hagiography of the modern era, the narratives being produced by the nuns and destined to propose effective models of surmounting all the difficulties and contradictory injunctions of monastic life, demoniac interventions are described as a way of unmaking the body, as a kind of discomposure of the nuns, making them look bedraggled, injuring themselves physically, forcing them to cry, to shout, to become agitated, and to break down. This self-decomposition became contagious only because these nuns could no longer hold their bodies together, because their emotions were no longer contained. Emotions and affects were the reason why the notion of contagion was brought to the center of the game. Contagion was a defeat; it marked the impossibility of a fight.

Somewhat paradoxically, this defeat allows demonic and devout contagion to be drawn closer, since the grace of God was also renown as inexorable. The narratives of religious ecstasy have a crucial significance in the attempts to transcribe on the bodies the unbearable necessity of ecstasy: bodies dried up through penitence and tears, ready to enflame and burned with charity, projecting sparks or a heat that spontaneously inflames other bodies. None of this belongs to the pure metaphorical register, either. This propagation of devout fire was considered a force that imposed itself from the exterior, even though some exercises and gestures—abundantly commented within the spiritual literature—were supposed to prepare the interior terrain for it. Hagiography, a literature of edifying entertainment, is obviously partial in its descriptions of ecstasy: the genre has its own codes and its obligatory passages (including sighs, tears, sudden flashovers): the strong emotivity emanated from all this was contagious and was supposed to be so, in order to edify the readers. There is a slight difference in the way the ecstatic and the possessed exerted their will. The desire of the ecstatic to imitate a saintly model allegedly sustained in itself a fire that ended up spreading around and contaminating others. Her will, supposed to have been sorely tested, was in the same movement rewarded and defeated by the force of grace. The weakness of the possessed was the cause of their being instrumentalized against their will to corrupt the whole community. One could say the difference is tenuous.

This type of categorization is not viable for giving us even a naively positive description of what went on in the bodies and minds of the nuns: it only constitutes an example for analytical frameworks used by those social actors of the time to interpret what went on. The contagious or the imitative nature of any spiritual event was, first of all, the fruit of the others' judgment. In this respect, monastic orders had prepared the field and theorized the mechanisms praising the "saint emulation" as an imitative competition between the nuns. This competition was supposed to spread a model of self-control conceived as purely artificial (the so-called composition of the self) which was meant to be reflected to the others as an edifying mirror to stimulate their reciprocal imitation. If the extraordinary occurred in one of the most zealous, this would then incite the perception of it as a rapture rather than as a demonic intervention.

translated by Zehra Gulbahar Cunillera

BIBLIOGRAPHY

Bergson, Henri. *Les deux sources de la morale et de la religion*. Paris: PUF, 2013.

Bouaniche, Arnaud. "Imitation et émotion: Bergson lecteur de Tarde." *Cahiers de philosophie de l'université de Caen* 54 (2017): 59–72. https://doi.org/10.4000/cpuc.313.

Karsenti, Bruno. *La société en personnes: Études durkheimiennes*. Paris: Economica, 2006.

Mucchielli, Laurent. "Tardomania? Réflexions sur les usages contemporains de Tarde." *Revue d'histoire des sciences humaines* 3 (2000): 161–184.

Rosental, Paul-André. "Où s'arrête la contagion? Faits et utopie chez Gabriel Tarde." *Tracés. Revue de sciences humaines* 21 (2011): 109–124.

Tarde, Gabriel. *Les lois de l'imitation (1895)*. Paris: Kimé, 1993.

Weber, Max. *Concepts fondamentaux de sociologie (1920)*. Edited and translated by Jean-Pierre Grossein. Paris: Gallimard, 2016.

SUICIDE

Moral Contagion versus Social Epidemic in the Development of Émile Durkheim's Sociology

Stéphane Baciocchi

Émile Durkheim developed his sociological work during a period said in European positivist circles to be a time when "the idea of moral contagion has become a *common belief*."[1] Set forth by a handful of alienist physicians, this idea of a possible "contagion" of minds and morals first flourished in a corpus filled with ancient philosophical and medical notions (*infectio*, *fascinatio*, *compassio*, but also *sympathy*). Around 1820, the concept was fully expressed in a sad anecdote that Dr. Jean-Étienne Esquirol had heard in a tale recorded by his old master Philippe Pinel: "Near Étampes a priest hanged himself, and within a few days two others killed themselves in the vicinity, and some other people imitated them."[2]

This was a typical case of moral contagion, then indiscriminately understood as a mimetic cascade of "bad examples," cause and consequence of morbid morals. Yet, the interpretative schema suggested by this anecdote loses its initial obviousness as the psychic meanings of the notion of moral contagion are refined and, on the margins of the microbial revolution, its metaphorical uses are developed.

Around 1900, the concept migrated from medical dictionaries to the heart of the encyclopedic *Dictionary of Philosophy and Psychology*: it now settled within a vast set of specialized but nevertheless related meanings—and, in this respect, common to and shared within the psychological and social sciences (figure 1).[3] Durkheim is particularly attentive to this polysemy, as it contributes to a disciplinary division and renewal in which he himself is engaged.

In light of this configuration, it is understandable that the author of *The Rules of Sociological Method* (1895) was keen to first "make the terminology

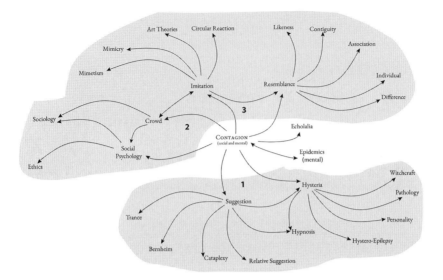

Figure 1

Notional environment of the entry "Contagion (Social and Mental)" in the *Dictionary of Philosophy and Psychology* (1901–1902). The figure shows entries in the *Dictionary of Philosophy and Psychology* (vertices) linked by a "See" reference (oriented arcs). Beginning from "contagion," all the entries and references located at an immediate distance of $n = 1$ were selected. Note that the notion of "contagion" develops into two large interrelated components (in gray) and three clusters (numbered). These clusters are directly related to the polysemic and multidisciplinary dimension of the term "contagion," specifically (1) psycho-pathology, (2) social psychology, and (3) individual psychology. The latter two fields of meaning being "based on the pathological analogy of the contagion of disease."

precise"[4] in his empirical work on suicide in Europe. Indeed, in this popular field of psychopathological studies (figure 1, cluster 1), there was no shortage of working hypotheses and perspectives competing with his own (notably figure 1, cluster 2). In a chapter of *Le suicide: Étude de sociologie* (*Suicide*, 1897), famous for its critique of "imitative contagion," which, according to Gabriel Tarde, is "social action par excellence,"[5] Durkheim again endeavors to "determine the meaning" of words to clarify a discussion where, he deplores, "contagion" is too often considered in a figurative manner. He strives to clearly define the mechanism of moral contagion before identifying, empirically, its real effects. To proceed otherwise is to condemn oneself to "mistaking a purely verbal expression for an explanation."[6]

He starts by explicating the terms and conditions of a rigorous analogy with "biological pathology." Indeed, as an admirer of Claude Bernard, Durkheim was able to follow the scientific progress of this field through assiduous use of the *Dictionnaire encyclopédique des sciences médicales* (1864–1889). The structuring of his reasoning is illustrative:

A disease is called contagious when it rises wholly or mainly from the development of a germ introduced into the organism from outside. Inversely, in so far as this germ has been able to develop thanks only to the active cooperation of the field in which it has taken root, the term "contagion" becomes inexact.

Likewise, for an act to be attributed to a moral contagion it is not enough that the idea be inspired by a similar act. Furthermore, once introduced into the mind, it must automatically and of itself have become an action. Then there *really is contagion*, because the external act is reproduced by itself entering into us by way of a representation.[7]

The reasoning thus laid out distinguishes, on the one hand, the normal from the pathological and, on the other hand, the inside from the outside. The analogy of physical contagion and moral contagion can then be based on the identity of the relationship between these pairs of elements, in this case a same vector (here an "active germ," there a "representation" of the action) identically oriented from an external and pathological point toward an internal and normal point. This vector notably runs exactly opposite to Tarde, for whom the passive and unlimited "imitative contagion" clearly radiated "*ab interioribus ad exteriora*."[8] The choice and mastery of this analogical reasoning are not surprising in the writings of a John Stuart Mill reader. Indeed, Durkheim wrote entire sections of his doctoral thesis (1879–1892) in the language of the biological science of organization. Taken within a naturalist analogy, the notion of contagion allows one to describe phenomena situated at the interface (at a "contact") of the morphology and physiology of the social world: "As the progress of the division of labour determines a greater concentration of the social mass, there is between the different parts of the same tissue, of the same organ or organ system, a closer contact that facilitates contagion phenomena. Motion originating at one point rapidly passes on to others."[9]

From this perspective, the biological analogy allows Durkheim to question, in a quasi-experimental way, the moral contagion of suicide. Furthermore, we know that these reflections take statistical and cartographic shape (figure 2): if suicides spread by moral contagion, their geography should reveal, hypothetically, pathological "foci" of contagion in capitals and large cities.[10]

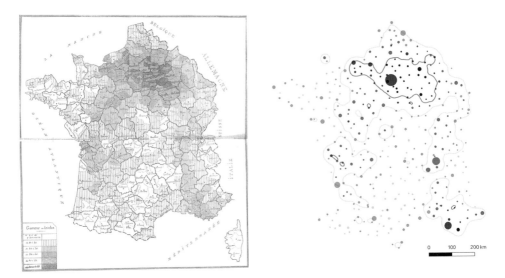

Figure 2

Spatial distribution of suicide rates in metropolitan France, by arrondissement and by size of main towns, 1887–1891. Sources and interpretation: The thumbnail on the left is a *facsimile* of the famous choropleth map of "Suicides in France, by arrondissements (1887–1891)" prepared by the schoolteacher Louis-Jean Ferrand based on individual data collected firsthand by Marcel Mauss from the Bureau of Statistics and Criminal Records within the Ministry of Justice. To draw up the map on the right, 354 main arrondissement towns were extracted together with the corresponding average suicide rates (six levels), enriched by the size of the population recorded in the said main towns in the 1891 census (points of proportional size). The different epidemic areas identified by Durkheim clearly emerge, calculated here using a kernel density estimation and represented by contour lines of decreasing density. Note the large epidemic area (*la grande tache*) covering the former Île-de-France, Champagne, and Normandy; and similarly, "to the south-east, along the Mediterranean coast" and "on the west coast," the two Charentes. Placed next to one another, the map published by Durkheim and its analytical modeling allow us to follow his reasoning and the critique of Tarde. Both of them combined the reading of the choropleth map with the individual data on which it is based: relative importance of the main arrondissement towns as point of origin of a possible spread of suicide rates and the possible limits of this diffusion.

Yet, the original map specially composed at the infradepartmental scale shows nothing of the kind: "suicide . . . occurs in great roughly (but only roughly) homogeneous masses and with no central nucleus."[11] For Durkheim, this is a valid rebuttal: "contagion consists only in more or less repeated repercussions of individual."[12] He therefore prefers, like physicians, to use the more neutral term "epidemic" to describe the constitution of those areas where suicide rates are the highest. Indeed, as Hippolyte Bernheim wrote, unlike the word contagion, "the word epidemic does not prejudge the cause; it only implies an observation."[13] If "the epidemic is a social fact," Durkheim intends to demonstrate, with his cartographic experiment, that its cause is less likely to be found in an unobservable moral contagion than in the sociological description of socially homogeneous environments.

translated by Maya Judd

NOTES

1. Scipio Sighele, *La foule criminelle: Essai de psychologie collective*, Bibliothèque de philosophie contemporaine, trans. from Italian by Paul Vigny (Paris: Félix Alcan, 1892), 39.

2. Jean-Étienne Esquirol, "Suicide (pathologie interne)," *Dictionnaire des sciences médicales, par une société de médecins et de chirurgiens*, vol. 53 (Paris: C. L. F. Panckoucke, 1821), 247.

3. James M. Baldwin et al., "Contagion (social and mental)," "Crowd," "Imitation," "Resemblance," "Suggestion" and "Social Psychology," in *Dictionary of Philosophy and Psychology: Including Many of the Principal Conceptions of Ethics, Logic, Aesthetics, Philosophy of Religion, Mental Pathology, Anthropology, Biology, Neurology, Physiology, Economics, Political and Social Philosophy, Philology, Physical Science, and Education; and Giving a Terminology in English, French, German and Italian*, ed. James M. Baldwin, vols. 1–2 (New York and London: Macmillan, 1901–1902), 222–224, 246–247, 305, 330, 494–496, 519–520, and vol. 2 (1902), 466–467, 619–620, 538.

4. Émile Durkheim, *Le suicide: Étude de sociologie* (Paris: Félix Alcan, 1897), 119; *Suicide: A Study in Sociology*, translated by John A. Spaulding and George Simpson (New York: Taylor and Francis, 2005), 83. Citations refer to the 2005 translation.

5. Gabriel Tarde, *La philosophie pénale* (Lyon-Paris: A. Storck/G. Masson, 1890), 24, 325, 429. The expression is old and quite central to the sociological work of the provincial philosopher from Sarlat. ("Qu'est-ce qu'une société?" *Revue philosophique de la France et de l'étranger* 18 [November 1884]: 491). Tarde explains this in his best-known opus, particularly in the reprint of his 1884 article (*Les lois de l'imitation: Étude sociologique* [Paris: Félix Alcan, 1890], 23–24, 82–98).

6. Durkheim, *Suicide*, 81.

7. Durkheim, *Le suicide*, 116, my translation.

8. Tarde, *Les lois de l'imitation*, 212.

9. Émile Durkheim, *De la division du travail social: Thèse présentée à la Faculté des Lettres de Paris* (Paris: Félix Alcan, 1893), 245 (my translation).

10. Figure 2 is from Durkheim, *Le suicide*, 124–125, plate ii (original: 20.4 × 22.2 cm) and, to credit the two contributors to the book, xi–xii. The original map presents a mold in inverted form of the Boussac/Bourganeuf main arrondissement towns. See also Gabriel Tarde, "Contre Durkheim à propos de son Suicide," unpublished text prepared and submitted by Philippe Besnard and Massimo Borlandi, in *Le suicide un siècle après Durkheim*, ed. Massimo Borlandi and Mohamed Cherkaoui (Paris: Presses Universitaires de France, 2000), 228.

11. Durkheim, *Suicide*, 128.

12. Durkheim, *Suicide*, 119.

13. Hippolyte Bernheim, "Contagion," in *Dictionnaire encyclopédique des sciences médicales*, ed. Amédée Dechambre, first series, vol. 20 (Paris: G. Masson and P. Asselin, 1877), 49.

SELECTED BIBLIOGRAPHY

Besnard, Philippe. "Des Règles au Suicide: Durkheim critique de Tarde." In *Les Règles de Durkheim un siècle après*, edited by Massimo Borlandi and Laurent Mucchielli, 221–243. Paris: L'Harmattan, 1995.

Borlandi, Massimo. "Durkheim et la psychologie." In *Durkheim fut-il durkheimien?*, edited by Raymond Boudon, 55–80. Paris: Armand Colin, 2011.

Castel, Pierre-Henri. *La Querelle de l'hystérie: La formation du discours psychopathologique en France (1881–1913)*. Paris: Presses Universitaires de France, 1998.

Goldstein, Jan. "'Moral Contagion': A Professional Ideology of Medicine and Psychiatry in Eighteenth and Nineteenth-Century France." In *Professions and the French state 1700–1900*, edited by Gerald L. Geison, 181–222. Philadelphia: University of Philadelphia Press, 1984.

Guillo, Dominique. "La place de la biologie dans les premiers textes de Durkheim: Un paradigm oublié?" *Revue française de sociologie* 47, no. 3 (2006): 507–535.

Karsenti, Bruno. "L'imitation: Retour sur le débat entre Durkheim et Tarde." In *La régularité, Habitude, disposition et savoir-faire dans l'explication de l'action*, edited by Christiane Chauviré and Albert Ogien, 183–205. Paris: Éditions de l'EHESS, 2002.

Mucchielli, Laurent, and Marc Renneville. "Les causes du suicide: Pathologie individuelle ou sociale? Durkheim, Halbwachs et les psychiatres de leur temps (1830–1930)." *Déviance et société* 22, no. 1 (1998): 3–36.

Rosental, Paul-André. "Où s'arrête la contagion? Faits et utopie chez Gabriel Tarde." *Tracés: Revue de Sciences humaines*, no. 21 (2011): 109–124.

SWAMPS
Drying Fever in Modern Europe

Raphaël Morera

In the modern era, wetlands, and swamps specifically, are commonly associated with noxious environments carrying dangerous germs. The inquiries of the nineteenth century still described them as vectors of illness, weakening the population living around them. This negative image, passed down from antiquity and Hippocratic thought, was first mobilized and then consolidated in the Renaissance. The rediscovery of the ancients within the context of Christianity had a profound impact on the images of the environment and nature. Extensively exploited until the end of the Middle Ages, and in some cases entirely manmade, wetlands have become coveted spaces. They are types of nature to be transformed. Between the sixteenth and eighteenth centuries in Europe, the draining of wetlands to create profitable territories was intense and almost constant. This resulted in a profound transformation not only of littorals and estuaries but also the valley floors of more continental zones. In the beginning, the intent of the drying was prophylactic: its aim was to sanitize and to combat swamp fever. But it was also motivated by economic reasons. The practice of drainage itself began to spread like a fever, a drying fever.

The draining of swamps and their conversion into arable lands and pastures was part of an ancient tradition. In the context of modern Europe, the practice gained a renewed popularity in the "water country" of Northern Italy and the Netherlands. During the sixteenth century, the deltas of the Po and the Rhine underwent fundamental transformations. In Italy, cities supported large-scale drainage sites by way of the help they gave to *consorzi.* The latter were a type of company consisting of landowners and urban elites joining together for purposes of agricultural improvements. The economic elites took control of lands considered empty and undeveloped. In the Netherlands, nobles in the south first took the initiative of vast drainage efforts, particularly in the Escaut estuary. Further north, the urban bourgeoisie intensified this movement starting in the 1570s. The twinned implementation of mechanical techniques, windmills, and vast hydraulic infrastructures allowed the Netherlands, and particularly the United Provinces, to support a population that had doubled during this period.

The Netherlands, the United Provinces, and the Duchy of Milan differ from each other, both in their institutional systems and their political and religious cultures. They share, however, a flourishing culture of water. Though founded on very different postulates for each state, all promoted the separation of land from water, as the mixing and joining of these two elements were understood as signs of a physical world as yet unfinished. In Italy the Counter-Reformation and fashionable Neo-Platonic thought conferred a very strong religious dimension to drainage efforts. Indeed, those implementing the drainage were working at perfecting creation and the renewal of its underlying mathematical language. In the United Provinces, the triumph of the Reformation, national independence, and hydraulic works also went hand in hand. In Holland, the separation of land and waters signified the divine election of both a territory and a people. This notion only intensified as the drainage guaranteed prosperity to its promoters. In Northern Italy as in the United Provinces, drying and agricultural development were signs of a strong power, giving rise to a political project that would be the expression of modernity.

In the sixteenth century, these two regions, representing two matrices of political and economical modernity, transformed into models and sources of inspiration. They became, in a manner of speaking, *foci* of contagion. And it is indeed in this way that they were perceived by European powers who were quickly contracting this drying fever. The internal expansion, due to this technique, of these two regions, characterized by both wetlands and dry, inspired the French and British monarchies in the 1580s. In 1585, Queen Elizabeth adopted the General Drainage Act to support such efforts in England. If these were not immediately successful, still the English monarchy pursued this policy throughout the seventeenth century, even during troubled times. In France, in 1599, Henry IV promulgated an edict for the drying of French marshes and lakes. From this date, and nearly without interruption until the French Revolution, the monarchy constantly upheld drainage works. It enlisted its entire judicial apparatus to encourage and facilitate capitalist investments throughout the kingdom.

Out of such laboratories, drying fever underwent a kind of mutation. Religious considerations did not disappear, but political and economical dimensions clearly came to the fore. In France and in England, the drainage works served as an underlying support to a kind of internal colonization of the country: to gain land from the water contributed to pushing back the borders of the realm. In France, the connection with sedentarization, the control of peoples, and the affirmation of sovereign power were particularly strong. In this sense the framework of the theory of climates, as formulated by Jean Bodin in the *Six Books of the Commonwealth* played a decisive role. According to Bodin, the kingdom of France is a climate defined by the existence of a strong sovereign power and a settled population. This political dimension was also present in England, but enriched by the Baconian framework of improvement, pairing economic progress with scientific and technical advances. Afterward, in the seventeenth century, drainage efforts were anchored to a culture of progress, embedded in projects of social regeneration.

The Dutch model was also spread widely in Northern Europe following the paths of urbanization. Copenhagen and Saint Petersburg were created by enlisting the building techniques of from the Netherlands, radically transforming the environment and permitting solid construction on unstable sands. Everywhere, the setting of these milestones joined together with the victories of the bourgeoisie and the states in question.

In the seventeenth century, drying fever experienced a rapid spread from several points of origin, although irregular in nature and failing to take root in a sustained fashion. The expansion depended upon economic and political reasoning. In the eighteenth century, however, the diffusion intensified. It was no longer a question of small groups supporting the spread of drying fever, but the different states encouraging these efforts to the greatest number. Draining projects became the norm and the common objective of landowners. Drying fever became endemic.

In England, the drainage works were fully part of the vast movement of parliamentary enclosures. The great projects of the seventeenth century, which did not always meet with the success expected of them, disappeared in favor of projects of a more limited and local nature but also much more efficient. This resulted in substantial land gains. There was a comparable tendency in France, where the monarchy ceased to support only one group of investors capable of acting on the whole of the realm. After the great liberal laws of the 1760s, drainage efforts needed no more than a simple declaration to the intendant, the local representative of the king, and as a result, the practice became generalized. Demographic growth also made the conquest of new arable lands necessary. While all the local means of implanting drying practices are not known, the convergence of interests between local bourgeoisie, nobles, and the tate often explains how practices endured. On the French Atlantic littoral, the bourgeois and the nobles invested while the state monitored, controlled, and supported investors.

At the end of the eighteenth century, drying fever was taking hold. Pockets of resistance did, however, appear. When economies declined and demographics dropped, water took back its rights. Environmental changes, social crises, and the dysfunction of the draining companies allowed the reed beds to regain terrain and grow anew. This is what happened in Provence when the disinvestment of the drainers allowed the Rhone to regain the land that had been taken from it before. In the United Provinces, comparably, the global shrinking of the economy forced the drainers to double their efforts for slighter and slighter gains.

In Europe, the drying fever grew stronger in the nineteenth and twentieth centuries, and the greed for wetlands even constantly intensified. While this greed was relatively contained in Europe, the colonial dynamics of the nineteenth and twentieth centuries offered new terrain for expansion where the renewed alliance between state support and agricultural development multiplied the capacities for action on wetlands, to the detriment of local populations. It has only been since the end of the twentieth century that drying fever has died out in the face of understanding the value of wetlands in their natural state, even if they continue to shrink worldwide.

translated by Vicki-Marie Petrick

BIBLIOGRAPHY

Ciriacono, Salvatore. *Building on Water: Venice, Holland and the Construction of the European Landscape in Early Modern Times.* New York: Berghan Books, 2006. First published in 1994 as *Acque e agricoltura: Venezia, l'Olanda e la bonifica in età moderna* (Milan: Franco Angeli).

Leveau, Philippe. "Mentalité économique et grands travaux hydrauliques: Le drainage du Lac Fucin, aux origines d'un modèle." *Annales ESC* 48, no. 1 (1993): 3–16.

Morera, Raphaël, and John Morgan. "Les desséchements modernes: Des projets coloniaux? Comparaison entre la France et l'Angleterre." *Études rurales* 203 (2019): 42–61.

Morera, Raphaël. "Mise en valeur des zones humides et associations de gestion: Naissance et affirmation de nouveaux pouvoirs territoriaux (France, XVIe–XVIIIe siècles)." *Siècles* 42 (2016). http://journals.openedition.org/siecles/2946.

Rippe, Gérard. *Padoue et son contado, Xe–XIIIe siècle. Société et pouvoirs.* Rome: École française de Rome, 2003.

Schama, Simon. *The Embarrassment of Riches: An Interpretation of Dutch Culture in the Golden Age.* New York: Knopf, 1987.

Van Cruyningen, Piet. "Dealing with Drainage: State Regulations of Drainage Projects in the Duthc Republic, France and England during the Sixteenth and the Seventeenth Centuries." *Economic History Review* 68, no. 2 (November 2015): 420–440.

Van Dam, Petra J. E. M., and Milja Van Tielhof. *Waterstaat in hetstedenland: Het hoogheemraadschap van Rijnlandvoor 1857.* Utrecht: Mathijs, 2006.

THEATER

From Poison to Patriotic Electricity: Eighteenth-Century Conceptions of the Spectacle

Thibaut Julian and Suzanne Rochefort

Considering the notion of contagion from a historical point of view allows for exploration of the broad range of discourse on the theater during the Enlightenment and later revolutionary turn of the eighteenth century. A period of stage mania and sweeping changes, both in conditions of performance and theories of acting and spectacle, the eighteenth century appears as a key moment in the history of theater. Applied to the theatrical space, the metaphor of contagion can express the dangers of moral contamination as well as point to the propagation of new ideas and civic feeling. This ambivalence as to the circulation of emotions highlights the complexity of contemporary inquiries into the power of spectacles, where the co-presence of actors' and spectators' bodies during a performance fascinated as much as it troubled.

As early as antiquity, a spectacle's inherent power to transmit emotions provoked sharp condemnations of the theater, even as the notion of catharsis outlined mainly by Aristotle in the *Poetics* supposed a purgation of passions, bestowing a medico-moral value upon mimetic representation. But its effectiveness became the object of enduring debates, and the spectacle, a site of simulacra and pleasure, was condemned by Plato and then by the early Christians. So it was with Tertullian in his *De Spectaculis*, or with Saint Augustine who writes in *The City of God*: "Comedy seduces the mind and provokes in it a communicable madness: it affects a few then spreads to all, like a pestilence of souls."[1]

In the latter half of the seventeenth century, when critiques of the theater are more sharply made, the metaphor of contagion returns in full force. Indeed, while a new theory of the passions is being elaborated, the process of emotional contagion in the theater attracts attention: since the human body is recognized as the site that produces the passions, that of the spectator finds itself particularly implicated in this dynamic.

The Age of Enlightenment is marked by the emergence in Paris of the *théâtre de la Foire*, then of the *théâtre des boulevards*, the provincial stages, and the private *théâtres de société*: this development fuels new denunciations of the supposed indecency of these spaces. In the preface to *The Marriage of Figaro*, Pierre-Augustin Caron de Beaumarchais—positioning himself as a defender of "theatrical decency"—thus dismisses "that polluted heap of stages raised to our shame."[2] The same note is struck by Nicolas-Joseph Sélis, who spins the epidemic metaphor in his *Lettre à un père de famille* (1789). The author describes the small theaters as "poisons" that corrupt morals, particularly those of the young who attend them. The risks may be limited with minimal exposure to the contagious agent (i.e., infrequent attendance of spectacles), but those infected, irrepressibly drawn to the source of their evil, cannot resist returning often.

The critique is thus mainly founded upon moral discourse, though one must not obscure its engagement in the debates over acting and stage reality. Jean-Jacques Rousseau, despite being himself a playwright and disgruntled theater enthusiast, systematically extends his censure to the theatrical apparatus. Spectacles are places of moral decline, and the actress is the primary contagious agent. Exposed onstage to the public's gaze, likened to a courtesan, she exercises a power of seduction that exceeds the duration of the performance. The theater, then, is not only associated with the threat of debauchery, but it also promotes an overturning of social and gender hierarchies, as actresses speak prominently in the public space. Even more originally, Rousseau explains the alienation of the spectator by the imaginary process of denial opened by the distance of fiction. To this phantasmal mediation, he opposes another contagion, which is sincere and healthy: that of the participative spectacles of the civic fête, according to Swiss and Spartan models. If he condemns the simulacrum of the actor, Rousseau protects the ethical transparency of the orator.

These hostile critiques become particularly noteworthy during the stormy period of the Revolution. The theatrical frenzy, heightened by the 1791 law on the freedom of theaters, provokes virulent diatribes and attempts—once the Terror has begun—to control and purify the dramatic world. Inventor of the classical melodrama, René-Charles Guilbert de Pixerécourt argues, in his *Observations sur les théâtres et la Révolution* written in the aftermath of the Thermidor, that if in the theater "all feelings are transmitted by injections, so that both the good and the ill always spread like wildfire,"[3] one requires an enlightened legislation that would survey and channel its course. Preventive and repressive censorship, as well as the legislation of theatrical life that grew stronger from the Directory to the French Empire, are a legal and political response to this aesthetic-moral thought.

But contrary to such mistrust, the contagious power of the theater is also valued during the Enlightenment. Voltaire makes of the theater a weapon for philosophical ideas, an "enduring school of poetry and virtue," as his suggests in *Tancrède* (1760).[4] Under the growing influence of sensualism, the theater is perceived as a moral tableau from which the public benefits by experiencing pleasure at the performance and whose spectacle enables the efficient circulation of emotions between stage and audience. Actors are the primary means of such circulation. In his treatise *Le Comédien* (1747), Rémond de Sainte-Albine affirms that one of the main qualities of interpreters is "having fire," that is, an unfeigned stage energy able to transmit a truth of action to the public. The fire spreads to the spectators, much like the fever provoked in 1765 by *The Siege of Calais*, a tragedy by Pierre-Laurent De Belloy that provoked lively argument between the *philosophes* and their opponents. To describe it, Melchior Grimm resorts to natural metaphors: "An unexpected storm breaks almost as soon as it has formed: a sudden catastrophe brings combustion to the parterre, the boxes, the entire theatre hall; and, after suddenly raising the curtain on *The Siege of Calais*, this fire begins to spread outside with the same speed, slipping into all circles, reaching all dining rooms, and communicating to all minds a heat that produces a universal wildfire."[5] The theater is not only an object of corrupting entertainment but also a political and polemical arena, whose signs could be put into service of opposing ideologies.

In the later eighteenth century, the metaphor of electricity reconfigures the thinking on contagion in a new "society of the spectacle." As Michel Delon has emphasized, the image of electro physics evokes a rapid, step-by-step transmission, especially palpable in the parterre of theaters, another forum for the expression and debate of "popular" or "public" opinion. The positioning of the spectators in the hall turns out to be crucial for the circulation of a spectacular electricity, hence the regrets of certain playwrights, enthusiasts, and theorists of the theater over the architectural renovations that, during the 1780s, favored seating in the parterre. Louis-Sébastien Mercier complains in his *Tableau de Paris* that "the electricity has been cut since the seats no longer allow heads to touch and mingle."[6]

On the eve of the Revolution, the theater's contagious power thus becomes the crucible of a new civic and political promotion of the art. The metaphor of electricity suggests a synergy of the collective, manifest in political assemblies as well as in theaters, privileged platforms for the fostering and expression of patriotism. This is what Marie-Joseph Chénier maintains by opposing solitary reading to the "quick, ardent, unanimous" sensation of dramatic representation. *Charles IX ou l'École des rois*, his first "national and patriotic tragedy,"[7] constitutes a notable political and cultural event in 1789, bringing to the stage, not without difficulty, the contagion of fanaticism during the St. Bartholomew's Day massacre. The "national" theater that consecrates the Revolution is based upon the drive to moralize, redress, and purify the spectators by offering them models of patriotism appropriate to the new times. Thus theatrical events are conducive to polemics and the battle of public opinion. In 1805, the success of *Les Templiers*, François-Just-Marie Raynouard's historical tragedy, provokes the hostile judgment of the conservative critic Geoffroy, who laments the "fervours of the enthusiasts" and resigns himself to waiting for "the fever of *Les Templiers* to run its course like any other epidemic disease."[8]

The theater of the eighteenth century offers a passionate and "electric" field of inquiry where one may understand the ideological fermentation peculiar to the age, along with continuities and transformations in the representations of the theater's role and practical reality, of its moral and utilitarian conceptions in society: theater as poison or as the remedy found in the disease itself.

translated by Jeffrey Burkholder

NOTES

1. D'Hippone, Augustin. *La Cité de Dieu*, book 1, edited by Pierre Lombert, 306–307 (Bourges: chez Gille, 1818).

2. Pierre-Augustin Caron de Beaumarchais, *Œuvres*, edited by Pierre and Jacqueline Larthomas (Paris: Gallimard, Bibliothèque de la Pléiade, 1988), 355.

3. René-Charles Guilbert de Pixerécourt, *Observations sur les théâtres et la Révolution*, edited by Gauthier Ambrus, in *Orages: Littérature et culture 1760–1830*, no. 14: "Le tragique moderne," ed. M. Melai, 147–165, at 159 (Neuilly: Atlande, 2015).

4. Voltaire, *Tancrède*, edited by John S. Henderson and Thomas Wynn, in *Les Œuvres complètes de Voltaire*, vol. 49B (Oxford: Voltaire Foundation, 2009), 129.

5. *Correspondance littéraire, philosophique et critique de Grimm et de Diderot depuis 1753 jusqu'en 1790*, edited by Maurice Tourneux (Paris: Garnier frères, 1877–1882), book 6, 256.

6. Louis-Sébastien Mercier, *Tableau de Paris*, 2 vols., edited by Jean-Claude Bonnet (Paris: Mercure de France, 1994), vol. 2, 88.

7. Marie-Joseph Chénier, *Théâtre*, edited by Gauthier Ambrus and François Jacob (Paris: GF, 2002), 168.

8. *Journal de l'Empire*, August 18, 1805.

BIBLIOGRAPHY

Berchtold, Jacques, Yannick Séité, and Christophe Martin, eds. *Rousseau et le spectacle*. Paris: Armand Colin, 2014.

Bourdin, Philippe. *Aux origines du théâtre patriotique*. Paris: CNRS éditions, 2017.

Darmon, Jean-Charles, ed. *Littérature et thérapeutique des passions: La catharsis en question*. Paris: Hermann, 2011.

Delon, Michel. *L'idée d'énergie au tournant des Lumières (1770–1820)*. Paris: PUF, 1988.

Frantz, Pierre. *L'Esthétique du tableau dans le théâtre du XVIIIe siècle*. Paris: PUF, 1998.

Frantz, Pierre, and Sophie Marchand, eds. *Le Théâtre français du XVIIIe siècle: Histoire, textes choisis, mises en scène*. Paris: L'Avant-scène théâtre, 2009.

Marie, Laurence. *Inventer l'acteur: Émotions et spectacle dans l'Europe des Lumières*. Paris: Sorbonne Université Presses, 2019.

Poirson, Martial, and Guy Spielmann. "Avant-propos." *Dix-Huitième Siècle* 49 (2017): 5–25.

Thouret, Clotilde. "La contagion des affects dans les polémiques sur le théâtre au XVIIe siècle, en Espagne et en France." In *La Contagion: Enjeux croisés des discours médicaux et littéraires (XVIe–XIXe siècle)*, edited by Ariane Bayle, 57–68. Dijon: Éditions universitaires de Dijon, 2013.

TRADITION

Ancient Writings and Political Legitimation in China at the Beginning of the Twentieth Century

Pablo A. Blitstein

The Qing dynasty (1644–1912), the last dynasty to reign over China, believed like its predecessors that the emperor was a kind of "transmitter," whose mission was to pass on to his subjects the words of the sages of remote antiquity. Such "transmission" was not conceived as a simple "contagion" independent of the wills of those concerned. Rather, if the emperor wished to keep the favor of Heaven—the ultimate arbiter of his actions—he had not merely to familiarize himself with the "Confucian" classics, read the exegeses, encourage the emergence of learned men and embody the teachings of the ancient sages through his own measures. He also had to ensure his administrators actively follow these ancient teachings and that all his subjects might benefit from a virtuous reign. The harmony among humankind, heaven, and earth depended upon it. *Chuan* 傳 (transmission) was in fact one of the keywords of the neo-Confucian tradition that the dynasty made its own. One of the tradition's forerunners, Han Yu, had as early as the eighth century called for the ancient sages' Way (Dao) to be restored, which meant their particular ways of doing things and the criteria they used to make judgments. He explained that wise kings had "transmitted" the Way to Confucius, Confucius had "transmitted" it to Mencius, and the transmission had broken off after Mencius. The Qing dynasty, like those that went before, believed they had restored the ancient transmission of the Way.

What happened to this notion of transmission—both textual and moral—when the empire collapsed in 1912? The dilemma was not a wholly novel one in nineteenth- and twentieth-century Asia. As in the case of Japan to the East or the Ottoman world to the West, the country's elites reread the various texts of the past in the light of European political discourse and compared them to their own experiences of the modern world. A symptomatic example of this new attitude toward the transmission of ancient knowledge was Li Dazhao's "Minyi yu zhengzhi" ("The Standards of the People and Politics"), written in 1916. Li was a central character in early twentieth-century China. Having been a protagonist of the May Fourth Movement of 1919, he figured among founders of the Chinese Communist Party in 1921. In 1916, he was not yet a Marxist; he was known rather for his opposition to Yuan Shikai, who had tried to restore the monarchy, and for his defense of the young Chinese republic. His "Minyi yu zhengzhi" was written in classical Chinese and was conceived within this political struggle. Resorting to ancient and more recent texts, he discussed the transmission of ancient knowledge and the role that the words of the sages ought to play in the new republican order. He was thus representative of a broader process, whereby the words of the sages became those of the nation and moral transmission became national tradition.

The keyword of "Minyi yu zhengzhi" was *yi* 彝, meaning "implement" or "standard." The term referred back directly to the ancient sages. Li Dazhao took it from the Confucian classics and reformulated it on the basis of an exegesis of the *Book of Documents* and the *Book of Odes*. The term was useful to him because in the classics it was employed in both a concrete and metonymic sense. Concretely, it referred to physical objects or implements used in the context of ancestor worship; metonymically, these "implements" indicated predispositions, customs, rules, and criteria, that is, "standards" in the sense of customary rules of practice and judgment. The *yi* was an emblem of the enduring character of ancient transmission; like the implements used in the temple of the ancestors, it was transmitted from generation to generation and characterized the nation's history.

Li Dazhao set his face against using the term in an antiquarian way. His exegesis of ancient occurrences of *yi* aimed to show that "in Antiquity, the divine implement(s) of politics was/were based on the standards of lineage (*zongyi* 宗彝); today the divine implement(s) of politics is/are based on the standards of the people (*minyi* 民彝)."[1] He contrasted two lines of ancient transmission. The first, that of the standards of lineage, corresponded to the norms that each reigning family tried to impose on the whole empire over millennia. According to Li , these were based on exclusively family transmission, as distinct from the true needs of the "people," and served the selfish needs of each dynasty. These standards of lineage were not an entirely new concept for Chinese readers familiar with the literati traditions of the empire. In some respects, they recalled an idea that Huang Zongxi had formulated in the seventeenth century, opining that "[ever since the wise kings of antiquity], what is called 'law' is in fact the law of a single family and not the common law of all who exist under Heaven."[2]

Li Dazhao put a different spin on this idea. For Huang Zongxi, the only way to put an end to this "law of a single family" was to abolish the imperial system in place since the third-century BCE, restore preimperial "feudalism," and encourage mandarins and local societies to become more autonomous. For Li Dazhao, on the contrary, the solution would come through setting up a parliamentary system and creating a constitution on the basis of the second line of transmission, that of the "standards of the people."

What exactly did Li Dazhao understand by "standards of the people"? For him, they meant the norms and practices to which the people spontaneously had recourse. They were not imposed by external constraint but came from spontaneous behavior; they flowed from the essential nature of the people and were passed down through centuries. Closer to *narodnik* populism (fairly widespread in anarchist circles) than to republican constitutionalism, Li Dazhao suggested the people were spontaneously good and that the Chinese constitution should be based on its standards. While echoing the liberalism of John Stuart Mill and the constitutional theories of A. V. Dicey, he combined them with the ideas of Tolstoy and neo-Confucian teachings on the basic goodness of human nature.

Each of these two groups of "standards," those of the people and those of lineage, depended on differing forms of transmission. The standards of lineage were based on "theft" and "usurpation." Since each reigning family had its own lineage-serving standards, each one had different standards, and every change of dynasty amounted to stealing the *yi* of another family. In other words, these standards/implements of lineage could be imposed only by force; they were inevitably different from the "standards/implements of the people" and were at the root of "despotism" (*zhuanzhi* 專制). The standards of the people, on the contrary, being transmitted spontaneously, could be neither stolen nor usurped: they were inherent in the very nature of the people. They were a common property that might be suppressed or reduced to silence by the standards of lineage, but they could not be stolen or extinguished by them.

Were these popular standards common to all humanity, or did they differ from one nation to another? Li Dazhao was not clear on this point. His text gives the impression that they appertained to all humanity, but he says also that each nation "has confidence" in "the standards of its people" and seeks to "express" these standards in its actions and political institutions.[3] Be that as it may, the standards of the people were conceived as something that was transmitted and yet evolved: it was no longer the transmission of ancient knowledge but a national tradition embedded in the people's customs and subject to a process of unending reformulation. Regarded thus, the idea of national transmission is not far from that of "contagion," for, while the ancient idea of transmission implied active engagement to preserve ancient knowledge and, above all, to top-down enforcement, national tradition functioned through spontaneous transmission between successive generations of the same "people."

Li Dazhao's "Minyi yu zhengzhi" shows how textual and moral transmission of the classics became national tradition. The notion that made such evolution possible, that of the "nation," had not existed in China fifty years earlier; it won over minds only in the 1890s. By the 1910s, it was everywhere; it could be found even in certain anarchistic and revolutionary circles pursuing a quest for "the essence of the nation" and seeing the world as a society of nations. The words of the ancient sages thus changed their meaning. Throughout the greater part of the nineteenth century, they had been regarded as the basis of the institutions of the empire and the precondition for the cohesion of its subjects: without the sages, there would be no empire, and without the empire there would be no political unity. As soon as the "nation" emerged conceptually as an autonomous collective entity, as something preexistent to political institutions, the words of the sages became the historic expression of a "tradition" characterizing the nation and rendering it recognizable over time. The phenomenon is traceable in the history of the modern Chinese word for "tradition" itself: *chuantong* 傳統. Although founded etymologically upon the word for "transmission"—*chuan*—*chuantong* emerged as a neologism that was clearly different from *chuan* and that connoted the cultural continuity of a collective, in this case a national collective.

The "national tradition" served to attack monarchical institutions, as is shown by the use of the standards of the people in Li Dazhao's text. Others used it to attack the parliamentary institutions that Li sought to defend. But whatever oppositions formed around this concept, in the early 1910s, arguments over transmission were absorbed by a nationalist discourse on tradition. Even today, a sizable number of contemporary appropriations of the words of the sages sit within this framework.

translated by Graham Robert Edwards

NOTES

1. Li Dazhao 李大釗, "Minyi yu zhengzhi 民彝與政治," in *Li Dazhao xuanji* (Beijing: Renmin chubanshe, 1959), 38.

2. Huang Zongxi 黃宗羲, *Mingyi daifang lu* 明夷待訪錄, in *Huang Zongxi quanji*, vol. 1 (Hangzhou: Zhejiang guji chubanshe, 2012), 6.

3. Li Dazhao, "Minyi yu zhengzhi," 40.

SELECTED BIBLIOGRAPHY

Duan, Lian 段煉. "'Xinli', 'minyi' yu zhengzhi zhengdang xing—yi Minguo chunian Li Dazhao de sixiang wei zhongxin 心力, 民彝與政治正當性—以民國初年李大釗的思想為中心." In *Chong gu chuantong. Zai zao wenming: zhishi fenzi yu wusi xinwenhua yundong* 重估傳統. 再造文明: 知識分子與五四新文化運動, edited by Huang Kewu, 154–186. Taibei: Xiuwei zixun keji, 2019.

Matten, Marc. "China Is the China of the Chinese: The Concept of Nation and Its Impact on Political Thinking in Modern China." *Oriens Extremus* 51 (2012): 63–106.

Meisner, Maurice. *Li Ta-Chao and the Origins of Chinese Marxism*. Cambridge, MA: Harvard University Press, 1967.

Zarrow, Peter. *After Empire: The Conceptual Transformation of the Chinese State, 1885–1924*. Stanford: Stanford University Press, 2012.

Zhou, Yanqiong 周艷瓊. "Li Dazhao minyi sixiang ji qi dangdai jiazhi 李大釗民彝思想及其當代價值." *Shenyang gongye daxue xuebao* 10/6 (2017): 565–670.

TRANSNATIONALISM
Migration Fever and the Study of Mobility
Nancy L. Green

Migration is contagious. So are the terms used to analyze it.

We do not always know why the first pioneer made the move, but we do know that tens of thousands of people often follow—in "flows," "streams," or "waves." The liquid metaphors of migration date to the vast nineteenth-century transatlantic movements. The terms still designate a collective activity whereby large numbers of individuals leave their home-towns and strike out elsewhere. But not everyone sees such movement with equanimity, and disapproval is not just the province of fearful xenophobes in the countries of arrival. In the nineteenth century, politicians and pun-dits in the countries of origin worried about population loss, and they already had a term for the phenomenon: "migration fever."

Although there were those who were happy to see radicals or unwanted minorities leave, many others, from family members to social critics to political actors, seeing loved ones depart and whole villages depleted, described the move in fearful or critical terms. "Migration fever" has been used to designate everything from Irish emigration in the early nineteenth century to Germans and other Central Europeans moving en masse to North and South America from the mid-nineteenth century on to Afri-can Americans moving from the US South northward during the Great Migration of the early twentieth century. The phrase continues to be used today to refer to Latin Americans heading to the United States or Africans migrating toward Europe. Villages have been described as "plagued" by the massive departure of youth.

When is migration a disease, and when is it the collective agency of a series of individual choices? The "fever" can be contracted in a variety of ways. Ever since the nineteenth century, letters (and money) and soon photos sent home encouraged followers. The rotary telephone, in its time, was also a way of trumpeting triumphs at the point of destination and describing the paths taken to family back home. In the early twenty-first century, smartphones provide immediate route and other information for prospective followers. Newspaper articles and films depicting opportunities abroad have also abetted the movement, circulating information about destinations in sometimes specific but also more general ways.

Yet the fever is also transmitted by more or less scrupulous intermediaries. Migration agents were already viewed with suspicion in the nineteenth century. One of them, Georges de Pardonnet, special emigration agent for Kansas and Oregon, even denounced his competitors. He warned his French compatriots to beware of a danger in the United States even greater than that of crossing the desert or encountering Native Americans: devious fellow citizens who could fleece the unsuspecting newcomer along the migration trail. Today, the human smugglers along the US–Mexico border are called, ominously, "coyotes."

Political authorities in the nineteenth century tried to counter the massive movement overseas in two ways. Emigration agents were discredited and at times prosecuted. Today, both emigration and immigration countries try to clamp down on those intermediaries who make fortunes while enticing individuals to try their luck via increasingly dangerous crossings. Countries of departure have also tried to counter the fever with counterpropaganda or with dire descriptions of fearsome ordeals of life in the new country, highlighting stories of failure rather than success.

Yet if migration has been bleakly described as a contagious fever by those despairing and disparaging of departures, social scientists have found other terms to explain how migration trajectories take off, circulate, and mushroom: social networks in action. In 1964, John S. and Leatrice MacDonald first postulated the functioning of "chain migration" and "social networks" to explain how ethnic neighborhoods developed. The mysteries of what can be called "the destination question" can be largely understood by the flow of data among social groups. People follow kith and kin thanks to informal informational networks and intrafamily and community financial aid and loans. Word of mouth among peers is stronger than any official naysayer's doubts and disapproval.

Contagion furthermore is not just about the historical movement itself. Social scientists have themselves been struck with a form of analytic contagion: topics trend periodically through the pens and screens of scholars, and theories spread throughout research cohorts. Articles and tomes are devoted to one model of explanation until another comes along in a series of "historiographic 'turns.'" For migration history, the infectious "new social history" of immigration that developed in the 1960s in the United States, for example, first focused heavily on assimilation. Influenced by sociologist Milton Gordon's postulate of the different stages of assimilation, historians (like sociologists) sought to study immigrants' processes of adopting the language, dress, daily customs, values, and norms of the host society. They studied how minorities eventually integrated into the clubs and institutions of the host society, moved out of their ethnic enclaves into mainstream neighborhoods and jobs, and intermarried with the locals. It was considered just a matter of time until immigrants came to identify with the dominant culture and were successfully integrated into the host society, henceforth devoid of discrimination.

However, in the late 1960s and early 1970s, new scholars questioned and soon sought to reverse the assimilationist paradigm. Had the loss of all original identity in the quest to conform really taken place? A new wave of research came to focus on the opposite of assimilation, and the study of ethnic retention became "catching." Affected by the "ethnic renaissance," academics feverishly turned, often with the same sources, to highlighting that which immigrants had retained rather than what they had forsaken in the process of settling in to a new country. "Ethnic studies" became all the rage in the United States, and, even in ethnic-reticent France, individual community studies took off, well noting how groups of immigrants recreated their own clubs and religious and cultural activities in the new land. In the United States in particular, however, consonant with the more multicultural times, researchers were swept up in the ethnic fever, usefully pointing out that assimilation was not the only way to analyze migrant behavior. The persistence of social networks was brought to the fore as theory and research agenda.

Yet in 1992, while also relying on an understanding of social networks, a new term was launched by anthropologists who sought, once again, to overturn the previous historiographic modes. In a programmatic essay and edited book by Nina Glick-Schiller, Linda Basch, and Christine Blanc-Szanton, *Towards a Transnational Perspective on Migration: Race, Class, Ethnicity, and Nationalism Reconsidered*, the authors/editors proposed "transnationalism" as a better way of describing migrant destinies to point out the interactions that immigrants continue to have with their home countries. At the same time, Ian Tyrrell used the term to encourage an internationalization of US history. The term has been contagious, and it has come to be used not just to analyze the actions of historical actors but as a research perspective beyond migration studies, examining the circulation of ideas and goods as well as people.

Migration historians were, however, at first reticent, arguing that this was nothing new (nineteenth-century migrants were already transnational). But they (we) too got infected by the new concept. Re-mining our sources, we have found not just dual identities of migrants past (which were already the subject of ethnicity-focused studies) but extensive proof of actual movement and ties back and forth. Concrete examples of circulation have modified ideas about linear migration and settlement. Even in the past, the tenacity of ties between homeland and hostland was widespread, albeit circumscribed depending on time and place. Today's historiographic emphasis has thus largely turned around transnationalism. Interpreting old sources in new ways, the term has become a "must" for the description of migration—even if migrants have themselves been transnationals all along, going back and forth across the Atlantic even when the trip took a month by sailboat.

Historians who looked for assimilation found it, those who subsequently focused on community (re-)formation (in the hostland) and ethnicity found that too. Now the concept of transnationalism is the latest wave of description of migrant behavior in much of the literature. The spread of the term has affected editors and publishers alike. The word gets bold letters, highlighted even on the cover of books that question its limits.

Both history and historiography can be contagious. The contagion of mobility has perhaps only been outdone by that of the concepts used to discuss mobility. Migration fever and transnational fervor form a joint lesson in the propagation of historical and historiographic phenomena.

BIBLIOGRAPHY

American Historical Review. "AHR Forum: Historiographic 'Turns' in Critical Perspective." *American Historical Review* 117, no. 3 (June 2012): 698–813.

Glick-Schiller, Nina, Linda Basch, and Cristina Blanc-Szanton, eds. *Towards a Transnational Perspective on Migration: Race, Class, Ethnicity, and Nationalism Reconsidered.* New York: New York Academy of Sciences, 1992.

Green, Nancy L. *The Limits of Transnationalism.* Chicago: University of Chicago Press, 2019.

Green, Nancy L., and Roger Waldinger, eds. *A Century of Transnationalism: Immigrants and Their Homeland Connections.* Urbana: University of Illinois Press, 2016.

MacDonald, John S., and Leatrice MacDonald, "Chain Migration, Ethnic Neighborhood Formation and Social Networks." *Milbank Memorial Fund Quarterly* 42, no. 1 (January 1964): 82–96.

Zahra, Tara. *The Great Departure: Mass Migration from Eastern Europe and the Making of the Free World.* New York: W. W. Norton, 2016.

VOGUE

The Lambeth Walk and the "Folklorization" of Cockney Culture in 1930s Great Britain

Ariane Mak

The famous Lambeth Walk dance number closes the first act of *Me and My Girl*, a musical written by Arthur Rose and Douglas Furber, with music by Noel Gay, and first performed at the Victoria Palace Theatre in London in 1937. The show's hero is Bill Snibson, a cockney from Lambeth who discovers that he is in fact the heir to an earl. When a crowd from Lambeth disrupts a high society party, Bill Snibson defends the freewheeling spirit of his home territory. He segues into the Lambeth Walk, a demonstration of the particular strut of cockneys from Lambeth: a jaunty step and exaggerated roll of the shoulders, with elbows held high and thumbs turned up. The walk turns into a dance and is so irrepressibly catchy that the aristocrats in attendance shed their initial hesitation and fall in step—even punctuating their movements with the cockney cry of "Oi!"—to the tune of the Lambeth Walk. Britain's leading dance hall chain, Mecca, adapted the Lambeth Walk as a couples' dance and launched a one-month tour to teach it in its venues in Manchester, Birmingham, Brighton, Glasgow, and Edinburgh. Amid growing public concern about the Americanization of British culture, Mecca touted the Lambeth Walk as typically English, even describing it as a traditional dance by Lambeth costers—street sellers of fruit and vegetables, as embodied by Bill Snibson.

Within months, the Lambeth Walk became a social phenomenon. The song set record-breaking sales, exceeding 350,000 in Great Britain. People seemed to be dancing the Lambeth Walk everywhere: in workmen's pubs, in dance halls, and in fancy ballrooms across the country. By the summer of 1938, to the immense pride of the British people, both the choreography and the music had become international sensations—in Hungary, Czechoslovakia, France, and the United States, where it enjoyed immense success and was recorded by Duke Ellington. It is not unusual for cultural trends, given their apparent suddenness and rapid spread, to be examined within the paradigm of contagion. Is the concept operative—and in what forms—in the context of a historical analysis of the Lambeth Walk?

Mass-Observation (MO), a social science research organization founded in 1937, decided to investigate the Lambeth Walk craze as of the summer of 1938. Its study, published under the title "Doing the Lambeth Walk" in Britain by MO,[1] was applauded as a preview of "the first large stirrings of 'serious' interest in popular culture,"[2] two solid decades before the emergence of cultural studies as a field of research. Although a large portion of the study employed a multi-sited ethnographic approach (fieldwork investigations at dance halls, popular gatherings, dance competitions, and private parties), the information gathered by MO from questionnaires provided the most insight into the timeline and spread of the Lambeth Walk.

The responses show an increase in the popularity of both song and dance in the spring of 1938. The Lambeth Walk seems to have been relayed by fairly traditional means, with the radio being predominantly cited by 41 percent of respondents. However, the statistics disguise a wide variety of responses, which runs counter to the idea of a homogeneous diffusion of the phenomenon. The testimonials bring to light the multiple sources of the dissemination and the viral nature of the cultural trend, highlighting the need to distinguish between the dance and the song in studying the Lambeth Walk, since the two flourished in distinct ways. They also revealed that the expression "the Lambeth Walk" had become a part of everyday speech and a popular catchword.

As one observer noted, "My niece has just begun to walk, her pace is very faltering and flat-footed. My mother calls this the 'Lambeth Walk.'" Another reported, "When I got home for the holidays I was walking up the lane, occasionally doing little skips because it was a beautiful morning, and a yokel on a bike came up behind me. 'Doing the Lambeth Walk?' he remarked cheerily and departed."[3] MO thus strove to examine not only the contagious power of a dance trend but also the manner in which it became a shared cultural reference and a social phenomenon.

The collective investigation also took an interest in the choreographic inventions added by dancers of the Lambeth Walk and underscored the ways in which the performers' variations spurred the propagation of the craze. In November 1938, dancers at Locarno Hall mixed swing steps into the Lambeth Walk, and in March 1939, dancers in Streatham amused themselves by stepping as quietly as possible and whispering "Shh" instead of "Oi" at the end of each verse.[4] The cockney interjection also underwent regional and international variations: in Scotland, the dancers would often cry "Och Aye" and in France, "La!" or "Whoo!" In fact, many French newspapers commented, "We shall never know why we should be shouting 'Oi!' instead."

Although the Lambeth Walk phenomenon lost some of its original meaning in its cultural transfer, it was also enriched with new interpretations. In crossing the Channel, the happy, boxer-like swagger of the cheeky Lambeth cockney took on a macabre note. A false story about the roots of the Lambeth Walk frequently surfaced in the French press: it claimed that the dance derived from an 800-year-old method of torture in the London district, which consisted in forcing the victim to wade across the Thames, much shallower at the time, with heavy stones tied to their feet and a rope around their neck.

The Lambeth Walk—a full performance that included the walk, the attitude, and the exclamations—encouraged dancers to mimic the Lambeth cockney. As one dancer observed, "One thing that struck me was the way dancers seemed to throw themselves into the part, as though they were play-acting, especially the men, who seemed to fancy they were costers, imitating their mannerisms."[5] The attraction for the middle and upper classes of pretending to be a Lambeth cockney, as one of the sources of the dance's popularity, was of particular interest to MO. Its study also revealed objections from some respondents to what they saw as a romanticized, depoliticized portrayal of working-class life, reduced to simple clichés of Victorian costers or pearly kings. Various cockney costumes were associated with the Lambeth Walk dance: suits adorned with mother-of-pearl buttons, like the outfits of pearly kings, and the caps and kingsman neckerchiefs that formed the typical attire of costermongers. Mecca's marketing strategies gave an early boost to the craze: when the dance was launched, thousands of pounds were spent to make paper versions of the hats worn by Victorian costers and to distribute them to dancers.

In the working-class neighborhood of Lambeth, swamped with curious tourists, the hit song exasperated more than a few locals. The lyrics—sometimes taken literally—claiming that Lambeth residents could be found doing the Lambeth Walk any time of day or night, were annoying to many. "Silly the way people think we do nothing but dance here," confided an exasperated waitress. One man in his seventies set the record straight: "They never had the pearly kings down this way, they wore the ordinary clothes of that time. There was none of this 'ere 'Oi' what they sing out now."[6]

MO's ethnographic study of the Lambeth district has been very little analyzed by historians. However, as I have shown, turning the lens on Lambeth adds several layers of complexity to the study of the social circulation of working-class representations and raises questions about the hiatus between the music hall cockney and the authentic culture of the costermongers conveyed by the interviews conducted and observations made in the working-class neighborhood.[7]

The figure of the high-spirited cockney and the idea of an amiable fraternization between the social classes, both relayed by the Lambeth Walk, were widely exploited during the war. In the midst of the Blitz, as the air raids struck the working-class areas of London's East End, the authorities sought to maintain civilian morale and contain the anger brewing against the elite. Anecdotes illustrating the optimism of London cockneys abounded in newspapers, while propaganda posters portrayed them as model citizens and allusions to the Lambeth Walk, evoking carefree, prewar days, flourished: "In spite of the damage caused in the Lambeth area during the latest Nazi raids, the gallant Cockneys of Lambeth Walk refuse to be down hearted. They still keep up their famous dance, and they can smile."[8]

The exploitation of the Lambeth Walk during the war was made possible not only by its reputation as an English tradition but also by Nazi

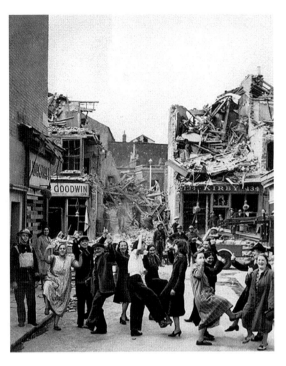

Figure 1

"In spite of the damage caused in the Lambeth area during the latest Nazi raids, the gallant Cockneys of Lambeth Walk refuse to be downhearted. They still keep up their famous dance, and they can smile." *Source: The Daily Sketch*, September 19, 1940.

Germany's highly publicized disapproval of the dance. After being forbidden at Heidelberg University, where it was deemed to be "incompatible with the National Socialist attitude of German students of both sexes," the Lambeth Walk would then be banned for all German soldiers in uniform. It was this prohibition that added spice to the best-known propagandized use of the Lambeth Walk. In 1941, the Ministry of Information produced a short film called "Lambeth Walk—Nazi style," designed to poke fun at the Wehrmacht: the clever remix of Leni Riefenstahl's *Triumph of the Will* sets the stiff troops of German soldiers dancing to the music of the Lambeth Walk. The film, which is said to have enraged Goebbels, was a roaring success among the Allies. One of the coups by the Danish resistance was to gain entry into movie theaters and force projectionists to show the short film, while in France, certain Parisian cinemas screened "Hitler's Lambeth Walk" upon the liberation of the capital.

Far from a contagious transmission of the Lambeth Walk to dancers, who passively relayed a phenomenon that they could not resist—much like the aristocratic party guests in *Me and My Girl*—the material gathered by MO calls for a broader interpretation of the concept of contagion. This larger reading would factor in the strategies consciously employed by participants, Mecca in particular, and the carriers who propagated and publicized the phenomenon. In contrast to the idea of an identical reproduction, the Lambeth Walk study gives weight to the importance of cultural transfer and its adaptations as well as to the inventions of the dancers as active participants. Last, the spread of the dance and music, and the various practices associated with them, also helped to disseminate a certain cliché of the cockney that would be appropriated and transformed, notably for political purposes.

translated by Elaine Holt

NOTES

1. Charles Madge and Tom Harrisson, *Britain by Mass-Observation* (Harmondsworth: Penguin Books, 1939).

2. Angus Calder, "Introduction," in *Britain by Mass-Observation* (London: The Cresset Library, 1986).

3. Madge and Harrisson, *Britain by Mass-Observation*, 165.

4. Mass Observation Archive, University of Sussex Special Collections. MOA TC 38/1/A, field notes by Alec Hughes; MOA TC 38/1/J, field notes by Stella Schofield.

5. Madge and Harrisson, *Britain by Mass-Observation*, 173.

6. MOA TC 38/2/D, field notes by Francis Cole, July 22, 1938; field notes by Joe Wilcock, August 13, 1938.

7. Ariane Mak, "Danser la Lambeth Walk ou les formes de folklorisation de la culture cockney. Étude et revisite de l'enquête du Mass Observation," *Mil Neuf Cent. Revue d'histoire intellectuelle* 35 (2017): 117–158.

8. See *The Daily Sketch*, September 19, 1940.

SELECTED BIBLIOGRAPHY

Abra, Allison. *Dancing in the English Style: Consumption, Americanisation and National Identity in Britain, 1918–1950*. Oxford: Oxford University Press, 2017.

Abra, Allison. "Doing the Lambeth Walk: Novelty Dances and the British Nation." *Twentieth Century British History* 20, no. 3 (2009): 346–369.

Hinton, James. *The Mass Observers: A History, 1937–1949*. Oxford: Oxford University Press, 2013.

Madge, Charles, and Tom Harrisson. *Britain by Mass-Observation*. Harmondsworth: Penguin Books, 1939.

Mak, Ariane. "Danser la Lambeth Walk ou les formes de folklorisation de la culture cockney: Étude et revisite de l'enquête du Mass Observation." *Mil Neuf Cent. Revue d'histoire intellectuelle* 35 (2017): 117–158.

Mak, Ariane. "Worktown. Les enquêtes fondatrices du Mass-Observation à Bolton (1937–1938)." In *Les enquêtes ouvrières dans l'Europe contemporaine*, edited by Éric Geerkens, Nicolas Hatzfeld, Isabelle Lespinet-Moret, and Xavier Vigna, 400–443. Paris: La Découverte, 2019.

Mak, Ariane. "Le Mass Observation: Retour sur un singulier collectif d'enquête britannique (1937–1949)." *Ethnographiques.org* 32 (September 2016). https://www.ethnographiques.org /2016/Mak.

Stedman Jones, Gareth. "The 'Cockney' and the 'Nation,' 1780–1988." In *Metropolis London: Histories and Representations since 1800*, edited by David Feldman and Gareth Stedman Jones, 272–324. London: Routledge, 1989.

WRITING
Textual Resemblance as a Historical Object
Dinah Ribard

Influence. Imitation. Compilation. Conference. Variation. Rewriting. Borrowing. Plagiarism. Adaptation. Parody. Pastiche. Quotation. Reuse. Misappropriation. Translation. Reading. Memory. Contagion. The possible names for the resemblance between writings from the same period are numerous. Many of these indicate intention, which would suggest some chronological interval between an original and later texts that incorporate passages of various lengths from this original, or that are modeled on it, whether with reverence (*imitation*), aggressivity (*misappropriation*), or potentially both (*parody, pastiche*). Others, on the contrary, imply that the resemblance is involuntary, diffuse, or even questionable (*influence, memory, contagion*). Each has its own history. Some (*rewriting, appropriation, reuse, influence*) convey an outside perspective on textual ensembles. They are chosen by historians to explain, according to the direction of their research, the proximity observed between writings of the past; those who have the means of seeing *reuse* are unlikely to see *influence*.

Conference, on the other hand, is an ancient term. It designated the act of reassembling texts—in particular legal or regulatory texts—so as to trace their underlying coherence, the previously invisible common spirit of the resemblances and redundancies now revealed. The word sometimes also referred to the book containing this collection, a type of bookshop product conducive to enriched subsequent editions. This usage is no longer common today. The word *compilation*, which also evokes an ancient and enduring intellectual technique—the search for passages in works accessible to

the compiler that are relevant to a given subject—took on negative connotations over the course of the eighteenth century. The development of the
printed book trade separated true authors from mere workers of the pen,
necessary to the production of books from other books, of new merchan-
dise made from writings already in circulation, divided up and stitched
back together, cut, and pasted: it galvanized and routinized practices of
compilation. And a number of writers who were well-practiced compil-
ers, or indeed self-compilers—one thinks of Voltaire for instance—worked
toward this de-intellectualization of the technique, no longer a quest for
meaning and knowledge in an ideal library.

Another sign of what Michel Foucault called the author function concerns *plagiarism*: as is well known, using this term to describe the resemblance between two writings implies that a group of utterances forming a
text belongs to the person who first assembled them, a principle that was
not recognized before the modern period. One might note that Charles
Fontaine, who adapted into French the term—originally from Roman law,
where it designated those who stole slaves and children—to denounce as
"Plagiarist Poets" Ronsard and du Bellay with his *Défense et illustration de
la langue française*, as well as Pierre Bayle, the first to use *plagiat* in his *Dictionnaire historique et critique* (1697, entry "Arétin, Léonard"), were both
targeting unacknowledged translations. In both cases, the translations were
of authors from classical antiquity. Plundering a common treasure was not
worthy of a man of letters, and the plagiarist was initially a boor, a hack, who
fed off the ignorance of his readers. Bayle is aware that he is using a neologism, which he says is preferable to *plagianisme*, used to describe the same
disguised translation of Procopius by Leonardo Bruni (*Aretinus*) in one of
the authors (Le Gallois) cited in his note, because one after another they
read, copied, and mislead each other about this story. The critic-compiler,
bookshop drudge turned hero of intellectual labors, brings new things to
other books. He reproduces texts to expose their faults and errors, to stop
their propagation in the ocean of printed books, or at least to accompany
them with corrections that themselves will unfailingly be reproduced. The
critic-compiler could be a journalist, as Bayle was. For journalism, one of

the typically modern activities productive of closely related pages, could also allow one to become an expert in controlling discourse put into circulation. *Conference, compilation*, and *plagiarism* tell different yet converging stories about the availability of written texts and about the work related to this availability.

Might the historian have something to learn from the diffuse, debatable resemblances between one very well-known text and others far more obscure? Influence, contagion: the words purport to, but do not actually, explain the presence of movements of thought, of expressions, of utterances that are seemingly Baconian or Cartesian, for example, but that are not quotations, in nonphilosophical writings of the seventeenth century. But what is a nonphilosophical text, and what is a philosophical text, in the seventeenth century? Whatever there is to learn by investigating of this type of resemblance begins with this question.

In 1652, in the context of civil war and, in Paris, political violence, a little book called *La Manière de cultiver les arbres fruitiers* (*The Manner of Ordering Fruit Trees*) appeared by the Sieur Le Gendre, the Vicar of Hénonville. It is a work on arboriculture, among the first ever to appear in French, and discusses how to select varieties and espalier fruit trees. It opens with a rather long preface, which begins thus: "It is certain that politeness of mind, the knowledge of beautiful things, and the study of philosophy, had no sooner entered the culture of the Persians and the Greeks than were followed by agriculture, as by their most faithful and innocent companion."[1]

This curious genealogical account, which against all custom has agriculture originating from philosophy, quickly takes on a theoretical sense: "Their foremost authors who have given men the rules for living well . . . have, at the same time, and in the same writings, taught them the art of cultivating the earth, and of soliciting her as she desires to be, so as to enrich us with the abundance of her fruits . . . believing that there was nothing more befitting and proper to a true philosopher, than reasoning with the earth, in order to learn how to reason well with men."

Agriculture proceeds from philosophy, because it is a way of understanding how to conduct oneself in society, how to act with men *by soliciting them as they desire to be*—it is a way of learning about government and politics. The lesson is further clarified when, having lingered over ancient Rome and Renaissance Europe, Le Gendre's account comes to seventeenth-century France:

> I remember that in my youth my curiosity led me to go see all the gardens of high repute. . . . I could not look at them without compassion . . . when the plants began to grow, some cut them . . . while others left them to grow freely, so that . . . all the branches bearing fruit received no advantage from it. . . . At the same time, I reflected a bit on what trees of themselves desire, in order to grow well; it seemed to me as I saw them maimed in this way that they groaned under the tyranny of their masters, and complained to me of their cruelty.

In the author's youth—the time of Louis XIII and of Cardinal Richelieu—the French did not reason well with the earth, which is to say with men, and did not attempt to understand their needs, and from this tyranny came no fruits. New principles were needed: "*Guiding myself by reason in a matter where as yet I had no example*, I soon found that it was impossible to get the satisfaction that one ought to expect from a beautiful tree abundant in fruit, by forcing it thus against its nature."

The formulation in italics, quite Cartesian in its manner, makes it quite clear that this fable is a discourse on the method—a discourse on political method, if one accepts the analogy put forth by the author. A bit further on, there is also the matter of those people who "profess that they will have no trees save those whose fruits and appearance were known in the time of their forefathers days." To speak of influence, to see in these passages a sign of the penetration of the new Cartesian spirit, in the most diverse of writings, would be to miss the use that Le Gendre makes of philosophy. He does not actually apply Cartesianism, or even its spirit, to politics, nor, for that matter, to the cultivation of fruit trees. He adopts the guise of a modern philosopher, at once bold and prudent in his approach, guided by a trust in his own good sense, to evoke a position of calm, aloof, rational and politically free speech, in a moment of crisis.

Moreover, the signs of modernity come to complete the signs of tradition, that is, the introduction of Greek reason to arboriculture: both the former and the latter are there as signs of philosophy. They are there as resources for writing about politics in a manner visibly different to the innumerable publications discussing and shaping the political crisis for the benefit of the various forces involved. They seek to show, in other words, that the right way to act at the moment is to stay outside of the arena where the political powers exercise their strength against one another and to prove that it is possible to do so by ostensibly speaking of, for instance, fruit trees.

To give oneself the means to understand this case is, among other things, to touch upon the question of authorship: that the sense of this publication is a political action that one could sum up as being disinterestedly progovernment constitutes an argument in favor of the attribution of the book, or of the preface, or of the process generally, to a specialist of publishing operations, Robert Arnauld d'Andilly. It is also to see the appearance of a deliberate practice of superficial resemblance between a very well-known book—the *Discourse on the Method* 1637—and an obscure and circumstantial work: not exactly a reuse, certainly not an influence, but rather a use of modern philosophy. It is to grasp modern philosophy as a historical fact, in the development of a politics of the book.

translated by Jeffrey Burkholder

NOTE

1. *La Manière de cultiver les arbres fruitiers, par le Sieur Le Gendre, curé d'Hénonville* (Paris: Antoine Vitré, 1652), with preface; all quotations that follow are translations of this unpaginated preface.

SELECTED BIBLIOGRAPHY

Boureau, Alain. *Le Feu des manuscrits: Lecteurs et scribes des textes médiévaux.* Paris: Les Belles Lettres, 2018.

Chartier, Roger, ed. *Les Usages de l'imprimé (XVe–XIXe siècle).* Paris: Fayard, 1987.

Chartier, Roger. *Les Origines culturelles de la Révolution française*. Paris: Le Seuil, 1990.

Décultot, Élisabeth. *Lire, copier, écrire: Les bibliothèques manuscrites et leurs usages au XVIIIe siècle*. Paris: CNRS Éditions, 2003.

Foucault, Michel. *L'Ordre du discours*. Paris: Gallimard, 1971.

Grihl. *Écriture et action XVIIe–XIXe siècle: Une enquête collective*. Paris: EHESS, 2016.

Jouhaud, Christian, and Dinah Ribard. "Événement, événementialité, traces." *Recherches de Science Religieuse* 102, no. 1 (January–March 2014): 63–77.

YAWNING

Why Is Yawning Catching? Fourteenth-Century Medicine and Natural Philosophy

Béatrice Delaurenti

In January 2015, the artist Sebastian Errazuriz erected a huge video screen in Times Square, New York, which lit up every evening at three minutes to midnight, showing him yawning.[1] The aim was to prompt visitors to stop awhile and yawn in their turn. It echoed several current preoccupations—the contagious character of yawning, distant suffering, empathy, and shared involvement in another's experience. Questions like these both perplex and focus the minds of those working nowadays in such fields as biological research, neuroscience, and the social sciences. Yet they have a long and enduring history. They already occurred to Aristotle, who, in his *Problems*, asked: "Why is that when men yawn others usually yawn in sympathy?"[2] Aristotle's reflections were a source of rich debate in the Middle Ages; he raised a particular form of line of enquiry regarding contagion, of which yawning is the exemplary *topos*.

The *Problems* is a compilation of original texts by Aristotle, Hippocratic writings, and later texts put together between the first and fifth centuries of our era. It contains 890 briefly raised problems in natural philosophy and medicine, divided into thirty-eight sections, which were translated as a whole into Latin in the 1260s by Bartholomew of Messina. The volume then circulated in European universities. Fifty years later, the physician and philosopher Pietro d'Abano wrote the first complete commentary on the *Problems*. The efforts of these two Italian scholars introduced the work to medieval educated culture. Pietro d'Abano's text even spurred others to emulate him; by the fourteenth century, five fresh commentaries appeared.

Section 7 of the *Problems*, which is authentic to Aristotle, is entitled in the Greek "On Sympathy." It contains the question about yawning together with a series of cases in which involuntary movements of the body or soul are implicated. Some of these consist in imitation of bodily movements that relieve oneself. In addition to the urge to yawn, the desire to urinate, desire to indulge in sexual activity, or urge to eat are also described as contagious. Other cases concern tiresome physical movements that involuntarily give rise to a disagreeable sensation. Thus a grating sound, sour taste, or biting cold all produce disagreeable shudders, as does the spectacle of someone else reacting to such sensations. A third type of reaction concerns the soul. Thus someone witnessing physical torture suffered by another person experiences from it a distress that Pietro d'Abano calls *condolor* (literally, "hurting in company with").[3] A final fourth category brings together diseases transmitted by a look, a breath, or contact.

Section 7's title became, in Latin, *De compassione* ("On Compassion"). The Greek notion of "sympathy" gained resonances that were specifically Christian and provided a matrix for philosophical and medical argumentation. Medieval commentators followed Aristotle in holding that it was legitimate to study these different cases together. They did not employ the term *contagio*, which was at the time predominantly employed in moral and political contexts; they preferred the term *compassio*. Like "contagion," "compassion" was a construction with imprecise boundaries and was not restricted—far from it—to the medical sphere. It played the part of a unifying label that covered phenomena of a particular type. According to Pietro d'Abano's definition, "compassion" was the result of a passive and involuntary interaction that assumed a likeness between the two parties. The term, above all, suited commonplace reactions consisting in an emotional contagion that was both physical and psychic and that everyone might experience in their daily lives.

For commentators on the *Problems*, the most important issue was understanding what caused these manifestations. How could a *passio* (something *passive* rather than *active*) be transmitted from one person to another? It seemed to contradict a central axiom of Aristotelian physics, that all natural movements are movements through contact. Was this similar to a form of action at a distance? If not, how could they be explained? Three sorts of explanation were proposed.

The first explicative model was philosophical. It relied on the natural concordance that linked people with one another and made it possible for individuals to participate in the behavior of others. Sharing in suffering could therefore be explained by a status common to all human beings, a complicity among the living that alone could enable the transfer of behaviors. Man was a microcosm subsumed in the macrocosm; he perceived the vibrations of a world of correspondences and harmonies. The example of yawning equally invited pondering on the distance between human beings and animals: both were subject to "compassion," but their difference in sensitivity provoked reactions that were also different.

The second explicative model was physiological. It emphasized the mobility of physical flows within the body: fumes, vapors, and steam circulated. Breath in particular was a substance that was easily mobilized. Yawning therefore readily occurred if something was provided to trigger it. This might be a perceiving of likeness or a memory of pleasure felt in yawning. The inner senses of the soul played a role in this process. Thus when a person saw another yawn, their imagination reactivated the sense-perceived impressions they had stored, and these provoked their body to yawn. The soul's external senses were also mobilized. The sense of sight was able to take over from the other senses and concentrate in the soul sensory impressions of varied nature. That explained why a person might shudder at *seeing* a scraping piece of chalk while not necessarily hearing the actual sound it produced.

The third model applied specifically to contagious diseases. The case of epidemics was both integrated with thinking about *compassio* and treated separately. Commentators referenced the Galenic conception of sickness, seeing it as a movement, an overflow of unhealthy humors outside the body, while health by contrast was a situation of balance. They also emphasized the role of the air, an explanation that went back to Hippocrates and was revived from the thirteenth century; after the Black Death of 1348, the argument from corruption of the air became commonplace both in medical literature and other writing.

In the fourteenth century, the contagious nature of yawning also interested educated men who taught philosophy, medicine, or theology but who had not written commentaries on the *Problems*. These men introduced a new tone. They associated yawning with cases that Aristotle had not mentioned: seeing someone eat something sour could set another's teeth on edge; the maternal imagination could leave a mark on a child's body; the flow of blood increased when red things were viewed; an excess of yellow bile could be purged when yellow things were observed. Some of these things were seen as pathological, in which case specific therapies were proposed. Jacopo da Forlì, master physician at Padua in the 1400s, recommended that women suffering from measles or children with smallpox should be wrapped in red cloth or lodged in a red-painted house. Being surrounded by the color red, he explained, would stimulate the imagination, which would stir up the body's spirits and enable the patient to expel unhealthy red substances.[4] The mechanism of imitation was thus sufficiently well known to the medical profession to encourage them to advance therapeutic procedures. However, such writers did not regard the phenomenon as a transfer or interaction but rather as a purely internal reaction. The yawner was a lone entity; he or she acted in isolation. The reaction therefore belonged to the realm of self-stimulation and could be triggered simply by the yawner's imagination. It was not really a matter of contagion but rather one of self on self.

Scholastic intellectuals thus did not have a unified conception of emotional contagion. The same phenomenon was understood as sometimes a transmission and sometimes a psychosomatic mechanism. The frontier between "compassion" and the transmission of disease remained imprecise. But in spite of this heterogeneity, all interpretations came together on two points: likeness and imagination. Likeness came into play sometimes at the start of the process, where there was a previous link that provided a favorable medium for the interaction to occur. At other times, such likeness served as a tool that the observer involuntarily made use of. He or she remembered the relief afforded by yawning, and the "reminiscence from what is alike" (*reminiscentia a simili*) prompted them to yawn in their turn.[5] The imagination meanwhile was "the chief among the other faculties and commands them in many instances."[6] All movements of emotional contagion and even the transmission of diseases depended in one way or another on activity by the imagination. Its place was central for the articulation of body and soul as well as for the human being's connection to the external world. Hence the power of the imagination emerged as the key factor in manifestations of contagion. It was central to explaining how one person could be activated by the emotions of another.

translated by Graham Robert Edwards

NOTES

1. "A Pause in the City That Never Sleeps," dir. Sebastian Errazuriz, Times Square, New York, NY, January 1–31, 2015.

2. Aristotle, *Problems*, Book 7, 1, 886a 24–887b 7, here 1, 886a24-25, transl. W. S. Hett (London: Heinemann, Cambridge, MA: Harvard University Press, 1970, 1st ed. 1926), 171.

3. Pietro d'Abano, *Expositio problematum*, 7.6, Paris, Bibliothèque nationale de France, MS lat. 6540, fols. 80v–84r.

4. Jacopo da Forlì, *Questiones in Tegni*, 3.11, in *Beyond Diet, Drugs, and Surgery: Italian Scholastic Medical Theorists on the Animal Soul 1270–1400*, ed. Kurt M. Boughan (Iowa City: University of Iowa, 2006), 638.

5. John of Spello, *IInda palestria*, quoted in Paul J. J. M. Bakker, "Les Palestrae de Jean de Spello: Exercices scolaires d'un maître en médecine à Pérouse au XIVe siècle," *Early Science and Medicine* 3 no. 4 (1998): 289–322, here 321.

6. Évrart de Conty, *Problemes*, 7.1, Paris, BnF, MS fr. 24281, fol. 136r.

SELECTED BIBLIOGRAPHY

Boureau, Alain. "Miracle, volonté et imagination: La mutation scolastique (1270–1320)." In *XXVe congrès de la SHMES (Orléans, 1994)*, 159–172. Paris: Publications de la Sorbonne, 1995.

Delaurenti, Béatrice. *La contagion des émotions: Compassio, une énigme médiévale*. Paris: Garnier Classiques, 2016.

Delaurenti, Béatrice. "L'action à distance est-elle pensable? Dynamiques discursives et créativité conceptuelle au XIIIe siècle." In *Histoires pragmatiques*, edited by Francis Chateauraynaud and Yves Cohen, 149–178. Paris: Éditions de l'EHESS, 2016.

Fossier, Arnaud. "La contagion des péchés (XIe–XIIIe siècle): Aux origines canoniques du bio-pouvoir." *Tracés* 21 (2011): 23–40. https://doi.org/10.4000/traces.5128.

Goyens, Michèle, and Pieter De Leemans, eds. *Aristotle's Problemata in Different Times and Tongues*. Leuven: Leuven University Press, 2006.

Jacquart, Danièle. "La scolastique médicale." In *Histoire de la pensée médicale en Occident*, vol. 1: *Antiquité et Moyen Âge*, edited by Mirko Dražen Grmek, 175–210. Paris: Seuil, 1993.

Van der Lugt, Maaike. "Genèse et postérité du commentaire de Pietro d'Abano sur les *Problèmes* d'Aristote: le succès d'un hapax." In *Médecine, astrologie et magie entre Moyen Âge et Renaissance: Autour de Pietro d'Abano*, edited by Jean-Patrice Boudet, Franck Collard, and Nicolas Weill-Parot, 155–182. Florence: Sismel, 2012.

Weill-Parot, Nicolas. "Pouvoirs lointains de l'âme et des corps: Éléments de réflexion sur l'action à distance entre philosophie et magie, entre Moyen Âge et Renaissance." *Lo Sguardo* 3, no. 10 (2012): 85–98.

AFTERWORD

Contagions, Ideologies, Economies: Thoughts in the Time of COVID-19

Thomas Piketty

When, in the spring of 2020, we were putting the final touches on this collective work devoted to the notion of contagion and the ways in which it has been used historically, a majority of the planet's inhabitants suddenly and simultaneously found themselves confined in their own homes to counter a previously unknown world pandemic. By mid-April, according to estimates reported by the international media, over 4.5 billion people were locked down throughout the world. Like all social statistics of this nature, this figure was the outcome of complex and controversial calculations, being based on dubious assumptions of uniformity and equality. In reality, people's experiences have been very different one from another, ranging from those of homeless people, migrants, and rural folk driven unceremoniously from urban areas of the global South to certain urbanites in the global North who deliberately opted to isolate themselves in the countryside.

The fact remains that the breadth and simultaneous nature of this worldwide lockdown has turned it into a unique experience with no parallel in human history. It can be analyzed in part as the consequence of the exceptionally fast-moving contagion caused by a coronavirus (SARS-CoV-2), a virus spread by the sort of transnational flows of goods and people that are now more intense and rapid than ever before. The unprecedented acceleration of human and commercial exchanges is what, in just a few weeks toward the end of 2019 and the beginning of 2020, put the main outbreaks of infection in central China into contact with northern

Italy. The same rapidity of exchanges similarly enabled members of an international evangelical gathering in Mulhouse (France) to share the virus unintentionally in a worldwide process of contagion, which unsurprisingly quickly hit Manhattan, an epicenter of planetwide globalization. Meanwhile, retired Spaniards returning from the Canaries spread the virus into Castile—at least that is one theory that was current in spring 2020, though it was quickly contested and complemented by any number of other tales of journeys and contagions, all as plausible and realistic as one another.

But if the lockdown phenomenon has quickly assumed worldwide application, it has done so also (perhaps preeminently) because of the contagious spread of ideas and practices concerning the best way to deal with the health crisis together with specific modes of production and transmission of knowledge and experience that themselves call for questioning and analysis. Such is particularly true for the central role played by epidemiological models in decision-making at the global level as well as for the superfast way in which the practice of lockdown was transmitted from North to South in spite of extremely different socioeconomic and sanitary circumstances that might have justified more balanced and diversified responses. But going beyond the question of lockdown, I shall try here to look briefly at the epidemic's impact on the development and spread of new socioeconomic ideologies.

To capture the different processes that contagiously spread ideas and practices I here use the term "contagion" in the broad sense analyzed in the introduction to this book, in particular taking it to include the "transmission of anything good or bad by frequentation, influence, or imitation." Like many of the contributors to this work, I stress the limitations of the notion of contagion, inasmuch as its mechanistic and unstoppable character can lead to the downplaying of human responsibility. In reality, the processes governing the spread of ideologies always entail a multiplicity of possible choices, sociopolitical trajectories, and opportunities that rely on numerous physical and intellectual connections among the human agents and social groups concerned and on the way in which they draw on past experiences to face present challenges.

THE INVENTION OF LOCKDOWN: EXPERTISE AND MIMICRY

In just a few days, roughly between the 10th and 20th of March 2020, a generalized lockdown strategy seemed an obvious step for virtually all governments on the planet. At the beginning of 2020, this was an option limited to a few hotspots in China and subsequently Italy. But suddenly, from March 10, major western European countries (Italy, France, Spain, Germany) extended a general lockdown to all their populations. The United Kingdom and the United States, which were initially hesitant, followed suit a week or so later. Conditions were then in place for a worldwide spread of lockdown to occur: India, South Africa, Brazil, the countries of West Africa and the Middle East, followed by dozens of others, used the law to lock down their populations. By the end of March, more than half the world's population were in a state of lockdown.

What processes led to this quasi-contagious spread of a such an unprecedented and coercive practice? It is too early to write its history, and it is very clear that multiple international networks and health monitoring procedures gradually developed and organized over the past hundred years played an essential role. But it is already possible to discern the specific importance of certain university centers with leadership in these areas, in particular Imperial College, London, with its "COVID-19 Reports" issued from January 2020 by Imperial's researchers in epidemiology.[1]

At the end of February and early March 2020, forecasts based on Imperial College's epidemiological models went round the offices of all the governments of the planet like a trail of digital gunpowder. They estimated that, if unimpeded, COVID-19 would cause the deaths of some forty million of the world's seven billion, including four hundred thousand in France, or 0.6 percent of France's seventy million. This would be almost the equivalent of an additional whole year's worth of mortality (which in an average year would be around 550,000 *morts* per annum in France, 55 million worldwide). In practice, it would mean that in the worst affected areas and during the darkest months, the number of coffins could be five or ten times higher than ordinarily seen (which is something we have unfortunately begun to see in certain Italian centers of infection, even if it is too soon to get a complete picture). However imprecise they may have been, in a matter of days these predictions were able to convince almost all the world's governments that we were not confronting a simple influenza epidemic and it was urgently necessary to lock down populations.

It is not my role to evaluate the plausibility of these forecasts and models, which some physicians judge wholly fanciful and whose authors themselves emphasize the standard deviations that surround them. As soon as epidemiological models existed, and where the best available models (or those regarded as such by health professionals and authorities) seemed to accredit such figures, it was inevitable that those in power would feel compelled to take exceptional measures and, above all, to copy almost immediately the measures adopted by other governments. Otherwise, the risk of stigma, even criminal prosecution, would have appeared considerable. According to Imperial College's report of March 26, 2020, the only policy that would substantially reduce losses would be a one of massive testing and isolating of individuals found to be contaminated. This would entail mobilizing considerable resources in terms of public health and accommodation. Conversely, lockdowns might, in the end, have only a limited impact on human losses.[2]

THE RETURN OF THE SOCIAL STATE: CONTAGION AND AUTONOMY

In the face of the uncertainties of epidemiology and its associated models, one of whose numerous limitations is extensive ignorance of the inequalities between social classes and between levels of development, it is undoubtedly useful to revisit historical experiences. One of the rare precedents available is the "Spanish flu" epidemic of 1918–1920. We now know there was nothing Spanish about it and that it caused fifty million deaths worldwide (about 2 percent of the then world population). From examination of civil records of the time, researchers have shown that the average mortality masked immense disparities: between 0.05 percent and 1 percent in the United States and Europe, as opposed to 3 percent in Indonesia and South Africa, and over 5 percent in India.[3]

There is no doubt that we need to contemplate as a priority the possibility that, in poor countries whose health systems are ill equipped to bear the shock, the epidemic could reach astronomical figures, and not least because those countries have undergone policies of austerity imposed through the prevailing antistate ideologies of recent decades. Lockdowns could moreover show themselves to be wholly out of place when applied to such fragile ecosystems. With no minimum wage, the poorest people quickly have to seek work, which risks relaunching the epidemic. The Indian lockdown has, above all, consisted in driving rural people and migrants from the cities, leading to violence and displacing large numbers of inhabitants and thereby worsening the spread of the virus. To avoid such carnage, we need the social state model, not that of the imprisoning state. In absolute terms and in the long run, the right response to the crisis is undoubtedly to relaunch the social state in the global North and, above all, to speed its development in the global South.

Here we reach again the limits of the notion of contagion, whose use without precautions as a tool to represent reality runs the risk of effacing power relationships and the autonomy of participants. The social state's spread in the South over the last few decades has been uneven, partly because of the desire of countries of the North to impose market deregulation and partly because of the sort of resistance put up by elites in the South that in the twentieth-century North encountered powerful movements to break it. Yet it would be wrong to characterize the South as eternally subject to prescriptions laid down by rich countries. Everything will depend on what movements arise. Other trajectories are and will be possible. During the electoral campaign in India in 2019—which looked extremely tight before the violence in Kashmir at the start of the year gave Hindu nationalists a chance to employ adept manipulation—the Congress Party and especially the socialist parties and lower castes were proposing an ambitious federal system of basic income. Had the elections turned out differently, such a system would doubtless be in place today. Other opportunities will certainly come about in the future.

In West Africa, for example, there could be an opportunity to reconsider the new common currency and put it to work in favor of a development project based on youth and infrastructure (rather than serving mobility of capital for the richest). Ideally, everything should be based on a more successful democratic and parliamentary architecture offering greater transparency than is current in the eurozone (which continues to rejoice in meetings of finance ministers behind closed doors, with the same inefficiency in the age of COVID-19 as in the financial crisis). In her novel *Rouge impératrice* (literally, "Red Empress"), Leonora Miano imagines an African federation that is finally united and has succeeded in inventing a new model capable of circumventing the impasses of the market-led, financial globalization of the West. She sees it ending up offering help to European refugees, thereby giving the lie to all those Africans who fear the contagion of the old racist and domineering ideas of the descendants of the white man.[4] One of the strengths of literature is its capacity to show that contagion is not inescapable. Let the social sciences and social players take inspiration from it!

translated by Graham Robert Edwards

NOTES

1. These reports are available online: http://www.imperial.ac.uk/mrc-global-infectious-disease-analysis/covid-19/.

2. COVID-19 report 12: "The Global Impact of COVID-19 and Strategies for Mitigation and Suppression," https://www.imperial.ac.uk/mrc-global-infectious-disease-analysis/covid-19/report-12-global-impact-covid-19/.

3. Christopher Murray, Alan D. Lopez, Brian Chin, Dennis Feehan, and Kenneth H. Hill, "Estimation of Potential Global Pandemic Influenza Mortality on the Basis of Vital Registry Data from the 1918–20 Pandemic: A Quantitative Analysis," *Lancet* 368, no. 9554 (2006): 2211–2218, https://doi.org/10.1016/S0140-6736(06)69895-4.

4. Leonora Miano, *Rouge impératrice* (Paris: Grasset, 2019).

Acknowledgments

This book is the fruit of collective research conducted at the Paris-based Center for Historical Research (Centre de recherches historiques). Aiming to bring together research from scholars whose diverse areas of expertise span a variety of geographies, objects, and periods, we chose to examine the common theme of *contagion*, understood as a historical process. The idea of the volume was born out of informal conversations within the laboratory and evolved gradually into a large-scale collective project. We warmly thank all of our colleagues who took up the challenge by contributing an original, synthetic text and by agreeing to think about issues often different from their usual research preoccupations.

From the writing of each original article to the publication of the final texts in English, the production of this volume required the cooperation of a connected group of colleagues. We would like to thank Mickaël Wilmart for proofreading the final French texts; Valérie Gratsac-Legendre for transforming the English articles into a standardized form; Joao Morais for setting up the contracts with the translators, the rights holders of the illustrations, and our editor; and finally, the eleven academic translators who were mobilized to create this English edition. Our thanks also go to all of those colleagues and friends who encouraged us to carry out the project; their enthusiasm supported us at every stage of the editorial work.

Contributors

The current volume is composed of recent work by researchers associated in various capacities with the French Center for Historical Research (CRH, Centre de recherches historiques), a Paris-based laboratory for historians covering all historical periods and a variety of research themes, located at the School for Advanced Studies in Social Sciences (EHESS, École des hautes études en sciences sociales) and the French National Center for Scientific Research (CNRS, Centre nationale de la recherche scientifique).

Stéphane Baciocchi is a research fellow at the EHESS. He is the coeditor of Émile Durkheim's *L'évaluation en comité* (with Jennifer Mergy, 2003) and Robert Hertz's *Sociologie religieuse et anthropologie* (with Nicolas Mariot, 2015). He is working on the history and theory of social science investigation.

Jean Baumgarten is a professor emeritus of research at the CNRS. He is also a specialist in the history of Jewish literature, Ashkenazi culture (Middle Ages–eighteenth century), and Hasidism. His latest published book is *Le Besht, mystique, magicien et guérisseur* (2020).

Pablo A. Blitstein is an associate professor at the EHESS. He conducts research on both medieval and late imperial China. His interests are global and intellectual history, with a special focus on writing practices and political institutions.

Olof Bortz is a Swedish historian and postdoctoral researcher at the EHESS in Paris. His PhD dissertation analyzed the work of Holocaust historian Raul Hilberg. His postdoctoral project focuses on scholarly interpretations of Nazism in France, the United Kingdom, and the United States before the Second World War.

Patrice Bourdelais is a retired professor at the EHESS. A historian and demographer, he has worked on population aging, the history of epidemics, and public health. He has published numerous articles in journals and several books including *Une Peur bleue: Histoire du choléra en France* (with Jean-Yves Raulot, 1988), *Les Hygiénistes, enjeux, modèles et pratiques* (2001), and *Epidemics Laid Low: A History of What Happened in Rich Countries* (2006).

Diane Carron received her PhD in history at the University of Burgundy where she studied Christian shrines of pilgrimage. After practicing as an archaeologist, she is currently a research fellow at the EHESS.

Jean-Pierre Cavaillé is an associate professor and teaches historical anthropology at the EHESS (Toulouse). His research focuses mainly on the history of irreligion and on religious dissent in early modern Europe.

Elizabeth Claire is an associate professor of gender history at the CNRS. She teaches the Cultural History of Dance at the EHESS and is currently completing a manuscript on medical theories of the powers of the imagination and social dancing in Europe after the French Revolution.

Yves Cohen, a professor at the EHESS, studies the history and present of influencing practices (advertising, marketing, propaganda, public relations, communication, fake news). In 2013 he published *Le siècle des chefs: Une histoire transnationale du commandement et de l'autorité (1890–1940)*.

Vincent Debiais is an associate professor of research at the CNRS. His research interest focuses on medieval epigraphy and on the relations between texts and images in medieval art. He recently published *Le silence dans l'art: Théologie et liturgie du silence dans les images médiévales* (2019).

In his new project, he explores abstract thinking and nonfigurative images in the visual culture of the Middle Ages.

Béatrice Delaurenti is an associate professor at the EHESS and director of the CRH. Her research interests focus on medieval intellectual controversies at the crossroads of religion, science and magic, dealing specifically with the question of action generated at a distance. She recently published *La contagion des émotions: "Compassio," une énigme médiévale* (2016).

Pierre-Olivier Dittmar is an associate professor at the EHESS. His work focuses on interfaces between humans and other life forms during the long Middle Ages, including animals, invisible beings, and artifacts. He cowrote *Image et transgression au Moyen Age* (2008), *Le monde roman par-delà le bien et le mal, Les images dans l'occident médiéval* (2015) and "Matérialiser les désirs: Techniques votives," *Techniques & Culture* (2018).

Maria Cecilia D'Ercole is a professor at the EHESS. A historian and archaeologist, she specializes in the economic and cultural history of the ancient Mediterranean. She is the author of several books and since 2019 has led the research center AnHiMA (Anthropology and History of the Ancient Worlds).

Marie-Élizabeth Ducreux is a professor emeritus of research at the CNRS. Her research interests focus on early modern history of the Habsburg Monarchy, especially bohemian and Hungarian political and religious history, including book culture, liturgy, chant and hymnody, and crypto-Protestantism. Among her works is *Dévotion et Légitimation: Patronages sacrés dans l'Europe des Habsbourg* (2016).

Catherine Fhima is a historian and PhD student at the EHESS. Her research focuses on the identities of writers, both Jewish and French, at the turn of the twentieth century. She recently published "Identity Face to Face: What Identity Does and Makes Do in the Mirror of Otherness," in *Questions de communication* (2019).

Jean-Baptiste Fressoz is a historian and associate professor of research at the CNRS. He has published *L'Apocalypse joyeuse: Une histoire du risque technologique* (2012), *The Shock of the Anthropocene* (with Christophe Bonneuil, 2016), and *Les révoltes du ciel: Une histoire du changement climatique XVe–XXe siècles* with Fabien Locher (2020).

Nancy L. Green, professor at the EHESS, is a specialist of migration history and comparative methods. Her recent publications include *A Century of Transnationalism: Immigrants and Their Homeland Connections* (coedited with Roger Waldinger, 2016) and *The Limits of Transnationalism* (2019).

Benoît Grévin, professor of research at the CNRS, is a researcher of medieval history. He has been a member of the French Institute for Italian History (École française de Rome) for four years and focuses on the comparative study of medieval linguistic cultures, contacts between Latin and Arabic world, and the study of medieval state rhetoric.

Sebastian V. Grevsmühl is an associate professor of research at the CNRS in history of science and environment. He specializes in environmental history and visual studies. He has mainly written on the geophysical sciences, polar history, and the role of images in science. He is the author of *La Terre vue d'en haut: l'invention de l'environnement global* (2014).

Florence Hachez-Leroy is an associate professor of modern history at Artois University and a researcher at the CRH. Her work crosses the economic, technical, social, cultural, and heritage aspects of entrepreneurial history and the history of modern industrial materials. Her most recent book focuses on environmental history, particularly the regulation of food additives and their relation to public health.

Élise Haddad defended in 2019 (EHESS, Paris) a PhD thesis on medieval images of the Apocalypse, with an iconographic dimension centered on the Romanesque portal of Beaulieu-sur-Dordogne as well as the social history of the theme and anthropological analysis of the evolution of apocalyptic images throughout the Middle Ages.

Marcela Iacub is a professor of research at the CNRS.

Thibaut Julian holds a PhD in French literature from Sorbonne Université and focuses on the connections between performance, history, and emotions in the eighteenth and nineteenth centuries. He coedited *Fièvre et vie du théâtre sous la Révolution française et l'Empire* (2019).

Christiane Klapisch-Zuber is a professor, now retired, at the EHESS. Her research was in the fields of demographic history, history of the family, and social history of art, particularly in Italy. She published various books since *Les maîres du marbre, Carrara, 1300–1600* (1969), such as *Tuscans and Their Families* (with David Herlihy, 1978) and, more recently, *Se faire un nom* (2019).

Thomas Le Roux is a CNRS associate professor of research in history and is director of the CRH. His work deals with the impact of early industrialization on the environment from 1700 to 1900, focusing on pollution, nuisance, risk, and occupational health. His publications include *The Contamination of the Earth: A History of Pollutions in the Industrial Age* (with François Jarrige, 2020).

Judith Lyon-Caen is a professor of contemporary history at the EHESS. Her research focuses on the connections between history and literature in modern times (nineteenth and twentieth century). She has published *La lecture et la vie: Les usages du roman au temps de Balzac* (2006) and *La Griffe du temps: Ce que l'histoire peut dire de la littérature* (2019).

Catarina Madeira-Santos is an associate professor at the EHESS. She conducts research on the history of the Portuguese empire and on the societies of West Central Africa. Her publications focus on imperial capital cities (Goa and Luanda), the Enlightenment and Empire periods, African writing, and archives of Angola and the Kongo. Her forthcoming book focuses on slavery in West Central Africa in the *longue durée*.

Ariane Mak is an associate professor in twentieth-century British history at the Université de Paris (LARCA, UMR 8225) and is affiliated with the Center for Historical Studies (EHESS). Her main areas of research expertise are in labor history and the social history of knowledge, with a particular focus on Mass-Observation.

Sébastien Malaprade is an associate professor at the Université Paris Est-Créteil/CRHEC, France. He is a specialist of the social and economic history of Spain in the early modern period. He recently published *Des châteaux en Espagne. Gouvernement des finances et mobilité sociale au XVIIe siècle* (2018).

Perrine Mane is a professor emeritus of research at the CNRS, specializing in medieval material and iconographic culture. She is the author of *La vie dans les campagnes au Moyen Âge d'après les calendriers* (2004) and co-editor of *La culture matérielle: un objet en question: Anthropologie, archéologie et histoire* (2018).

Davide Mano holds a PhD in history from Tel-Aviv University. A postdoctoral researcher at the EHESS-Paris, he is currently a lecturer at the University of Strasbourg. He is the author of numerous articles on the history of Italian Jews with specific regard to the Revolutionary and Napoleonic periods.

Niccolò Mignemi is an associate professor of research at the CNRS and a member of the research group ERHIMOR. His work focuses on the policies and the (local, national, and international) organizations that participated in the development of the farming systems and agri-food markets in Europe in the nineteenth and twentieth centuries.

Raphaël Morera is an associate professor of research at the CNRS and an editor of the journal *Études Rurales*. He works on European early modern environmental history and mainly focuses his research on water management. In 2011 he published *L'assèchement des marais en France au XVIIe siècle.*

Natalia Muchnik is a professor at the EHESS. Her research focuses on religious minorities and diasporas in early modern Europe, including Sephardi Jews, Moriscos, Recusants, and French Huguenots. She also examines the various dimensions of confinement in England, France, and Spain. Among her recent books is *Les prisons de la foi: L'enfermement des minorités, XVIe–XVIIIe siècles* (2019).

Ron Naiweld is a historian of Judaism and associate professor of research at the CNRS. His research focuses on the ethical and political dimension of rabbinic religion and the history of the biblical myth in Jewish and Christian societies.

Sofia Navarro Hernandez is a PhD student at the EHESS. Her research focuses on colonial Mexican material culture and the circulation of artistic objects in the Spanish Empire. Her latest article, "La pintura de castas como 'maravilla americana': Las estrategias del pintor tras el discurso oficial" (Pablo de Olavide University, 2019), is a comparative study on two casta paintings.

Hugo Perina has defended a PhD thesis at the EHESS entitled "Renaissance italian organ (1400–1550). Art commissions, practical knowledges and liturgical usage" (2018). He is currently pursuing his research in Rome as an affiliated member of the CRH on the uses of bell and organ sound in Italian Renaissance cities.

Thomas Piketty is a professor at the EHESS and at the Paris School of Economics. He studies the interplay between economic development, the distribution of income and wealth, and political conflict. He is the author of the international bestsellers *Capital in the 21st Century* (2014) and *Capital and Ideology* (2020).

Marie Anne Polo de Beaulieu is a professor of research at the CNRS in medieval history, didactic literature, and predication. She recently published *The Art of Cistercian Persuasion in the Middle Ages and Beyond: Caesarius of Heisterbach's Dialogue on Miracles and Its Reception* (with Victoria Smirnova and Jacques Berlioz, 2015).

Dinah Ribard is a professor at the EHESS. She specializes in the history of writing practices and of the intellectual labor of workers. In 2016, she co-authored *Ecriture et action XVIIe–XIXe siècle: Une enquête collective* (EHESS) and has recently published *1969: Michel Foucault et la question de l'auteur* (2019).

Suzanne Rochefort is a former student of the ENS de Lyon and is currently pursuing a PhD thesis at the EHESS on the profession of actors and actresses in Paris (1740–1799). Her research is at the crossroads of a social history of artistic work and a cultural history of the visibility of artists in the public space.

Paul-André Rosental is a professor in modern history at Sciences Po in Paris. He studies the making and implementation of social, demographic, and health policies in nineteenth- and twentieth-century Europe. Among his works are *A Human Garden: French Policy and the Transatlantic Legacies of Eugenic Experimentation* (2020) and *Population, the State, and National Grandeur: Demography as a Political Science in Modern France* (2018).

Antoine Roullet is an associate professor of research at the CNRS in early modern history, dedicated to the economic, social, and religious history of convent life in Spain and America and especially to the history of penance. He is the author of *Corps et pénitence: Les Carmélites déchaussées espagnoles (ca. 1560—ca. 1640)* (2015).

Sergi Sancho Fibla is a postdoc researcher in UCLouvain. His interests focus on the female monasticism of the late Middle Ages in Southern France and the Iberian Peninsula. He particularly works on literacy, writing and reading practices, spirituality, and the construction of holiness and memory. Since completing his PhD at the Universitat Pompeu Fabra, he has worked at Aix-Marseille Université and the EHESS (Paris).

Nicolas Sarzeaud is a PhD student at the EHESS. As an associated researcher of the project "CNRS-Notre-Dame," he studies the power of holy images, especially the Holy Shroud, and their reproducibility through the Middle Ages and Early Modernity as well as the facsimile in contemporaneous cultural heritage.

Jean-Claude Schmitt is a retired professor at the EHESS. In 2003, he received the CNRS silver medal for his work, which promotes an anthropological approach to the culture of the medieval West, for example, on rituals, images, and dreams. He recently published *Rhythms in the Middle Ages* (2016).

Silvia Sebastiani is an associate professor at the EHESS. A specialist of the Scottish Enlightenment, she works on the questions of race, gender, and history writing. She is now completing a book on the boundaries of humanity in the Enlightenment, focusing on how the great apes contributed to the shaping of human and social sciences.

Alessandro Stanziani is a professor at the EHESS and a professor of research at the CNRS. His main interests cover global history, labor history, and social history, eighteenth to twentieth century, in Russia, Europe, and the Indian Ocean. Among his works are *Rules of Exchange: French Capitalism in Comparative Perspective* (2012), *Bondage: Labor and Rights in Eurasia* (2014), and *Labor on the Fringes of Empire* (2018).

Frédéric Vagneron, historian, is an associate professor at the University of Strasbourg (DVHS, SAGE). His research focuses on the history of medicine and health since the nineteenth century, and on the history of the relationship between human and animal health and the environment. His doctoral research has examined the history of influenza in France.

Sebastian Veg is a professor of intellectual history of twentieth-century China at the EHESS in Paris and is an honorary professor at the University of Hong Kong. His most recent book is *Minjian: The Rise of China's Grassroots Intellectuals* (2019).

Mickaël Wilmart is a research fellow at the EHESS. He works on social history and material culture in France between the thirteenth and fifteenth centuries. He coedited *La culture matérielle: Un objet en question* (2018) and *Le vêtement au Moyen Âge, de l'atelier à la garde-robe* (forthcoming).